Arthritis
FOR
DUMMIES®
2ND EDITION

by Barry Fox, PhD
Nadine Taylor, MS, RD
Jinoos Yazdany, MD

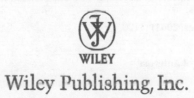

WILEY
Wiley Publishing, Inc.

Arthritis For Dummies,® 2nd Edition

Published by
Wiley Publishing, Inc.
111 River St.
Hoboken, NJ 07030-5774
www.wiley.com

Copyright © 2004 by Wiley Publishing, Inc., Indianapolis, Indiana

Published by Wiley Publishing, Inc., Indianapolis, Indiana

Published simultaneously in Canada

For general information on our other products and services or to obtain technical support, please contact our Customer Care Department within the U.S. at 800-762-2974, outside the U.S. at 317-572-3993, or fax 317-572-4002.

Wiley also publishes its books in a variety of electronic formats. Some content that appears in print may not be available in electronic books.

Library of Congress Control Number: 2004111126

ISBN: 0-7645-7074-9

Manufactured in the United States of America

15 14 13 12

2B/RT/QZ/QU/IN

WILEY

About the Authors

Barry Fox and Nadine Taylor are a husband-and-wife writing team living in Los Angeles, California.

Barry Fox, PhD, is the author, coauthor, or ghostwriter of numerous books, including the New York Times number-one bestseller, *The Arthritis Cure* (St. Martin's, 1997). He also wrote its sequel, *Maximizing The Arthritis Cure* (St. Martin's, 1998), as well as *The Side Effects Solution* (to be published by Broadway Books in 2005), *What Your Doctor May Not Tell You About Hypertension* (Warner Books, 2003), *What Your Doctor May Not Tell You About Migraines* (Warner Books, 2001), *Syndrome X* (Simon & Schuster, 2000), *The 20/30 Fat and Fiber Diet Plan* (HarperCollins, 1999), and *Cancer Talk* (Broadway Books, 1999). His books and over 160 articles covering various aspects of health, business, biography, law, and other topics have been translated into 20 languages.

Nadine Taylor, MS, RD, is the author of *Natural Menopause Remedies* (Signet, 2004), *25 Natural Ways To Relieve PMS* (Contemporary Books, 2002) and *Green Tea* (Kensington Press, 1998), as well as co-author of *Runaway Eating* (to be published by Rodale in 2005), *What Your Doctor May Not Tell You About Hypertension* (Warner Books, 2003), and *If You Think You Have An Eating Disorder* (Dell, 1998). After a brief stint as head dietitian at the Eating Disorders Unit at Glendale Adventist Medical Center, Ms. Taylor lectured on women's health issues to groups of health professionals throughout the country. She has also written numerous articles on health and nutrition for the popular press.

Jinoos Yazdany, MD, MPH, is a board-certified internist and a Rheumatology Fellow at the University of California, San Francisco. She completed her undergraduate education at Stanford University, where she received the Deans' Award for Academic Achievement and graduated with Honors and Distinction. She completed medical school at the University of California, Los Angeles, where she received a Humanism in Medicine award from the Health Care Foundation of New Jersey and graduated Alpha Omega Alpha. Dr. Yazdany also studied public health at Harvard University. Her research involves examining health disparities in the care of patients with chronic diseases. This is her first book.

Dedication

Dedicated to Nina Ostrom Taylor, world's greatest mom and mom-in-law.

Authors' Acknowledgments

Nadine and Barry thank Arnold Fox, MD, for providing us with a great deal of information on arthritis; Jinoos Yazdany, MD, for her invaluable contributions; Anthony Padula, MD, for his careful review of the manuscript; and of course, Natasha Graf, Traci Cumbay, and the editorial staff at Wiley.

Jinoos thanks the many patients who have shared with her their lives and wisdom regarding living with arthritis.

Publisher's Acknowledgments

We're proud of this book; please send us your comments through our Dummies online registration form located at www.dummies.com/register/.

Some of the people who helped bring this book to market include the following:

Acquisitions, Editorial, and Media Development

Project Editor: Traci Cumbay

Acquisitions Editor: Natasha Graf

Copy Editor: Jennifer Bingham

Technical Editor: Anthony S. Padula, MD

Editorial Manager: Jennifer Ehrlich

Editorial Assistants: Courtney Allen, Melissa Bennett

Cover Photo: ©Abbie Enneking/2004

Cartoons: Rich Tennant, www.the5thwave.com

Composition

Project Coordinators: Maridee Ennis, Courtney MacIntyre

Layout and Graphics: Andrea Dahl, Lauren Goddard, Joyce Haughey, Stephanie D. Jumper, Michael Kruzil, Barry Offringa, Melanee Prendergast, Heather Ryan

Proofreaders: Carl William Pierce, Dwight Ramsey, TECHBOOKS Production Services

Indexer: TECHBOOKS Production Services

Special Help
Sherri Pfouts, Trisha Strietelmeier

Publishing and Editorial for Consumer Dummies

Diane Graves Steele, Vice President and Publisher, Consumer Dummies

Joyce Pepple, Acquisitions Director, Consumer Dummies

Kristin A. Cocks, Product Development Director, Consumer Dummies

Michael Spring, Vice President and Publisher, Travel

Brice Gosnell, Associate Publisher, Travel

Kelly Regan, Editorial Director, Travel

Publishing for Technology Dummies

Andy Cummings, Vice President and Publisher, Dummies Technology/General User

Composition Services

Gerry Fahey, Vice President of Production Services

Debbie Stailey, Director of Composition Services

Contents at a Glance

Table of Contents

Introduction

● ●

*W*hether it appears as a little bit of creaky stiffness in the hip or knee or as a major case of inflammation that settles in several joints, arthritis is an unwelcome visitor that knocks on just about everybody's door sooner or later. Although we don't have an out-and-out cure for arthritis, there are many techniques for *managing* this disease — that is, controlling its symptoms so that you can get on with your life! Arthritis does *not* mean that you must spend your days relegated to a rocking chair or shuffling from your bed to an easy chair and back again. Most of the time, you can take charge of your disease, instead of letting it take charge of you. By following the simple techniques outlined in this book, you can do much to control your pain, exercise away your stiffness, keep yourself on the move, and slow down or prevent progression of your disease. All you need is a little know-how — and that's what we provide in these chapters.

About This Book

When writing this book, our goal was to provide you with the best and most up-to-date information on arthritis treatments in an easy-to-read format that you could simply thumb through. We have included the best-of-the-best of many different healing systems — ranging from standard Western medicine (including medications and surgery), to Eastern hands-on healing methods (including acupuncture, acupressure, and reiki), to alternative therapies (including homeopathy, herbs, dehydroepiandrosterone (DHEA), dimethyl sulfoxide (DMSO), methylsulfonylmethane (MSM), and such far-out approaches as bee venom therapy). If you like, you can read this book straight through from cover to cover, but it's not absolutely necessary. We do suggest that you read the first chapter as an introduction, and then zero in on the description of your particular kind of arthritis, found in Chapters 2, 3, 4, or 5. After that, feel free to flip through the book and read whatever catches your fancy.

Because arthritis impacts your life in so many different ways, we have chapters that address the many complex issues that you may face, including the technical aspects of arthritis (tests, medicines, and surgeries), the practical aspects (diet, exercise, and day-to-day living), and the emotional aspects (depression and anger). We also give tips on how to assemble your healthcare treatment team, how to talk to your doctor, and what to do about chronic pain.

Foolish Assumptions

In writing this book, we made certain educated guesses about you, the reader, so that we could figure out what might be most interesting and useful to you and write our book accordingly. We've assumed the following:

✔ You either have arthritis yourself or you're close to someone who has it.

✔ You're interested in finding out more about arthritis and its treatments.

✔ You want to do something to ease arthritis pain and other symptoms.

✔ You want to play an active part in managing the disease, rather than just going along with whatever your doctor tells you.

✔ You're interested in finding out about some alternative ways to treat arthritis.

✔ You'd like to find out how to handle the emotional issues that go hand-in-hand with the disease.

How This Book Is Organized

The organization of *Arthritis For Dummies,* 2nd Edition, is meant to correspond with the way that you may experience arthritis in your daily life. When you first realize that you have arthritis, you probably want to know what it is, what the common symptoms are, and what you can expect as the disease progresses. Next, you'll visit your doctor for tests. Medicines may be prescribed, pain management strategies discussed, and surgery (if applicable) may be mentioned.

But after you've made it through all that, you'll go back to living your life. Suddenly, the everyday things that you used to take for granted will become important parts of your arthritis management — like diet, exercise, and the way that you use your joints. Stress and depression may be new and confounding problems, and getting through the day may be a tougher prospect, both physically and mentally, than it was before.

Eventually, you may start wondering about alternative healing methods and have an urge to explore them. And you may become curious about certain myths that you've heard repeated about super foods that can be used to help ease arthritis symptoms and cutting-edge medical treatments that are on the horizon. This book will answer all of your questions.

Part 1: Getting a Grip on Types of Arthritis

These five chapters give an overview of arthritis in its many forms — the symptoms, disease processes, causes, and likeliest victims. Chapter 1 discusses arthritis in general, Chapter 2 tackles osteoarthritis (the type of arthritis that most people get), Chapter 3 explains rheumatoid arthritis (another fairly common kind of arthritis), Chapter 4 discusses the other forms the disease may take, and Chapter 5 is dedicated to other conditions that are linked to arthritis. We also explain what doctors do for each type of arthritis and what you can do for yourself.

Part 11: Tests and Treatments: What to Expect from Your Doctor

Chapters 6 through 10 walk you through the maze of medical treatments, beginning with a trip to the doctor's office. We explain how doctors diagnose the many forms of arthritis and discuss the high-tech and low-tech tests that they may use. Equally important, we show you how to work with your doctor to make the treatment decisions. Chapter 8 outlines the medicines that may be prescribed and the surgeries that may be applicable. Finally, strategies that you can use at home for managing pain are thoroughly explained.

Part 111: The Arthritis Lifestyle Strategy

Many of the keys to arthritis management lie in the little things that you do every day, such as what you eat, the kind and amount of exercise you get, and how you use your joints. In this part, we tell you how to fight arthritis pain through diet and supplements; how to keep your joints in shape through exercise; how to protect your joints by walking, sitting, and moving correctly; and how to deal effectively with depression and anger. Plus, we provide loads of tips on how to make day-to-day living with arthritis easier.

Part 1V: Is Alternative Medicine for You?

Alternative medicine has become incredibly popular in the past twenty years, and scientific studies are beginning to show that many of these methods have merit. In this part, we discuss the most popular alternative therapies for arthritis, including massage, herbs, homeopathy, acupuncture, reflexology, and others. We also give you tips on finding a reputable alternative practitioner and identifying false claims.

Part V: The Part of Tens

In this part, we concentrate some of the key information on managing your arthritis into five lists, each containing ten "information bites." We include ten tips for traveling with arthritis, ten ways to save money on prescriptions, ten health professionals that can help you fight arthritis, ten crackerjack new treatments that you may not have heard about yet, and ten myths about arthritis.

Part VI: Appendixes

Appendix A contains a glossary of arthritis terms to help keep you straight as you wend your way through the information in this book. Appendix B lists lots of interesting organizations that may help you find the treatment you seek. We give detailed information on the foundations associated with most kinds of arthritis or arthritis-related conditions, as well as major medical associations. We list the certifying boards or associations for each alternative therapy we discuss, so you can request practitioner referrals or more information. Information on support groups, mail-order catalogues featuring assistive devices, books, and videotapes are all included in Appendix B. In Appendix C, we discuss strategies for losing weight the safe and healthy way, because getting rid of extra pounds can be one of the best things you do for your weight-bearing joints.

Icons Used in This Book

The icons tell you what you must know, what you should know, and what you may find interesting but can live without.

When you see this icon, it means the information is essential, and you should be aware of it.

This icon marks important information that can save you time and energy.

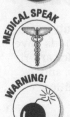

The Medical Speak icon marks a more in-depth medical passage or gives you further information about confusing medical terms.

The Warning icon cautions you against potential problems.

Where to Go from Here

Someone once said, "Knowledge is power." You have the power to take charge of your arthritis; all you have to do is educate yourself and apply what you discover. This book is a good place to start, but you'll have to commit and recommit yourself to maintaining your health on a daily basis. Remember, it's the little things that you do every day that count. As you embark on your journey, we wish you luck, strength, and many active, pain-free years!

Part I
Getting a Grip on Types of Arthritis

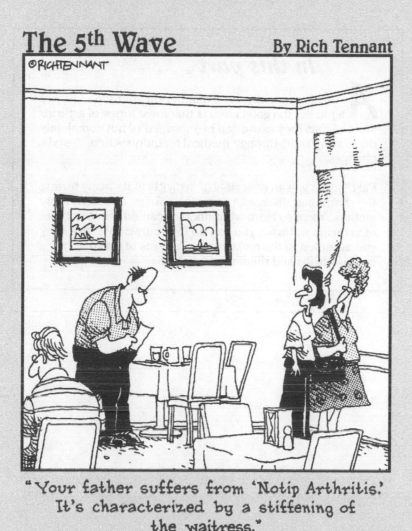

The 5th Wave   By Rich Tennant

©RICHTENNANT

"Your father suffers from 'Notip Arthritis.'
It's characterized by a stiffening of
the waitress."

In this part . . .

Arthritis can really put a damper on your life . . . if you let it. But the good news is that most forms of arthritis and the pain they cause can be managed (if not completely done away with) through medical techniques and lifestyle changes.

Part I gives you an overview of arthritis in its many forms: the symptoms, diseases, processes, causes, and most likely victims. You also learn what doctors can do for each type of arthritis and what you can do for yourself. We give special attention to the most common forms of this disease: osteoarthritis and rheumatoid arthritis.

Chapter 1

What Is Arthritis?

*O*uch! There it goes again! That grinding pain in your hip, those aching knees that make walking from the kitchen to the bedroom a chore, the stiff and swollen fingers that won't allow you to twist the lid off a sticky jar or even sew on a button. Arthritis seems to get to everybody sooner or later — slowing us down, forcing us to give up some of our favorite activities, and just generally being a pain in the neck (sometimes literally!). In more advanced cases, the disease can seriously compromise quality of life as sufferers surrender their independence, mobility, and sense of usefulness while being relentlessly worn down by pain.

The good news is that you can manage your arthritis, if not cure it, with a combination of medical care, simple lifestyle changes, and good old common sense. You don't have to spend your life sitting at home in an easy chair, gritting your teeth from pain, or hobbling around the backyard with a cane. Although you may not be able to run a marathon or do back-flips like you did when you were 13, if you follow the program outlined here, you should be able to do the things you really want to do — such as take a brisk walk in the park, carry a sleeping child upstairs to bed, or swing a golf club with the best of them. Arthritis may affect a lot of people, but thanks to intensive research over the past several years, we now know a lot more about how to handle it.

Understanding How Arthritis Affects Your Joints

So what exactly is arthritis, this disease that brings us so much misery and pain? Unfortunately, we can't provide one easy answer to that question, because arthritis involves a group of diseases — each with its own cause, set of symptoms, and treatments. However, these diseases do have the following in common:

✔ They affect some part of the joint.

✔ They cause pain and (possibly) loss of movement.

✔ They often bring about some kind of inflammation.

As for the causes of these different kinds of arthritis, they run the gamut from inheriting an unlucky gene to physical trauma to getting bitten by the wrong mosquito.

The word *arthritis,* which literally means joint inflammation, is derived from the Greek words *arthros* (joint) and *itis* (inflammation), and its major symptom is joint pain. Although the same group of ailments is sometimes called *rheumatism,* it's usually referred to as arthritis, so that's what we call it in this book. The word *arthralgia,* a term that's used much less frequently, refers to joint pain alone. According to the Arthritis Foundation, arthritis affects some 70 million Americans (one out of every three people). That's a big chunk of the population.

Saying hello to your joints

Before you can understand what's wrong with your joints, you need to understand what a joint is and how it works. Any place in the body where two bones meet is called a joint. Sometimes those bones actually fuse; your skull is an example of an area with fused bones. But in the joints that can develop arthritis, the bones don't actually touch. As you can see in Figure 1-1, a small amount of space exists between the two bone ends. The space between the ends of the bones keeps them from grinding against each other and wearing each other down.

Bones are living tissue — hard, porous structures with a blood supply and nerves — that constantly rebuild themselves. Bones protect our vital organs and provide the supporting framework for the body. Without bones, we would be nothing more than blobs of tissue — like tents without supporting poles!

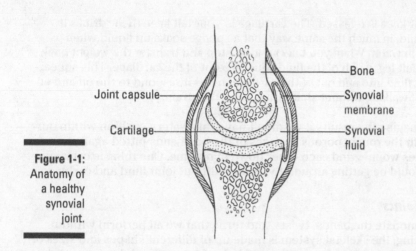

Joint capsule

Cartilage

Bone

Synovial membrane

Synovial fluid

Figure 1-1:
Anatomy of
a healthy
synovial
joint.

But bones are more than broomsticks that prop us up; fortunately, they don't leave us rigid and awkward. The 200-plus bones that reside in our bodies are connected together in some 150 joints, giving us remarkable flexibility and range of motion. If you don't believe it, just watch a gymnast, ballet dancer, or figure skater execute a handspring, arabesque, or triple axel. But you don't have to be an athlete or contortionist to enjoy the benefits of joint flexibility. Just think about some of the things you do regularly — such as twisting around while you sit in the front seat of your car to grab something off the backseat floor. Now imagine how limiting it would be if you had fewer joints or if they didn't move the way they do!

Other structures surrounding the joint, such as the muscles, tendons, and *bursae* — small sacs that cushion the tendons — support the joint and provide the power that makes the bones move. The joint capsule wraps itself around the joint, and its special lining, the *synovial membrane* or *synovium,* makes a slick, slippery liquid called the *synovial fluid.* This liquid fills that little space between the bone ends. Finally, the bone ends are capped by *cartilage* — a slick, tough, rubbery material that is eight times more slippery than ice and a better shock absorber than the tires and springs on your car! Together, these parts make up the joint, one of the most fascinating bits of machinery found in the body.

Cartilage: The human shock absorber

Cartilage is extremely important for the healthy functioning of a joint, especially if that joint bears weight, like your knee. Imagine for a moment that you're looking into the inner workings of your left knee as you walk down the street. When you shift your weight from your left leg to your right, the pressure on your left knee is released. The cartilage in your left knee then "drinks in" synovial fluid, in much the same way that a sponge soaks up liquid when immersed in water. When you take another step and transfer the weight back onto your left leg, much of the fluid squeezes out of the cartilage. This squeezing of joint fluid into and out of the cartilage helps it respond to the off-and-on pressure of walking without shattering under the strain.

Can you imagine the results if we didn't have this watery cushion within our joints? With the rough, porous surfaces of the bone ends pitted against each other, bones would grind each other down in no time. One thing is certain: Nobody would be getting around too easily without joint fluid and cartilage.

Types of joints

To accommodate the bends, twists, and turns that we all perform without even thinking, the skeletal system is made up of different shapes and sizes of bones, which connect to form different kinds of joints. The joints are categorized according to how much motion they allow:

- **Synarthrodial joints** allow no movement at all. You can find these in the skull, where the bones meet to form tough, fibrous joints called *sutures*. Because they don't move, arthritis doesn't affect them.

- **Amphiarthrodial joints,** such as those in the spine or the pelvis, allow limited movement. Generally, these joints aren't attacked by arthritic conditions as often as others. (A slipped disc is not arthritis.)

Strange-but-true joint points

Here are a couple of things you may not know about your joints:

- By the time a fetus is four months old, its joints and limbs are in working order and ready to move.

- A newborn baby has 350 bones, many of which fuse to form the 206 bones of the adult body.

- Cartilage is 65 percent to 85 percent water. (The amount of water in your cartilage generally decreases as you get older.)

- When you run, the pressure on your knees can increase to ten times that of your body weight.

- Not a single man-made substance is more resilient, a better shock absorber, or lower in friction than cartilage.

✓ **Synovial joints** allow a wide range of movement; most of our joints fall into this class. Synovial joints come in all kinds of interesting variations including those that glide, hinge, pivot, look like saddles, or have a ball-and-socket type structure. (For more on these joints, take a look at the section "Looking at the types of synovial joints" later in this chapter.) Because of the synovial joints, you can bend over and pick a flower, kick up your heels while swing dancing, reach for a glass on a high shelf, and turn around to see what's going on behind you. Unfortunately, these joints are also the ones most likely to be hit with arthritis, precisely because they do move!

Looking at the types of synovial joints

Because of their tendency to become arthritic, synovial joints are the ones that we discuss the most throughout this book. Synovial joints come in a wide variety of shapes and sizes to accommodate a wide variety of movements.

Gliding joints

A gliding joint contains two bones with somewhat flat surfaces that can slide over each other. The vertebrae in your spine are connected by gliding joints, allowing you to bend forward to touch your toes and backward to do a back-bend (well, maybe!). See Figure 1-2 for an example of a gliding joint.

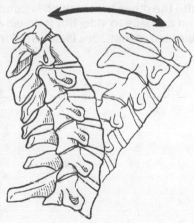

Figure 1-2: A gliding joint. The gliding joint helps keep your vertebrae aligned when you bend and stretch.

Hinge joints

You can find hinge joints in your elbows, knees, and fingers. These joints open and close like a door. But just like a door, hinge joints only go one way — you can't bend your knee up toward your face, only back toward your rear. See Figure 1-3 for an example of a hinge joint.

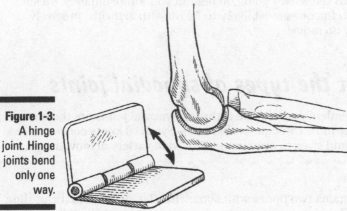

Figure 1-3: A hinge joint. Hinge joints bend only one way.

Saddle joints

This joint looks like a horse's back with a saddle resting on it. One bone is rounded (convex) and fits neatly into the other bone, which is concave. The saddle joint moves up and down and side to side, but it doesn't rotate. Your wrist and your thumb have this kind of joint. See Figure 1-4 for an example of a saddle joint.

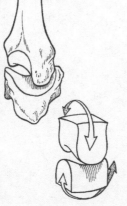

Figure 1-4: A saddle joint. The saddle joint moves up and down and side to side.

Ball-and-socket joints

This is truly a freewheeling joint — it's ready for anything! Up, down, back, forth, or around in circles. The bone attached to a ball-and-socket joint can move in just about any direction. The end of one bone is round, like a ball, whereas the other bone has a neat little cave that the ball fits into. Your shoulders and hips have ball-and-socket joints. Swimming the backstroke is a perfect example of the kind of range of motion made possible by these joints. See Figure 1-5 for an example of a ball-and-socket joint.

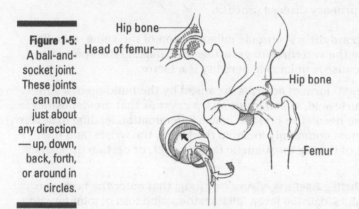

Figure 1-5:
A ball-and-socket joint. These joints can move just about any direction — up, down, back, forth, or around in circles.

Hip bone
Head of femur
Hip bone
Femur

Distinguishing Between Arthritis and Arthritis-Related Conditions

Some organizations define arthritis as a group of more than 100 related diseases, ranging from bursitis to osteoarthritis. But in this book, we use the following classifications, which conform to those widely accepted by the medical community:

- ✔ "True" arthritis
- ✔ Arthritis as a "major player"
- ✔ Arthritis as a "minor player"
- ✔ Arthritis as a "companion condition"

In the following subsections, we go over the various types of arthritis and arthritis-related diseases and their classifications. We also discuss each disease in greater detail in Chapters 2, 3, 4 and 5.

Defining "true" arthritis

True arthritis isn't a medical term; it's just a convenient way of referring to the group of ailments in which arthritis is the primary disease process and is a major part of the syndrome. Osteoarthritis and rheumatoid arthritis are the best-known members of this group, which can cause problems ranging from mild joint pain to a permanently bowed spine.

The following include conditions in which arthritis is the major part of the syndrome and the primary disease process:

- **Ankylosing spondylitis:** A chronic inflammation of the spine, this disease can cause the vertebrae to grow together, making the spine rigid. Although the cause is unknown, heredity is a factor.

- **Gout:** This "regal" form of arthritis is caused by the build-up of a substance called uric acid, which forms sharp crystals that are deposited in the joint. These needlelike crystals cause inflammation leading to severe pain and are most commonly found in the knees, the wrists, and the "bunion" joint of the big toe. Genetic factors, diet, or certain drugs may cause gout.

- **Infectious arthritis:** Bacteria, viruses, or fungi that enter the body can settle in the joints, causing fever, inflammation, and loss of joint function.

- **Juvenile arthritis:** This is a catchall term for the different kinds of arthritis that strike children under the age of 16, the most common of which is *juvenile rheumatoid arthritis* (JRA). Pain or swelling in the shoulders, elbows, knees, ankles, or toes; chills; a reappearing fever; and sometimes a body rash are the typical symptoms of JRA. The cause is unknown.

- **Osteoarthritis (OA):** In this, the most common type of arthritis, the cartilage breaks down, exposing bone ends and allowing them to rub together. The result can be pain, stiffness, loss of movement, and sometimes swelling. Osteoarthritis is most often found in the weight-bearing joints, such as the hips, knees, ankles, and spine, but it can also affect the fingers. It may be the result of trauma, metabolic conditions, obesity, heredity, or other factors.

- **Pseudogout:** Like gout, pseudogout is caused by the deposition of crystals into the joint, but instead of uric acid crystals, they're made from calcium. Pain, swelling, and sometimes the destruction of cartilage can result.

  Note: This deposition of calcium crystals is not related to the dietary intake of calcium.

- **Psoriatic arthritis:** This form of arthritis occurs in people who have the inherited skin condition called *psoriasis,* which causes scaly, red, rough patches on the neck, elbows, and knees, as well as pitting of the nails. Often settling in the joints of the fingers and toes, psoriatic arthritis can cause the digits to swell up like little sausages.

✔ **Rheumatoid arthritis (RA):** In this, the second-most common form of arthritis, the immune system turns against the body, causing inflammation and swelling that begins in the joint lining and spreads to the cartilage and the bone. It often affects the same joint on both sides of the body (for example, both wrists).

Classifying arthritis as a "major player"

In the following conditions, arthritis is present and is usually a major part of the syndrome but is not the primary disease process:

✔ **Lyme disease:** Caused by a certain type of bacteria transmitted to humans via tick bites, Lyme disease brings about fever, a distinctive red skin lesion in the shape of a bull's-eye, problems with the nerves and/or heart, and arthritis. Antibiotics are the treatment of choice for this disease.

✔ **Reactive arthritis:** An inflammation of the joints, reactive arthritis strikes along with or shortly after the onset of a sexually-transmitted or intestinal infection. The three problems generally associated with reactive arthritis are arthritis, conjunctivitis (inflammation of the eyelid's lining), and urethritis (inflammation of the urethra).

✔ **Scleroderma:** The word *scleroderma* means hard skin. When tiny capillaries and blood vessels become inflamed and the body responds by overproducing collagen, the skin, blood, internal organs, and joints can suffer. The joint stiffness in scleroderma is actually due to the hardening of the skin. An autoimmune disease, scleroderma usually attacks adults rather than children.

✔ **Systemic lupus erythematosus:** Yet another disease caused by an immune system gone wrong. In lupus, the body attacks its own tissue, causing inflammation, joint pain, stiffness, permanent damage to the joints, and exhaustion. Although lupus most often affects women of child-bearing age, it *does* strike some men and can occur at nearly any age, including childhood and post-menopause.

Describing arthritis as a "minor player"

In these conditions, arthritis may appear but is a minor part of the syndrome.

✔ **Bursitis and tendonitis:** Caused by overusing or injuring a joint, *bursitis* is the inflammation of the fibrous sac that cushions the tendons. *Tendonitis* is the irritation of the tendons, which attach the muscles to the bones.

✔ **Paget's disease:** With Paget's disease, the breakdown and rebuilding of bone speeds up. The resulting bone is larger but also softer and weaker, making it more likely to fracture. These weakened and deformed bones cause arthritis to develop in their respective joints, which typically include those of the hip, skull, spine, knee, and ankle. The cause is unknown.

✔ **Polymyalgia rheumatica:** Seemingly overnight, severe stiffness may strike in the lower back, hips, shoulders, and neck, making it difficult even to get out of bed, a condition known as polymyalgia rheumatica or PMR. The pain is similar to that of RA, but there's no evidence of any active arthritis. PMR can occur by itself or together with a life-threatening inflammation of the blood vessels called giant cell arteritis (GCA). Symptoms of GCA can occur before, after, or at the same time as PMR, and include headaches, scalp tenderness, hearing problems, jaw pain, difficulty swallowing, and coughing. Anyone experiencing these symptoms should be evaluated by a medical professional immediately.

✔ **Sjögren's syndrome:** Another autoimmune disease, Sjögren's syndrome brings about inflammation of the tear glands and saliva glands, causing dryness of the eyes and mouth, hazy vision, cracks at the corners of the mouth, and problems chewing and swallowing. Inflammation of the brain, nerves, thyroid, lungs, liver, kidneys, and, of course, the joints may also be present.

Hypersensitive fingers and toes

Raynaud's phenomenon, a condition that can turn the fingers, toes, and other areas blue or red and cause tingling, numbness, burning, or a pins-and-needles sensation, sometimes occurs in conjunction with (or as a result of) certain arthritis-related conditions (lupus, scleroderma, rheumatic arthritis, and polymyositis to name a few). Prompted by arterial spasm, Raynaud's can cause the hands and feet to become extremely sensitive to cold and to emotional upsets.

Raynaud's can be caused not only by an underlying disease or medical problem but also by repetitive trauma or injuries to the nerves serving the hands or feet, smoking, certain medications, or chemical exposure. Typical attacks include tingling, numbness and whitening of the fingers (without affecting the thumb), and pain or redness when blood circulation returns (usually within 30 minutes to 2 hours).

There's no single blood test to diagnose Raynaud's: Most doctors diagnose this disease based on a description of your signs and symptoms. Your doctor might try to bring about an episode of Raynaud's by putting your hands in cool water or exposing you to cold air. Treatment of the disease generally involves protecting yourself against the elements (wearing gloves and socks and staying warm) and avoiding workplace triggers, such as vibrating tools. In severe cases of Raynaud's, doctors prescribe medication to dilate the blood vessels. See Chapter 5 for more on Raynaud's phenomenon.

Experiencing arthritis as a "companion condition"

These following conditions are linked to arthritis; that is, arthritis may be present, but it constitutes another separate disease process:

✔ **Carpal tunnel syndrome:** This syndrome results when pressure on a nerve in the wrist makes the fingers tingle and feel numb. This syndrome is usually caused by overuse of the wrist. Permanent muscle and nerve damage can occur if carpal tunnel isn't treated.

✔ **Fibromyalgia:** Also known as fibromyalgia syndrome (FMS), this condition involves pain in the muscles and tendons that occurs without a specific injury or cause. Fibromyalgia can make you "hurt all over," particularly in certain tender points in the neck, upper back, elbows, and knees. Those with fibromyalgia can suffer from disturbed sleep, fatigue, stiffness, and depression. The cause is unknown. Physical or mental stress, fatigue, or infections may trigger this disease.

✔ **Myositis:** This disease causes inflammation of the muscles, which can take one of two forms: *polymyositis* — an inflammation of the muscle that causes muscle weakening and breakdown, as well as pain, and *dermatomyositis* — polymyositis plus rashes that can lead to skin scarring and changes in pigmentation.

Deciding Whether It's Really Arthritis: Signs and Symptoms

With all the different kinds of arthritis, how do you know whether you have one of them? Remember two things: Arthritis can strike anyone at any time, and many times you may find it difficult to tell whether the pain you're experiencing is serious enough to warrant medical attention. Almost everyone has had an ache or pain at some time or has overextended herself physically, but you need to know what is minor and temporary, and what may be serious and long term. Knowing what to watch for can make a difference in your treatment and physical comfort. Typical warning signs of arthritis include:

✔ **Joint pain:** This not only includes steady, ever-present pain, but also off-again-on-again pain, pain that occurs only when you're moving or only when you're sitting still. In fact, if your joints hurt in any way for more than two weeks, you should see your doctor.

✔ **Stiffness or difficulty in moving a joint:** If you have trouble getting out of bed, unscrewing a jar lid, climbing the stairs, or doing anything else that involves moving your joints, consider it a red flag. Although difficulty moving a joint is most often the result of a muscular condition, it could be a sign of arthritis.

✔ **Swelling:** If the skin around a joint is red, puffed up, hot, throbbing, or painful to the touch, you're experiencing joint inflammation. Don't wait. See your doctor.

The warning signs may come in triplicate (pain plus stiffness plus swelling), two together, or one all alone. Or, as you find out in Chapters 3 and 4, you may experience other early signs, such as malaise or muscle pain. But if you experience any of these or other symptoms in or around a joint for longer than two weeks, you should see your doctor.

You may be tempted to read this book's descriptions of various diseases, pick out the one with symptoms most closely matching yours, and make your own diagnosis. Some people may make the right diagnosis. But a lot of people make the wrong one, because the symptoms of many forms of arthritis overlap with those of other forms of the disease — they can even be confused with entirely different ailments. Making the wrong diagnosis can lead to the wrong treatment, which can be dangerous. Do not self-diagnose. No matter how obvious the situation seems, go to a medical doctor, have a complete examination, and get an "official" diagnosis.

Considering the Causes of Arthritis

Just as many different kinds of arthritis exist, many different causes also exist — and some of them are still unknown. But in general, scientists have found that certain factors can contribute to the development of joint problems:

✔ **Heredity:** Your parents gave you your beautiful eyes, strong jawline, exceptional math ability, and, possibly, a tendency to develop rheumatoid arthritis. Scientists have discovered that the genetic marker HLA-DR4 is linked to rheumatoid arthritis, so if you happen to have this gene, you're more likely to develop the disease. Ankylosing spondylitis is linked to the genetic marker HLA-B27, and although having this gene doesn't mean that you absolutely *will* get this form of arthritis, you *can* — if conditions are right.

✔ **Age:** It's just a fact of life that the older you get, the more likely you are to develop arthritis, especially osteoarthritis. Like the tires on your car, cartilage can wear down over time, becoming thin, cracked, or even wearing through. Bones may also break down with age, bringing on joint pain and dysfunction.

✔ **Overuse of a joint:** What do ballerinas, baseball pitchers, and tennis players all have in common? A great chance that they'll develop arthritis due to the tremendous repetitive strain they put on their joints. The dancers, who go from flat foot to *pointe* hundreds of times during a practice session, often end up with painful arthritic ankles. Baseball pitchers, throwing fastballs at speeds of more than 100 mph, regularly develop arthritis of the shoulder and/or elbow. And you don't need to be a tennis pro to develop *tennis elbow,* a form of tendonitis that has sidelined many a player.

✔ **Injury:** Sustaining injury to a joint (from a household mishap, a car accident, playing sports, or doing anything else) increases the odds that you may develop arthritis in that joint in the future. Football players are well-known victims of arthritis of the knee, which is certainly not surprising: They often fall smack on their knees or other joints when they're tackled — then have a ton of "football flesh" crash down on top of them. What's most amazing is that they ever walk away uninjured.

✔ **Infection:** Some forms of arthritis are the result of bacteria, viruses, or fungi that can either cause the disease or trigger it in susceptible people. Lyme disease comes from bacteria transmitted by the bite of a tick. Infectious arthritis can arise following surgery, trauma, a needle being inserted into the joint, bone infection, or an infection that's traveled from another area of the body.

Arthritis by the numbers

Arthritis affects a surprisingly large number of us, as you can see by the following numbers:

✔ Seventy million Americans currently suffer from arthritis, or 1 in 3 of us.

✔ Women are nearly twice as likely as men to suffer from arthritis, which currently affects 41 million women and 29 million men.

✔ Arthritis is the reason behind 39 million doctor visits and over a half million hospitalizations.

✔ Osteoarthritis leads the pack in prevalence, affecting more than 21 million Americans, most of whom develop the disease after the age of 45.

✔ Rheumatoid arthritis (RA) and gout are tied for third, at 2.1 million Americans. But RA strikes mostly women, whereas gout tends to favor men.

✔ Gout is twice as likely to strike African-American men as Caucasian men, possibly because African-American men are more likely to use medicines to lower blood pressure. Some blood pressure medications increase production of uric acid, which can crystallize and settle painfully in joints.

✔ The number of children under the age of 17 who have arthritis is an astonishing 285,000, including 50,000 who have juvenile rheumatoid arthritis (JRA).

✔ The lower your income, the more likely you are to develop arthritis. According to the Arthritis Foundation, 20.3 percent of those with an annual income of less than $10,000 had arthritis, as opposed to 13.4 percent of those who made $50,000 or more.

✓ **Tumor necrosis factor (TNF):** TNF is a substance the body produces that causes inflammation and may play a part in initiating or maintaining rheumatoid arthritis. Although scientists are unsure exactly what triggers rheumatoid arthritis, they have found that drugs that counteract the effects of TNF, called *TNF antagonists,* are often helpful in managing the symptoms of this disease.

Understanding Who Gets Arthritis

Statistically speaking, the typical arthritis victim (if there were such a thing) would be a middle-class Caucasian woman between the ages of 65 and 74 who has a high school education, is overweight, is a city-dweller in the southern United States, and has osteoarthritis.

But arthritis isn't all that picky and doesn't worry too much about statistics. It strikes young and old, male and female, and rich and poor and doesn't seem to care where you live. Arthritis, in one form or another, can affect just about anybody.

However, arthritis does seem to hit women particularly hard. Nearly two-thirds of those who get the disease are women — an estimated 41 million Americans. Some facts about women and arthritis:

✓ Arthritis affects about 37 percent of the female population and 28 percent of males.

✓ Arthritis limits the daily activities of an estimated 4.6 million women.

✓ Some 16 million women are currently affected by osteoarthritis, a disease that strikes women nearly three times more often than men. To make matters worse, women usually develop the disease at a younger age.

✓ Seventy-five percent of rheumatoid arthritis patients (about 1.5 million) are women.

✓ Ninety percent of those who have either lupus or fibromyalgia are women.

✓ Twice as many girls as boys develop juvenile rheumatoid arthritis.

Additionally, arthritis affects some 4 million African Americans, making it the third most prevalent health condition affecting them, topped only by high blood pressure and chronic sinus problems. It was placed ahead of heart disease, diabetes, and asthma, among others. African Americans are also more likely than others to limit their activities due to arthritis.

African-American women are at particular risk for arthritis. There's a higher rate of arthritis reported among African-American women after age 35 than in Caucasian women, and young African-American women are three times more likely to develop lupus than their Caucasian counterparts.

Assessing Your Treatment Options

The good news is that, in many cases, arthritis can be managed. It may take some time and effort to find the right treatment(s) for your particular version of the disease, but answers are out there. Medications and surgery are only a part of the answer. Following an arthritis-fighting diet, exercising, using joint protection techniques, controlling stress, anger, and depression, and organizing your life can offer relief from pain and a new lease on life. And the world of herbs, homeopathy, hands-on healing, and other alternative medicine treatments may offer you additional ammunition in the fight against arthritis pain and other symptoms.

Looking into medications

When you're in pain, your joints are hot or swollen, and you can hardly walk from one end of the house to the other, you want relief *now*. In many cases, the fastest way to relieve arthritis symptoms is to take medication. Arthritis medications fall into five main classes:

- **Analgesics:** Analgesics fight pain but do not interfere with the inflammation process, so they're easier on the stomach than the NSAIDs. The best-known and most commonly-used analgesic is acetaminophen.

- **Biologic response modifiers (BRMs):** The BRMs help fight stubborn cases of inflammation by inhibiting or shoring up certain components of the immune system called cytokines. The cytokines play a part in the inflammation seen in rheumatoid arthritis, and BRMs inhibit their inflammatory action. Enbrel, Humira, Remicade, and Kineret fall into the category of BRMs.

- **Corticosteroids:** These are manmade versions of naturally-occurring hormones in the body that help quell inflammation. Although they're a powerful anti-inflammatory, they can also have powerful side effects, including elevated blood pressure, stomach ulcers, thinning of the bones and skin, and increased risk of infection.

- **Disease modifying antirheumatic drugs (DMARDs):** The DMARDs are usually used in inflammatory forms of arthritis (like RA, psoriatic arthritis or ankylosing spondylitis) that haven't responded to other medicines. They change the way the immune system works, slowing or stopping its attack on the body. Drugs like sulfasalazine, methotrexate, and anti-malarials fall into this category.

✔ **Nonsteroidal anti-inflammatory drugs (NSAIDs):** The NSAIDs help relieve pain and reduce inflammation by interfering with an enzyme called COX (cyclooxygenase). Milder versions (aspirin, ibuprofen) are available over the counter, and the more powerful ones (Anaprox, Feldene, Tolectin) require a prescription.

Chapter 8 gives you the complete lowdown on arthritis medications.

Considering surgery

If pain is interfering with your ability to lead a happy and productive life, you have to take the maximum amount of pain relievers just to get through the day, and you've tried all other pain-relieving methods with no luck, you may want to consider surgery. Although joint surgery is complex and not to be taken lightly, some people have enjoyed excellent results, to the point of feeling that they've gotten a new lease on life. Surgical techniques can involve flushing a joint with water, resurfacing rough bone ends or cartilage, removing inflamed membranes, growing new bone, or putting in a whole new joint. Turn to Chapter 9 to find out more about surgical treatments.

Making lifestyle changes

Chances are excellent that you can do much to ease your arthritis-related pain, stiffness, swelling, and decreased range of motion just by changing certain things you do every day. The following list goes over some options you may want to consider:

✔ **Eat an arthritis-fighting diet.** By this diet, we mean one that includes plenty of fish, fresh fruits and vegetables, and whole grains, with a minimum of processed meats and salad oil (corn, safflower, or sunflower). The Mediterranean diet fits the bill, while also warding off both heart disease and certain types of cancer. See Chapter 11 for the skinny on the elements of a good arthritis-fighting diet.

✔ **Consider taking joint-saving supplements.** Many supplements can help ease the symptoms of different kinds of arthritis, including antioxidants (beta-carotene, vitamins C and E, and selenium), boron, vitamin B6, niacin, vitamin D, zinc, grapeseed extract, flaxseed oil, green tea, glucosamine sulfate, chondroitin sulfate, SAMe, bromelain, and others. We discuss these at length in Chapter 11.

✔ **Exercise daily (whenever possible).** Countless studies have shown that exercise can help lubricate and nourish the joints by forcing joint fluid into and out of the cartilage. Underexercised joints don't get much of this in-and-out action, so cartilage can thin out and become dry. Brisk

Stargazing: Famous arthritis sufferers

Does the idea of having arthritis make you feel like you may as well just give up? Well, many people have felt the same, but persevered anyway. Take a look at what some people have done with their lives while coping with arthritis:

- **Lucille Ball** was diagnosed with rheumatoid arthritis at the age of 17, but she went on to live a long and healthy life, enjoying a top-notch career in movies and television.

- The famous French artist **Pierre-Auguste Renoir** developed RA in his late fifties, but painted nearly 6,000 pictures during his lifetime, many of them great masterpieces.

- Actress **Mary McDonough,** best known for her role as Erin on the TV show *The Waltons,* has lupus, yet is a wife and mother and continues a successful career as an actress and spokesperson for the Lupus Foundation of America.

- **Dr. Christian Barnard** developed rheumatoid arthritis as a youngster but went on to perform the world's first human heart transplant in 1967.

- **Billie Jean King** has osteoarthritis of the knees, probably the result of a car accident when she was 18 years old. Yet she won the Wimbledon singles title for the sixth time when she was in her early thirties and successfully took on Bobby Riggs in the "Battle of the Sexes" tennis tournament.

- **Norman Cousins,** editor of the *Saturday Review,* developed ankylosing spondylitis in 1964. As part of his then unheard-of treatment, he watched the Three Stooges, the Marx Brothers, and *Candid Camera* to make himself laugh and keep his spirits up. The book he later penned, called *Anatomy of an Illness,* became a bestseller, and he lived a long and productive life.

- **Rosalind Russell,** star of the silver screen, suffered from severe RA and did much to garner support for the advancement of research into this disease.

- **Wayne Gretzky,** possibly the greatest hockey player of all time, suffers from early signs of osteoarthritis.

- **Grandma Moses** had arthritis in her hands at age 76 when she began painting the folksy, whimsical scenes of American life that made her famous. Despite her condition, she created hundreds of paintings, many of which hang in major museums all over the world.

walking may be one of the best exercises for those with arthritis, because it doesn't put undue stress on the joints and is easy and fun to do. For a rundown of exercises that help ease arthritis symptoms, see Chapter 12.

- **Watch your joint alignment.** Making sure to stand, sit, walk, run, and lift correctly can help protect your joints from injury or excess wear and tear. We discuss the best joint-saving techniques in detail and describe how to make them a part of your life in Chapter 13.

- **Control stress, aggression, and depression.** The way you think and feel about your arthritis pain can actually make it worse. So can stress, anger, hostility, aggression, and depression. Luckily, you can reduce your pain just by reducing your stress levels and tapping into your natural potential for relaxation. In Chapter 14, we tell you all about positive thinking, biofeedback, controlling your breathing, laughter, prayer, and spirituality — all effective ways of improving your mood, easing your pain, and making you feel better all over.

✔ **Organize your life for maximum efficiency.** Studies have shown that people who actively manage their arthritis and find new ways to cope with physical problems feel less pain and fatigue. In Chapter 15, we give you helpful tips for managing arthritis on a day-to-day basis. Included are ideas for conserving your energy, getting a good night's sleep, using assistive devices, making household chores easy, and holding on to your sex life. An occupational therapist and a home health caregiver can offer valuable assistance.

Looking at alternative approaches

Because there isn't any one magic bullet that cures arthritis, a great many people are looking to alternative approaches — either as a substitute for traditional medicine or as that extra something that just may do the trick. In Chapters 16 through 19, we discuss the most popular alternative treatments for arthritis — from herbs to homeopathy, from acupuncture to reflexology, from aromatherapy to hydrotherapy. Included are sections describing the therapy, explaining what it can do for you, and giving you tips on how to find a reputable practitioner.

Chapter 2

Osteoarthritis: The Most Common Form

*W*hether you call it osteoarthritis, degenerative arthritis, or degenerative joint disease, osteoarthritis (OA) is the painful result of cartilage breakdown. When the tough, rubbery substance that cushions bone ends no longer does its job, the bone ends can't slide easily across each other within the joint. That's when pain and stiffness can settle into a joint. Suddenly, your knee aches, your hip burns, a finger joint swells and throbs, or your shoulder stiffens up. You can't bend and flex the painful joint like you used to; its range of movement is limited. Most of all, it just plain hurts!

But what happened to mess up your cartilage in the first place? To understand what went wrong, here's a look at how things work in healthy cartilage.

Considering Cartilage

Healthy cartilage is absolutely essential for joints to function properly and painlessly. Slick as polished marble and tough as galvanized rubber, cartilage protects the ends of your bones from wearing each other away where they meet inside a joint. It also provides a smooth, slick surface so bone ends can glide easily across each other. And cartilage is an excellent shock absorber, cushioning the bones and soaking up the impact created by movement and physical stresses. Without intact cartilage, bones grind away at each other and bear the brunt of the impact of movement. Eventually, the joint itself can be damaged or even destroyed.

Four elements help cartilage do its all-important job:

- ✔ **Water:** Sixty-five to 80 percent of cartilage is water — a crucial substance that lubricates the joints, cushions bones, and absorbs shock.

- ✔ **Collagen:** Elasticity and a superb capability to absorb shock make collagen an integral part of healthy cartilage. A connective tissue that helps hold bones, muscles, and other bodily structures together, collagen is the mesh-like framework that provides a home for the proteoglycans.

- ✔ **Proteoglycans:** These large, oblong molecules are covered with centipede-like "arms" that weave themselves securely into the collagen mesh and soak up water like a sponge. Then, when pressured, they release water. Thanks in part to the proteoglycans, cartilage can mold itself to the shape of the joint and respond to the ever-changing amount of pressure within the joint capsule.

- ✔ **Chondrocytes:** These cells follow the principle "out with the old and in with the new" as they break down and get rid of old proteoglycan and collagen molecules, forming new ones to take their place.

Water, collagen, proteoglycans, and chondrocytes all work together to keep your joints moving like well-oiled machinery. When the pressure is released from a joint, say your knee when you lift your leg to take a step, water rushes into the cartilage, nourishing, bathing, and plumping it up. The water-loving proteoglycans, woven securely into the collagen web, soak up water and hold on to it until pressure is applied to the joint (that is, you take another step). Then the water and wastes rush out of the cartilage. But as soon as the pressure is off, the proteoglycans thirstily soak up the water again. The resilient collagen stretches and shrinks to accommodate joint pressure and water content, so your cartilage can bounce back after being flattened out.

But if your cartilage loses its ability to attract and hold water, it becomes thin, dry, cracked, and unable to provide a slippery surface (see Figure 2-1). No longer plump and resilient, it makes a poor shock absorber and cushion for the bones, particularly affecting the weight-bearing joints.

You can visualize the action of the cartilage by thinking of two cans of soup facing each other end-to-end with an almost-filled water balloon in between them. As you press the soup cans together, the water balloon changes shape to accommodate the pressure, but never lets the cans actually touch. When you release the pressure, the water balloon (like your cartilage) resumes its old shape.

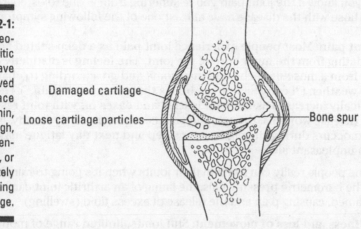

Figure 2-1: Osteoarthritic joints have narrowed joint space and thin, rough, broken-down, or completely missing cartilage.

Damaged cartilage

Loose cartilage particles

Bone spur

Identifying the Signs and Symptoms of Osteoarthritis

Don't assume that you have osteoarthritis just because you have one or more of the following symptoms. Get a thorough examination and diagnosis from a qualified physician. Figure 2-2 shows you the most common sites affected by osteoarthritis.

Figure 2-2: The neck, lower back, knees, hips, ends of the fingers, and the base of the thumbs are the sites most commonly affected by osteoarthritis.

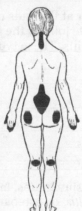

How do you know if the joint pain you're suffering from is due to osteoarthritis? Most of those with the disease have at least one of the following symptoms:

- **Joint pain:** Most people experience joint pain as a deep-seated ache radiating from the inner core of the joint. The feeling is distinctly different from a muscular ache and may come and go according to changes in the weather. ("I can feel it in my bones that it's going to rain.") The pain typically increases as the joint is used and eases off with joint rest. As the disease worsens, though, the pain can become fairly steady. If joint pain occurs during the night, poor sleep and next-day fatigue may be two unpleasant side effects.

    Some people really can feel it in their joints when it's going to rain, because as the barometric pressure falls, the lining of an arthritic joint can become inflamed, causing pain and the release of excess fluid (swelling).

- **Stiffness and loss of movement:** Stiff joints, limited range of motion, and, in later stages, joints that freeze into a bent position are all signs of osteoarthritis.

- **Tenderness, warmth, and swelling around the joint:** Although swelling is not usually a big problem with osteoarthritis, some joints do swell in response to cartilage damage and irritation, especially if they've been overused. The finger joints and the knees are most often affected.

- **"Cracking" joints:** If you hear popping or crunching sounds when you move a joint, you may have osteoarthritis. These cracking sounds (doctors call them *crepitus*) can be created by roughened cartilage. (This isn't the same thing as "cracking" your joints by applying pressure to them, which causes a harmless release of nitrogen bubbles and isn't associated with OA.)

- **Bony growths on the fingers:** Bony lumps, either at the ends of the fingers (called *Heberden's nodes*) or on the middle joint of the fingers (called *Bouchard's nodes*) are signs of osteoarthritis. These types of bony growths may be hereditary.i

Discovering What Causes Cartilage Breakdown

Sometimes, we really don't know why the cartilage disintegrates. In that case, we designate the problem as *primary osteoarthritis,* or osteoarthritis of unknown cause. Other times we know that the osteoarthritis has been triggered by another problem, in which case we call it *secondary osteoarthritis.*

Considering causes of primary osteoarthritis

The ultimate cause of primary osteoarthritis remains a mystery. Although scientists aren't sure why, the collagen mesh of the cartilage becomes scrambled; it weakens and can't hold its structure. The proteoglycans, once so cozily intertwined in the collagen mesh, suddenly find themselves evicted from their secure homes. As they float off into the joint fluid, they take their water-retaining abilities with them. The cartilage is left high and dry; it thins and may even crack. At the same time, the newly-freed proteoglycans draw excess fluid into the joint capsule, causing swelling. (Unfortunately, this fluid can't get back into the cartilage, where it's desperately needed. It's something like dying of thirst in the middle of the ocean.)

Although no one is absolutely certain what causes primary osteoarthritis, here are a few theories:

- **The chondrocytes become too efficient at breaking down the collagen and proteoglycan molecules.** In healthy cartilage, the amount of breaking down enzymes is equal to the amount of building up enzymes. An overabundance of destructive enzymes leads to weakened collagen and a lack of proteoglycans.

- **The chondrocytes go wild and start making too many proteoglycan and collagen molecules.** The opposite of the previous condition, these chondrocytes are too good at making new cartilage components. The excess proteoglycan and collagen molecules, in turn, pull extra fluid into the joint, flooding it and washing away most of the chondrocytes. The cartilage, then, is left bereft of cartilage-producing molecules.

Sorting out the sources of secondary osteoarthritis

Although the origins of primary osteoarthritis remain murky, experts are quite sure what causes secondary osteoarthritis: various types of trauma to the joints. That includes sudden, high-velocity trauma (the kind you'd experience in a car accident), as well as little insults to your joints that occur time and again, like repeated poor posture or running on a concrete surface every day for years. The causes of secondary osteoarthritis can be further broken down as follows:

- **Joint injury:** Weekend warriors beware! Once a joint has been injured, be it through a sports mishap, car accident, household slippage, or anything else, it is much more likely to develop osteoarthritis.

✔ **Repetitive motion injury:** Joints that are stressed over and over again in the same way (for example, a ballerina's ankles, a football player's knees, or a data processor's wrists) are more likely to experience a cartilage breakdown than joints subjected to normal use.

✔ **Damage to the bone end:** Usually due to trauma or continual stress, a bone may chip or sustain small fractures. In the body's zeal to repair the damage, it may cause an overgrowth of bone in the injured area. The result is a bone end that's bumpy, not smooth, and joint problems can ensue.

✔ **Bone disease:** A bone disease, such as Paget's disease, weakens the bone structure, making it more likely to fracture and develop bony overgrowth.

✔ **Carrying too much body weight:** The heavier you are, the more stress your knees, hips, and ankles must bear. Osteoarthritis of the knee has been clearly linked to excess body weight. That's not surprising considering that every time you take a step the stress on your knee is roughly equivalent to three times your body weight. Increase that figure to ten times your body weight when you run!

Regarding the repair problem

To make matters worse, once your cartilage is damaged, your body can compound the problem if it repairs itself in certain ways. Like injured bone, injured cartilage can overdo the repair process, piling too much new cartilage into a crack or tear. The result is a lumpy, bumpy surface that doesn't glide smoothly against the cartilage on the opposing bone end. On the other hand, sometimes the cartilage doesn't repair itself at all, and remains in its damaged state — cracked, pitted, frayed, and even worn-through. Pieces of loose cartilage and/or bone may break off and float freely through the joint fluid. The bone ends, no longer well cushioned, start to rub against each other and can develop bony spurs (osteophytes) that further interfere with smooth joint movement. The joint space narrows, and the entire shape of the joint can change. All this from a little damaged cartilage!

You may hear your doctor use some of these technical terms: *eburnation* (increased and abnormal bone density), *subchondral bone* (the bone right below the cartilage), or *subchondral cyst* (an abnormal pocket of fluid in the bone beneath the cartilage).

Recognizing Risk Factors for Osteoarthritis

Although osteoarthritis affects nearly 21 million Americans, not everybody suffers from it. Some people actually sail into their golden years with joints unaffected by pain, stiffness, or other symptoms, while others are hobbling around by the time they're 35. So how come one person gets osteoarthritis while another gets away scot-free? And how can you tell if you happen to be particularly susceptible to it?

Your chances of developing osteoarthritis are increased if:

- **You're past age 45:** Cartilage and other joint structures, like most bodily tissues, tend to degrade and become weaker over time. After decades of use, they start to wear out. Luckily, research has shown that osteoarthritis isn't inevitable as we age. The odds just go up.

- **You've had a joint injury:** If you've been in a car accident, have played rough-and-tumble sports, or have injured any of your joints in any way, you are more likely to develop osteoarthritis in the joints that were affected by those activities.

- **Your joints have been repeatedly stressed:** Ballet dancers, assembly line workers, baseball pitchers, grocery checkers, and anyone else who overuses and stresses a joint or joints can suffer from cartilage breakdown in those joints.

- **You're a woman:** Women are three times more likely than men to develop osteoarthritis. This may be due to smaller joint structures or some link to estrogen; nothing has yet been proven.

- **Your parents had it:** There appears to be a genetic component to osteoarthritis; in fact, one study concluded that genes were responsible for 50 percent of hip osteoarthritis cases. Osteoarthritis in the hands is also believed to be at least partially due to genetics. An inherited tendency toward defective cartilage or poorly structured joints can certainly put you on the road to osteoarthritis, although you won't necessarily develop it.

- **You're overweight:** Excess weight puts a great deal of strain on the weight-bearing joints — the hips, knees, and ankles. For every ten pounds of excess weight you carry, you increase the force exerted on these joints anywhere from three to ten times, depending upon the type of activity. Researchers have found a definite link between being overweight and osteoarthritis, especially involving the knee joints.

Using chopsticks can increase your risk of developing OA of the hand! Researchers studying 2,507 60-year-old residents of Beijing, China found significantly more OA in the first, second, and third fingers of the hand that used chopsticks than the non-chopstick-using hand. Repeated mechanical stress to these joints, via chopstick use, is believed to be the culprit.

Determining Whether It Really Is Osteoarthritis

Nearly 50 percent of those suffering from osteoarthritis don't know what kind of arthritis they have and therefore can't make good decisions about their treatment.

Say your knee hurts. The first time that you visit your doctor complaining of the pain, he puts you through the standard round of interviews, examinations, and tests. He reviews your medical history and makes a detailed list of the injuries you have sustained, especially to your knees. He may palpate your knee to see if it's painful to the touch, carefully bend your knee and straighten it several times (it may hurt a little and seem stiff), and listen for cracking or popping in the joint. If your arthritis appears to be inflammatory, your doctor may send you to the lab to get some blood drawn to rule out other forms of the disease. At this point, all your doctor has to go on is a history of knee injuries, some pain and stiffness upon movement, and a little cracking in the joint. Your symptoms may sound like osteoarthritis but may not yet be a sure thing.

The next step would be to order an X-ray of your knee to see if one or more of the following signs are present:

- ✔ Cartilage degradation
- ✔ Cartilage overgrowth
- ✔ Narrowing of the joint space
- ✔ Bone spurs
- ✔ Bits of cartilage or bone floating in the joint fluid
- ✔ Joint deformity

Treating Osteoarthritis

After a diagnosis of osteoarthritis is confirmed, you and your doctor can begin to devise a treatment program — confident that you're headed in the right direction. Although the symptoms may not disappear completely, you still have a good chance that, with proper treatment, your pain will diminish significantly and joint degradation can be kept to a minimum.

A good treatment plan for osteoarthritis should include the following elements to help you manage pain and discomfort on a daily basis.

Muting the pain with medication

Both prescription and over-the-counter remedies are commonly used to relieve osteoarthritis pain. Whether prescription or nonprescription, the drugs usually fall into one or two categories:

- ✔ **Acetaminophen:** These relieve pain and fever but don't reduce swelling (for example, Tylenol, Liquiprin, or Datril).

- ✔ **Nonsteroidal anti-inflammatories or NSAIDs:** These relieve pain and fever and *do* reduce swelling (for example, aspirin, Advil, Aleve, or Motrin).

If your joints are swollen, the doctor may prescribe an NSAID. If swelling isn't a problem, he or she may give you acetaminophen.

To avoid drug interactions, overdoses, or side effects, make sure you check with your doctor before taking any over-the-counter medications. (See Chapter 8 for more information on medicines.)

Lubricating your joints with exercise

If you're in pain, you probably want to *stop* moving, and it's certainly advisable for you to rest your joints when you're feeling achy. But too much sitting around can actually be the *worst* thing for you in the long run. Exercise is a great way to "oil and feed" the cartilage. Underexercised joints don't get the lubricating and nourishing benefits of the in-and-out action of the joint fluid, so cartilage can become thin and dry, losing its resilience and capability to cushion the bones.

Include three types of exercises in your overall physical fitness program:

- ✔ **Flexibility exercises:** You should do stretching, bending, and twisting exercises every day to increase your range-of-motion and reduce stiffness. Flexibility exercises help keep your joints loose and flexible.

- ✔ **Strengthening exercises:** Weight lifting or isometric exercises should be done every other day to build your muscles and help keep your joint-supporting structures stable. These types of exercises help increase your muscle strength.

- ✔ **Endurance (aerobic) exercises:** These should be done at least three times a week for at least 20 to 30 minutes each session to increase overall fitness, strengthen your cardiovascular system, and keep your weight under control. Brisk walking (especially up hills), jogging, cycling, dancing, jumping rope, and so on, all help to increase your fitness and capacity for exercise.

Before starting a new exercise program, check with your doctor to find out what kinds of exercise and which levels of activity are appropriate for you. Doing the wrong exercises — or doing the right exercises in the wrong way — can cause you further injury. (See Chapter 12 for more information on exercise.)

Protecting your joints through good alignment

Applying the techniques of body alignment, proper standing, sitting, walking and running, and correct lifting can go a long way toward sparing your joints from excessive wear and tear and protecting them from future injury. You may also find it helpful to wrap affected joints with elastic supports or take a load off with assistive devices, such as canes or crutches. Other joint-protective techniques include alternating your activities with rest periods, varying your tasks to avoid too much repetitive stress on any one area, and pacing yourself. Don't try to do too much at once. (See Chapter 13 for more information on joint protection.)

Heating and cooling the pain away

Some people prefer heat, others cold, but use whatever works for you. Hot baths, heating pads, electric blankets, and hot tubs can relax painful muscles, while ice packs can numb the affected area. To avoid damaging tissues, just make sure you don't use either method for longer than 20 minutes at a time. (See Chapter 10 for more information on physical therapy for pain relief.)

Always give your skin time to return to its usual temperature before reapplying hot or cold packs.

Taking a load off with weight control

If you're overweight, your hips, knees, and ankles are probably suffering. Not only are they subjected to a force equal to three times your body weight each time you take a step, they can be pummeled by ten times your body weight if you jog or run! So that extra 10 pounds around your middle may translate to an extra 100 pounds slamming away on certain joints at certain times. And that's only *one* reason why keeping your weight at an acceptable level is so important. (See Appendix C for more information on diet and weight control.)

Fifty percent of patients who develop knee osteoarthritis have been overweight for between three and ten years.

Knowing how to help yourself

Strategies for pain management, foods and supplements that can help heal, positive thinking, prayer, spirituality, massage, relaxation techniques, and alternative healing methods can add to your arsenal in the fight against pain and disability. Don't ignore their enormous potential to improve the quality of your life. (See Chapters 10, 11, and 15 through 19 for more information on these topics.)

Keeping OA at bay: Mark's story

Mark, a 35-year-old television executive, had been a hotshot college quarterback in his younger days. But after winding up at the bottom of one too many half-ton pileups, his knees were shot.

"I was a sitting duck for those guys," Mark says ruefully. "They just couldn't wait to pounce on me, no matter what the play. After two years of getting hit over and over again, my body just couldn't take it anymore. I was permanently sidelined."

Sidelined from football, perhaps, but not other sports. Over the next several years he took up jogging, karate, fencing, and weight lifting. "I tried to do something every day," Mark said. "But it wasn't just because I wanted to keep in shape. I would get itchy if I didn't get a certain amount of exercise on a daily basis." In spite of his efforts, though, he managed to pack an extra 20 pounds onto his once rock-hard body. ("Beer and nachos while watching football," Mark explained, smiling.)

Then one day, right in the middle of a fencing match, his right knee began to hurt. "It was a deep pain, way inside my knee, a pretty intense soreness that lasted through the match and really bugged me," Mark said. Afterward, he iced his knee, and the pain went away. But it began to bother him now and again, often during fencing, and also when he was jogging or in the bent-knee stance of karate. When the pain became present more often than not, Mark went to see a sports medicine doctor.

"Sounds to me like osteoarthritis," his doctor said. An X-ray confirmed that the cartilage in his knee was "rough" and quite thin. "Arthritis!" Mark exploded. "But that's for old people. I'm only 35!"

Two years later, Mark's osteoarthritis is pretty well under control. He rarely has pain, unless he stands in line for long periods of time. And although he has given up certain knee-thrashing sports (such as football, karate, and fencing), he has found that he's still physically able to do just about whatever he wants.

"I chalk my recovery up to two main things," Mark says. "Losing weight and switching activities. Once I dropped that extra 20 pounds I'd been lugging around, my knee pain also dropped about 50 percent. Then I started swimming every day — a real boon to my joints since I could keep them loosened up without the slamming impact of jogging or jumping rope. Yoga has also helped me gain some flexibility while getting rid of some tension. And I've been taking a few supplements that seem to help. All in all, I feel like a brand new guy."

Considering surgery

When you have a painful joint that isn't going to get better, and the pain is seriously compromising the quality of your life, you may want to consider surgery. These days, routine surgeries like arthroscopic surgery, cartilage transplants, and joint replacement surgery can make a huge difference for those who live in pain. (See Chapter 9 for more information on surgery.)

Chapter 3

A War Within: Rheumatoid Arthritis

*R*heumatoid arthritis (RA) is a case of the human body's good intentions gone awry. Your body is equipped with a very effective immune system that fights off bacteria and other foreign bodies. Specialized immune cells attack these invaders, surround them, paralyze them, and destroy them. A strong, intact immune system is absolutely essential to your survival — without it, you would quickly become consumed by infections and disease. But if your immune system should suddenly go haywire and start attacking your body's own tissues, it could become your worst enemy. Such is the case with rheumatoid arthritis (RA). When you have RA, your immune system attacks the tissues that cushion and line your joints, eventually causing entire joints to deteriorate.

Turning on Itself: The Body Becomes Its Own Worst Enemy

For reasons that aren't completely understood, in rheumatoid arthritis the white blood cells of the immune system attack the joint lining (synovial membrane) as if it were a foreign object. And pain, loss of movement, and joint destruction are the unhappy results. After the immune system goes to work on the joint lining, here's what happens:

1. The assaulted membrane becomes inflamed and painful, the entire joint capsule swells, and the synovial cells start to grow and divide in an abnormal way.

2. Almost as if they're launching a counterattack, these abnormal cells invade the surrounding tissue — mostly the bone and cartilage.

3. The joint space begins to narrow, and the joint's supporting structures become weak. At the same time, the cells that trigger inflammation release enzymes that start eating away at the bone and cartilage, causing joint erosion and scarring.

4. Reeling under this many-sided attack, the joint itself deteriorates, eventually becoming misshapen and misaligned.

See Figures 3-1 and 3-2 for comparison of a healthy joint to one with RA.

Rheumatoid arthritis insidiously makes its way through the body and (in more severe cases) can eventually spread to all of the joints. But the joints are not its only targets. RA is a systemic disease capable of triggering numerous problems in various parts of the body, not just the joints. It can cause inflammation of the membranes surrounding the eyes, heart, lungs, and other internal organs, generally wreaking havoc on the body as a whole.

If the tear and salivary glands partially "dry up," Sjögren's syndrome can develop in association with RA. See Chapter 4 for more on this "drying disease."

Some people have RA for just a short time — a few months or a couple of years — and then it disappears forever. Others suffer through painful periods (flares) that come and go, although they can feel quite well in between episodes. Those with severe forms of RA, however, may be in pain a good deal of the time, experience symptoms for many years, and suffer serious joint damage.

Figure 3-1:
In the healthy joint, the synovial membrane is thin and free from inflammation; the cartilage is smooth, thick, and even. The joint space is well defined, and the joint capsule assumes a normal shape.

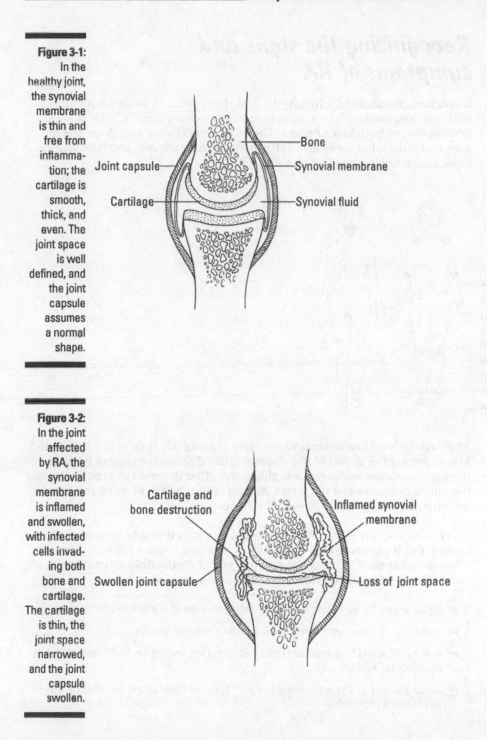

Joint capsule

Cartilage

Bone

Synovial membrane

Synovial fluid

Figure 3-2:
In the joint affected by RA, the synovial membrane is inflamed and swollen, with infected cells invading both bone and cartilage. The cartilage is thin, the joint space narrowed, and the joint capsule swollen.

Cartilage and bone destruction

Swollen joint capsule

Inflamed synovial membrane

Loss of joint space

Recognizing the signs and symptoms of RA

If you have rheumatoid arthritis, the first thing you may notice is a dull ache, stiffness, and swelling in two matching joints — for example, both elbows, both knees, or both index fingers. The most typical sites for RA are the fingers and wrists, but it can also settle in the hands, elbows, shoulders, neck, hips, knees, ankles, and feet. See Figure 3-3.

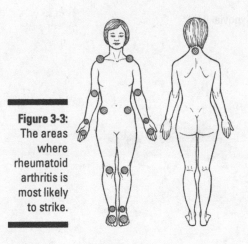

Figure 3-3: The areas where rheumatoid arthritis is most likely to strike.

Although pain and inflammation are early signs of RA, they're not always the first to herald the arrival of the disease. Still's disease is a type of RA in which the first indicators are fever, rash, chills, and other general symptoms affecting the entire body, not just the joints. Among children with juvenile rheumatoid arthritis, some 10 percent have Still's disease.

RA typically begins with minor symptoms and slowly makes its presence known. But it can also strike dramatically, causing several joints to become inflamed all at once. Although the symptoms of rheumatoid arthritis vary, most people with RA experience one or more of the following:

- Pain, warmth, redness, swelling, or tightness in a joint
- Swelling of three or more joints for six or more weeks
- Joints affected in a symmetrical pattern (for example, both knees, both shoulders, and so on)
- Joint pain or stiffness lasting longer than an hour upon arising or after prolonged inactivity

- ✔ Pea-shaped bumps under the skin (called *rheumatoid nodules*), especially on pressure points like the elbows or the feet. In bedridden patients, they may also occur at the base of the scalp or on the back side of the hip

- ✔ Evidence of joint erosion on an X-ray

- ✔ Loss of mobility

- ✔ General soreness, aching, stiffness

- ✔ A general "sick" feeling *(malaise)*

- ✔ Fatigue and weakness, especially in the early afternoon

- ✔ Periodic low-grade fever and/or sweats

- ✔ Difficulty sleeping

- ✔ Anemia

- ✔ Blood tests showing the presence of rheumatoid factor (an abnormal substance found in the blood of about 80 percent of RA patients)

As RA progresses, the joints enlarge and can become deformed. They may even freeze in a semicontracted position, making complete extension impossible. The fingers can start to curl up, pointing away from the thumb, as their tendons slip out of place. RA may also attack other parts of the body, causing the following conditions:

- ✔ **Pleurisy:** If RA attacks the lungs, it can cause *pleurisy* (inflammation of the membranes around the lungs), prompting difficulty in breathing, chest pain, and lung scarring.

- ✔ **Episcleritis:** If it attacks the tissues covering the white part of the eye (a condition called *episcleritis*), it can cause eye pain, sensitivity to light, and tearing of the eye.

- ✔ **Pericarditis:** If it settles in the membrane surrounding the heart (a condition called *pericarditis*), it can cause abnormal heart function.

- ✔ **Vasculitis:** If it affects the blood vessels *(vasculitis),* the blood supply to other parts of the body can be cut off, causing nerve damage and tissue death.

Even though rheumatoid arthritis can have some very serious consequences, this disease can be managed. Many people with RA live long, successful lives. But remember: Early treatment can make a big difference in RA, so don't wait to see a doctor.

The older you are when rheumatoid arthritis first strikes, the milder your case is likely to be.

Understanding the causes of RA

The truth is that nobody really knows what causes RA, although some believe it is linked to a defect in the immune system. Many people with RA have a particular genetic marker — HLA-DR4 — so it's reasonable to suspect that this gene may be to blame. Yet, not everyone with this gene ends up with RA, and not everyone with RA has this gene. And scientists are certain that more than just one gene is involved: Perhaps HLA-DR4 is only one of several genes that can tip the scales in favor of developing RA. Most likely, genetic markers play a part in the development of the disease but aren't the determining factor. Some researchers believe that RA may be triggered by a virus, or perhaps an unrecognized bacteria, that "wakes up" a dormant genetic defect and sets it in motion. As of yet, no such infectious agent has been discovered, and RA has not been found to be contagious.

Hormones or hormone deficiencies may also play a part, although their possible role is unclear. Women are more likely than men to develop RA, suggesting a possible link to estrogen. But, at present, doctors have more questions than answers about RA.

Overcoming RA: Lucy's story

Lucille Ball, the famous comedienne and zany star of the *I Love Lucy* television series, was just 17 years old and working as a model in Hattie Carnegie's internationally renowned dress shop when she suddenly developed a fiery pain in both her legs. "It was so bad, I had to sit down," she wrote in her autobiography, *Love, Lucy.* She had recently recovered from a bout with pneumonia and a high fever; now this!

Hurrying to her doctor, she received the terrifying news: She had rheumatoid arthritis, a crippling disease that becomes progressively worse over time. In fact, it was conceivable that she would spend her life in a wheelchair. Lucy's doctor sent her to an orthopedic clinic where she waited for three hours, nearly fainting from the pain, before the doctor informed her that there was no cure. He did ask if she would like to try an experimental treatment, though — injections of a kind of "horse serum." Lucy agreed and received these shots over the next several weeks until she finally ran out of money. Unfortunately, the pain continued.

Discouraged but not about to give up, Lucy went back home to her parents, who massaged her legs, gave her money to continue the horse serum injections, and encouraged her to take better care of her health. Finally, months later, the pain began to ease, and Lucy was able to stand up on weak and shaky legs. Her left leg had shortened a bit during the course of the disease, so she added a 20-pound weight to her corrective shoe to stretch the leg out.

Lucy's hard work and perseverance paid off. She was able to return to New York; she made several movies and eventually starred in her own television series, one that required vigorous physical comedy, stamina, and energy. She also starred in Broadway plays, performing eight shows a week while managing to sail through energetic song and dance numbers with a seemingly effortless grace and ease. Lucy remained active and healthy until her death in 1989, and in spite of her doctor's ominous prediction, never spent a single day in a wheelchair.

Describing the most likely victim of RA

Rheumatoid arthritis can strike just about anybody — children, the elderly, the middle-aged, and people of almost all racial or ethnic groups. But RA has a particular affinity for women, especially those between the ages of 20 and 50. Women account for 1.5 million of the 2.1 million Americans who suffer from RA, making them more than twice as likely as men to get the disease, although scientists have yet to determine why.

Diagnosing Rheumatoid Arthritis

Unfortunately, no one test can tell your doctor you definitely have RA. Instead, your doctor looks for a tell-tell pattern in the information taken from many sources, like your medical history, physical examination, laboratory tests, X-rays, a fluid sample taken from affected joints, and, if rheumatoid nodules are present, a biopsy of those nodules.

Searching for clues: The medical history and physical exam

During your initial examination, your doctor will ask about the onset of your symptoms, whether you're experiencing any morning stiffness, the kind and amount of pain you feel, the presence of swelling, whether or not joints are affected on both sides of your body, and so on. Looking into your medical history is a way to see if your symptoms fit the general pattern of RA or suggest another disease instead. During your physical exam, your doctor will also check for tenderness, range of motion, and the presence of rheumatoid nodules.

Taking tests

Three tests typically help diagnose rheumatoid arthritis, all of which involve taking a sample of your blood and sending it to the laboratory for examination:

- ✔ **Rheumatoid factor (RF) test** checks for the presence of a particular antibody that appears in the blood of the majority of people who have RA. But a positive RF test doesn't necessarily mean you have rheumatoid arthritis. The RF antibody can be caused by other rheumatic diseases as well as many other medical conditions.

- ✔ **Erythrocyte sedimentation rate (ESR)** checks for the presence of inflammation in the body.

> ✔ **Red blood cell count (RBC)** checks for anemia, a common symptom associated with systemic types of arthritis.

(See Chapter 7 for a complete description of these tests.) In addition to the preceding, your doctor may also perform the following tests:

> ✔ **Joint fluid sample:** The doctor inserts a needle into your affected joint(s) to remove some fluid, which is examined under a microscope for evidence of infection or inflammation.

> ✔ **Joint X-ray:** An X-ray of your joints is taken to detect early bone and cartilage loss or to serve as a baseline for future X-rays.

> ✔ **Biopsy of rheumatoid nodules:** If you have rheumatoid nodules, the doctor may want to excise a piece of tissue from one of them and examine it under a microscope to confirm the diagnosis. Here's how it's done: After carefully cleansing the skin and injecting a local anesthetic, the doctor makes a tiny cut near the nodule. If the nodule is easily accessible, the doctor may decide to reach in with a scalpel and shave off a piece of tissue. Or she may push a thin, hollow needle into the nodule and, using suction, pull out a sample.

Treating Rheumatoid Arthritis

Although RA is often a chronic disease, most people who have it respond well to treatment and lead active, productive lives. A few years back, a victim of RA could look forward to a dreary life spent bedridden or in a wheelchair. But today, those with rheumatoid arthritis have a better prognosis: Only about one patient in ten progresses to the point of disability (although one-third of patients leave work prematurely). In a full 70 percent of the cases, symptoms are relieved or controlled by treatment for long periods of time. And one out of ten people completely recovers from RA, usually within the first year, never to be bothered by it again.

Treatment usually begins with the least aggressive, most conservative measure — rest — and gradually moves on to more aggressive methods — medication and surgery — if necessary.

Relying on rest

Resting the affected joints during a flare is a must, because using them tends to increase inflammation. Regular rest periods should be worked into the daily schedule, and at times, total bed rest may be necessary. Immobilizing a severely affected joint with a splint may help, but the joint should be moved from time to time to keep it from locking up. You may want to wear a splint during the most active times of the day, and take it off during the least active times — for example, 12 hours on and 12 hours off.

Mental outlook appears to affect RA symptoms. Stress tends to make flares worse, whereas a positive outlook can help keep complications at bay.

Delving into your diet

What you do and don't eat can make a difference to the arthritis disease process and how much pain you feel. Because many forms of arthritis and arthritis-related conditions involve inflammation, eating foods that reduce the inflammation response (like fish, fish oils, flaxseed oil, black walnuts, and green soybeans) can make a positive difference. Eating plenty of fruits, vegetables, and whole grains supplies ample amounts of antioxidants like vitamins C and E and selenium, which can fight the cellular damage that contributes to arthritis. And taking the dietary supplements glucosamine sulfate and chondroitin sulfate can not only reduce pain, but in some cases can even stop the arthritis process in its tracks. (See Chapter 11 to find out more about how what you eat affects how you feel.)

Easing into exercise and physical therapy

A good overall exercise program helps strengthen joint-supporting structures, increases endurance, and maintains or improves flexibility. Even inflamed joints should be exercised a little to prevent them from freezing up. A physical therapist can provide exercises that gently take the joints through their full range of movement. Exercising in water, especially during flares, may be easier than exercising on land, because it's low impact and the cool water may help ease inflammation. (See Chapter 12.)

Protecting your joints

Not only do you make your mom happy when you stand up straight, but you reduce the pressure on your joints. Maintaining proper posture while walking, standing, and sitting can go a long way toward easing joint stress. And understanding how to lift or move heavy objects correctly is also a must. (See Chapter 13.)

Applying hot or cold compresses

Applying hot or cold packs to inflamed joints may ease the pain and help reduce inflammation. Use heat to ease sore muscles and increase circulation, and try cold to dull the pain and reduce inflammation. (See Chapter 10.)

Taking medication

Many drugs can be used to combat RA symptoms. The following subsections give you details on the five main types commonly prescribed.

Non-steroidal anti-inflammatory drugs (NSAIDs)

NSAIDs (pronounced n-seds) reduce swelling, relieve pain, and are the most commonly prescribed drugs for RA. Aspirin and ibuprofen are two well-known NSAIDs, but these drugs are typically prescribed in much larger doses than recommended when you buy them over the counter. A dose of 600 milligrams of ibuprofen taken three times a day is a standard treatment for pain for most newly diagnosed RA patients. (Naturally, you should not take this dosage of aspirin or any other medication unless your doctor prescribes it.)

As with all drugs, certain side effects can occur when taking NSAIDs, including upset stomach, nausea, diarrhea, and stomach bleeding. Take this type of medication with food to prevent these physical reactions.

Analgesics

Analgesic pain fighters don't relieve inflammation, which makes them less irritating to the stomach than NSAIDs. Acetaminophen, the best-known and most commonly used analgesic, is often recommended as a first-line treatment for RA pain. Analgesics are available in over-the-counter forms such as Tylenol, Excedrin, and aspirin-free Excedrin, and in prescription forms in such drugs as Vicodin, Percocet, Darvon, and codeine. Sometimes a combination of an analgesic and an NSAID is prescribed for intense pain.

Disease-modifying antirheumatic drugs (DMARDs)

If NSAIDs aren't effective, or if your disease seems to be progressing quickly, your doctor may want to prescribe DMARDs, which can potentially alter the course of the disease by reducing inflammation and joint damage, while preserving joint function. This category of drugs includes methotrexate, hydroxychloroquine sulfasalazine, and leflunomide, to name a few.

DMARDs are also known as *remittive drugs* and *slow-acting drugs*. They're called slow acting because you may not see results for weeks or months.

These drugs may influence the immune system — whose errant behavior can lead to RA — to slow the formation of bone deformities, affect cell growth, or otherwise slow the progress of RA. They can even send the disease into remission, at least temporarily. Depending upon which drug is being used, it may be given until symptoms improve, until unacceptable side effects appear, or until it's clear that the medicine isn't helping.

Potential side effects of DMARDs include increased infections, gastrointestinal distress (diarrhea, loss of appetite, vomiting, and so on), liver problems, rashes, and blood cell disorders.

Corticosteroids

Corticosteroids (or steroids), such as prednisone, are powerful weapons against inflammation. They work by suppressing the immune system, which is the trigger of the errant inflammation seen in RA.

These drugs work well because they're "souped-up" versions of cortisone, the body's natural immune suppressor, and the latest data suggests that they may indeed have disease-modifying properties. Two studies published in 2002 indicate that steroids reduced bone damage in early RA.

These strong drugs can trigger severe side effects, including high blood pressure, osteoporosis, an increase in blood glucose, cataracts, and bruising and thinning of the skin. When used for a month or longer, they may cause fluid retention in the face ("moon face"), the belly, the legs, and so on. Because of this side effect, corticosteroids are typically reserved for severe cases, and then used for only short periods of time. Because they work more quickly than most other therapies, they can serve as a bridge until other medications take effect.

If you suddenly stop taking corticosteroids, you may suffer from pain, swelling, critical illness, or even death from adrenal crisis. Always taper off your use of these drugs.

Biologic response modifiers (BRMs)

Four BRMs are currently approved to treat RA: infliximab, etanercept, anakinra, and adalimumab (all generic names). These new and promising therapies inhibit inflammation, shore up certain components of the immune system, and can alter the course of the disease. These drugs are quite expensive because they must either be injected or infused, but researchers are currently working on less expensive versions that can be taken by mouth.

Each BRM partially disables an "arm" of the immune system and therefore makes you more susceptible to certain infections. For example, the anti-TNF BRMs can increase your risk of tuberculosis and similar infections. Ask your doctor about these risks before taking BRMs.

Saving your joints via surgery

When all else fails and RA becomes severe or disabling, surgery may be an option. Surgeons have different approaches to relieving the symptoms. Some of the approaches are included in the following list:

✔ Diseased joint linings can be surgically removed.

✔ Joint replacement can correct deformities and ease pain.

✔ Fusing or removing joints in the foot may relieve the pain experienced when walking.

✔ Fusing vertebrae in the neck may prevent spinal cord compression.

✔ Fusing of the thumb joint can aid in grasping.

Other sophisticated surgical techniques that are on the horizon may ensure a healthier and less painful future for RA sufferers.

Modifying risk factors for heart disease

Many studies have shown that the risk of illness or death due to coronary artery disease is much higher in patients with RA; in fact, it's the number-one cause of death. This is most likely because the chronic inflammation caused by RA speeds up the progression of atherosclerosis. Most rheumatologists recommend that their RA patients exercise, watch their weight, eat a nutritious diet, keep their cholesterol and blood pressure under control, and stop smoking as part of their routine care. Check out *Heart Disease For Dummies* (Wiley) to find out more.

Predicting the outcome

Predicting how a person with RA will fare is difficult; after all, everyone is different. But certain factors can suggest that the course of the disease may be either easier or more difficult. For example, RA may be less severe if one or more of the following factors applies to you:

✔ **You're female.** Women are more likely to get RA, but the disease often takes a greater toll on men.

✔ **You have a college degree or better.** Educated people tend to seek help earlier, are more likely to follow doctor's orders to the letter, often have less physically strenuous jobs, and have better access to care.

✔ **You're middle-aged or older when stricken.**

✔ **Your cartilage and bone ends have not been worn away, and you don't yet have joint deformities.**

> ✔ **You don't have rheumatoid nodules.**
>
> ✔ **Your level of rheumatoid factor is low.** Remember, however, that some people who have little or no rheumatoid factor suffer severely.
>
> ✔ **You're pregnant.** Some women enjoy a nine-month period of time with fewer symptoms.

Perhaps as many as 10 percent of RA patients enjoy what doctors call *spontaneous remission,* or the disappearance of the disease for no apparent reason.

Looking to the future

Today, rheumatoid arthritis rarely manifests as the crippling, deforming disease of just a few years ago. Researchers in genetics and immunology are constantly uncovering new and fascinating parts of this puzzle, and some 15 new drugs have recently been introduced to treat RA. Great strides have also been made in surgical techniques, enabling surgeons to offer hope to those with deformed, painful joints. Through our rapidly expanding arsenal of knowledge, our medications, certain lifestyle changes, and new surgical techniques, we should soon be able to tame, if not conquer, the beast known as rheumatoid arthritis.

Understanding the Difference between Osteoarthritis and Rheumatoid Arthritis

RA and OA have two things in common: namely joint pain and damage to certain joint structures, such as the cartilage and the bone. Other than that, they're about as different as night and day. Table 3-1 outlines the differences between RA and osteoarthritis.

Table 3-1	Rheumatoid Arthritis Compared to Osteoarthritis
Rheumatoid Arthritis	*Osteoarthritis*
Joint inflammation and swelling are prominent symptoms.	Joint inflammation and swelling are less common.
Usually begins between the ages of 25 to 50, but can also strike children.	Usually begins after the age of 40. Rarely strikes children.
Settles in a majority of joints, especially fingers, wrists, shoulders, knees, and elbows.	Affects the weight-bearing joints primarily (for example, knees, hips, ankles, and spine).

(continued)

Table 3-1 *(continued)*

Rheumatoid Arthritis	Osteoarthritis
Affects joints symmetrically (for example, both wrists).	Affects isolated joints or one joint at a time.
Morning stiffness lasts more than one hour.	Brief periods of morning stiffness.
Often causes systemic symptoms, such as fatigue, fever, weight loss, and general malaise.	Does not cause systemic symptoms.

Chapter 4

Investigating Other Forms of Arthritis

● ●

In This Chapter

▶ Discovering the different forms of arthritis

▶ Understanding various disease processes

▶ Recognizing symptoms

▶ Finding out what doctors can do

▶ Knowing what you can do to help yourself

● ●

The various forms of arthritis all have one thing in common: They produce pain, swelling, and other problems in or near one or more joints. The symptoms may appear suddenly and obviously, or they may sneak up so gradually that you can't remember when they began. They may strike with the force of a jackhammer or feel more like a chilly breeze. Sometimes the diagnosis is obvious; other times it may elude doctors for a year or longer. The varied treatments can be quick and effective, produce delayed reactions or in some cases, not work at all.

Osteoarthritis and rheumatoid arthritis, the subjects of Chapters 2 and 3, are well-known forms of arthritis. This chapter examines some of the lesser-known and less prevalent, but still troublesome, forms of the disease, including gout, pseudogout, juvenile rheumatoid arthritis, infectious arthritis, gonococcal arthritis (a form of infectious arthritis), psoriatic arthritis, and ankylosing spondylitis.

Gaining Insight into Gout: It's Not Just for Royalty

Many people think that gout is a disease reserved for corpulent kings and beefy barons, but any one of us can be stricken, even if we're slim and never drink alcohol.

Summarizing the symptoms

Some two million Americans, mostly male, suffer from gout. Officially known as *acute gouty arthritis,* the problem usually begins with a sudden, overwhelming "assault" on a joint. You may go to bed feeling fine, with no inkling of trouble ahead, only to wake up in the middle of the night with excruciating pain in the bunion joint of your big toe. The joint is stiff and warm to the touch; swelling lends a shiny, tight, reddish or purplish look to the skin, which is severely stretched over the area. Sometimes the joint is so inflamed and painful that even the touch of a bed sheet causes agonizing pain. You may also have a fever, chills, a rapid heart rate, and a general blah feeling.

Gout is linked to excess uric acid in the blood. (Doctors call this *hyper-uricemia.*) When the blood has more uric acid than it can handle, the body may convert the excess into sharp, pointed crystals and store them in one or more joints. See Figure 4-1 for an example of what the crystal deposits look like in a joint.

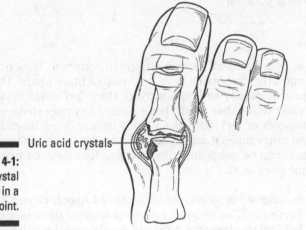

Uric acid crystals

Figure 4-1:
Crystal
deposits in a
gouty joint.

The big toe is quite often the first site that gout strikes. The elbows, wrists, fingers, knees, ankles, heels, and instep may also be attacked during the first or subsequent bouts, while the shoulders, spine, and hips are rarely touched. No matter where gout strikes first, the odds are three out of four that it will affect the big toe at some point.

Your first attack of gout may also be your last, for gout often disappears in several days without treatment and without lingering after-effects. Or, it may herald the beginning of a series of attacks on that joint and/or others, leading to progressive and irreversible joint injury. Fortunately, medical treatment can help ward off recurring attacks while preventing or minimizing permanent joint damage.

If you want to guard against gout, the best strategy is probably to be born female. Women's uric acid levels are lower than men's until menopause is reached. After menopause, women's uric acid levels start to rise, but up to 20 years may pass before they're equal to male levels.

Several situations can lead to an excessive amount of uric acid, including the following:

✓ Genetics — 6 to 18 percent of those with gout have a history of the disease in the family.

✓ Eating lots of organ meat and/or other meats, gravies, peas, anchovies, dried peas, and beans. These foods contain large amounts of purines, which can stimulate the body's production of uric acid.

✓ Blood cancer or other diseases that cause the rapid multiplication and destruction of body cells, leading to higher levels of purines and uric acid.

✓ Certain diseases that hamper the kidneys' capability to filter out uric acid.

✓ Drinking too much alcohol (which can upset kidney function).

✓ Taking drugs that can lead to increased uric acid.

Gout is also associated with high blood pressure, high levels of blood fats, and obesity.

Though the disease comes about when excess uric acid in the blood is converted into crystalline form and deposited in the joints, elevated uric acid alone doesn't cause gout. Many people with excess uric acid suffer nary a twinge, while others, with terrible pain, have fairly standard amounts of uric acid in their bodies. You can also have fully-formed uric acid crystals in a joint or two, yet feel no pain.

Diagnosing and treating gout

Sometimes the symptoms of gout "speak" loudly, making the diagnosis fairly easy. Other times, the symptoms can be vague, making the diagnosis difficult.

Microscopic examination of fluid taken from the stricken joint is an important diagnostic step. If needlelike uric acid crystals are visible, gout is the probable diagnosis. White blood cells may also be present, sent to the joint as part of the inflammation process. To diagnose gout, your doctor will order a blood test to check uric acid levels and to look for *tophi* (lumps of uric acid crystals stored under the skin). Your doctor may also X-ray the afflicted joint.

Gout has no surefire cure, although medications and lifestyle changes can help. Treatment often begins with high doses of nonsteroidal anti-inflammatory drugs (NSAIDs — see Chapter 8) for pain and inflammation, and a drug called colchicine may be given to prevent further attacks. This regimen is usually used only for the short term (12 weeks or so), due to side effects that may occur with long-term usage. If you have recurrent or disabling attacks of gout, tophi in your blood, your X-rays show evidence of joint destruction, or you have recurrent kidney stones, your doctor may give you urate-lowering drugs such as allopurinol and probenecid to keep your uric acid levels under control. Corticosteroids are sometimes injected into the afflicted joint to reduce inflammation.

In addition to offering medicines, your doctor can "tap" your joint by inserting a needle and drawing out the excess fluid. This procedure often helps relieve the pain and pressure, and sometimes is all that's needed to treat someone.

Helping yourself heal

You can help heal gout and prevent its recurrence by:

- ✔ Losing weight if you are overweight
- ✔ Eliminating alcohol intake, especially beer, which contains purines
- ✔ Eliminating foods containing purines (for example, organ meats, fatty meats, meat gravies, wild game, sardines, anchovies, herring, mackerel, and scallops) and limiting meat, fish, poultry, dried peas, and beans to one serving per day
- ✔ Working with your doctor to keep your blood pressure under control, if it's a problem
- ✔ Consulting with your doctor to make sure you're not taking any medicines or supplements that encourage gout or interfere with your treatment
- ✔ Exercising regularly

Studying Pseudogout: The Royal Pretender

Although gout is an ancient disease that ruined many a medieval VIP's days, pseudogout is a "new" affliction. Although it's probably been around as long as "regular" gout, doctors didn't realize it was a separate problem until about 40 years ago.

Summarizing the symptoms

The symptoms of pseudogout are similar to those of gout but without the needlelike uric acid crystals in the joint. Instead, pseudogout is characterized by rhomboid-shaped crystals made up of calcium pyrophosphate dihydrate. And although gout typically affects the big toe joint, pseudogout more often targets the knee.

The disease itself may be acute or chronic. Acute attacks are likely to strike suddenly, settle in, and last for several days or even weeks. (Fortunately, they are usually not as painful as acute attacks of "true" gout.) The chronic attacks last longer, typically target more than one joint at once and, over time, severely damage these joints.

The causes of pseudogout are unknown. Surgery, a hormonal imbalance, or a metabolic upset may touch it off. Sometimes it strikes in conjunction with other diseases or states, such as low blood magnesium or too much iron in body tissues. Pseudogout strikes men and women at about the same rate and prefers older folks, especially those over the age of 60.

Diagnosing and treating pseudogout

Because pseudogout can masquerade as gout, rheumatoid arthritis, or other ailments, diagnosis is usually made by inspecting fluid taken from the affected joint. If you have pseudogout, your fluid will contain calcium pyrophosphate dihydrate crystals. (These crystals can also be picked up on X-rays.)

Unfortunately, there's no way to cure the disease completely and no method for removing the offending crystals from the joints. Instead, doctors try to relieve the symptoms, typically prescribing NSAIDs to reduce the pain and inflammation. Other drugs may be used if necessary. Sometimes, simply "tapping" the joint and drawing out the excess fluid is enough. Treatment can bring relief during attacks but can't prevent joint damage. Still, most sufferers do well if their pain and inflammation are kept under control by medication.

Understanding Juvenile Rheumatoid Arthritis

Arthritis is bad for everyone, but somehow it seems worse when it strikes children. Youngsters can develop most of the forms that strike adults, and arthritis affects nearly 300,000 children. That's more children than are currently affected by cystic fibrosis, sickle cell anemia, and muscular dystrophy combined! Many of these children suffer from juvenile rheumatoid arthritis (JRA), which is similar to adult rheumatoid arthritis (see Chapter 3), except that many children outgrow the problem. Adults, unfortunately, don't.

An autoimmune disease, JRA causes the body to turn on itself and destroy its own tissue. No one knows just why the immune system goes wrong, but researchers suspect it's a two-part process. The child has a genetic tendency toward JRA to begin with; then something in the environment (like a virus) sets it off, allowing the disease to develop.

Summarizing the symptoms

Three kinds of juvenile rheumatoid arthritis exist and are differentiated by their symptoms:

✔ **Pauciarticular JRA:** The most common form of JRA, pauciarticular JRA, involves no more than four joints. About 50 percent of children with JRA have pauciarticular JRA, which usually strikes in the knees and other large joints, attacks mostly girls ages 8 and younger, and may only strike one of a pair of joints (one knee rather than both, one elbow instead of both, and so on).

In 20 to 30 percent of cases, pauciarticular JRA can trigger eye inflammation that if untreated, can become serious. This particular kind of eye inflammation, called *uveitis,* can occur even in the absence of any eye symptoms, so children with this form of JRA should be routinely screened by an ophthalmologist. Fortunately, many children outgrow this disease (although the eye problems can continue into adulthood).

✔ **Polyarticular JRA:** Polyarticular JRA attacks five or more joints. Striking some 40 percent of children with JRA, the polyarticular form usually settles in the fingers and other small joints, although large joints are not immune. The disease is typically symmetrical, which means it attacks the fingers on both hands, and so on. There may also be a fever and rheumatoid nodules. Girls are more likely than boys to develop polyarticular JRA, and Native American children are more likely to develop it than Caucasian children.

✔ **Systemic JRA:** The systemic form of JRA "travels" throughout bodily systems, causing trouble wherever it settles. The least common form of juvenile rheumatoid arthritis, systemic JRA may produce fever, pale red spots on various parts of the body, anemia, swollen lymph nodes, inflammation of the linings of the lungs and heart, and other problems.

Regardless of the form JRA takes, it causes joint stiffness, pain, and swelling that is usually worse upon awakening from a full night's sleep or even a nap. Symptoms usually come and go. Sometimes a child is lucky — the symptoms arise just a few times and then disappear forever — but a large percentage of children continue to have arthritis into adulthood. Luckily, most have only mild cases.

Diagnosing and treating JRA

To be considered JRA, the disease must produce joint inflammation and stiffness for at least six weeks in someone under the age of 17. JRA is similar to "adult" rheumatoid arthritis, except for a few key differences:

✔ Many children with JRA outgrow the problem, while most adults with RA don't.

✔ JRA may affect bone development and growth in children, causing slow, rapid, or uneven growth in the afflicted joints.

✔ Less than 50 percent of those with JRA test positive for rheumatoid arthritis factor, compared to 70 or 80 percent of adults.

Doctors diagnose and treat JRA in much the same way they do the adult version. In addition to the strict medical treatment, children with JRA need special emotional and social support.

Figuring Out Infectious Arthritis

Infectious arthritis is caused by viruses, bacteria, or fungi that enter the body and settle into one or more joints. Depending upon which germs have invaded, which joint(s) they inhabit, the strength of your immune system, and the speed and accuracy of the treatment, a bout with infectious arthritis can be brief and relatively painless, or serious and painful.

Technically speaking, infectious arthritis is an infection of the joint tissues and/or fluid. Several different germs, ranging from staphylococci to HIV to tuberculosis, can infect a joint. But remember, these are not specifically "arthritis germs;" they're "regular germs" that cause staph infections, mumps, hepatitis B, and other diseases. Only when they settle in the joints can infectious arthritis occur.

Summarizing the symptoms

The nature and extent of the symptoms depend on which germ has taken up residence in the joint(s). In the joint itself, you may experience pain to the touch or with movement, as well as swelling and stiffness. The skin around the joint may be red and puffy. If the infection spreads beyond the joint, a fever or other symptoms may accompany it (although fever can occur for other reasons). Some forms of infectious arthritis can hit strong and fast, so it's important that you see your doctor immediately if you have any symptoms. If left untreated, they may seriously damage joints within just a few days or weeks.

Diagnosing and treating infectious arthritis

If your doctor suspects infectious arthritis, she will quickly call for various tests to firm up the diagnosis. Blood, urine, and joint fluid samples will be analyzed for infectious organisms. But even before the lab results come back, your doctor may begin giving you antibiotics, starting with those that kill the "usual suspects." Other medicines may follow after the doctor is sure what's ailing you.

Antibiotics are effective against bacterial infections, and antifungal medicines fight fungus infections, but viruses are another story. Unfortunately, no effective antiviral medications exist. But don't despair if you have a virus; many viruses clear up on their own.

In addition to the medicines, your doctor may drain pus from your joint, splint the joint, if necessary, and arrange for physical therapy. Certain infections can require surgery to wash out the joint.

Getting a Grip On Gonococcal Arthritis

Caused by the *gonococci* bacterium — the same culprit responsible for gonorrhea — gonococcal arthritis is the most widespread of the infectious forms of arthritis.

Summarizing the symptoms

Gonococcal arthritis typically strikes hard and fast, and pain seems to move from one joint to another. Small blisters can appear on the skin over some or many parts of the body, and the tendons may swell and ache.

Diagnosing and treating gonococcal arthritis

Both men and women can develop gonococcal arthritis. Men are much more likely to know that something is wrong because of penile discharge and painful urination. Thus, they're more likely to receive treatment for gonorrhea before it progresses to gonococcal arthritis. Women, who don't have such obvious symptoms, are less likely to receive early treatment for gonorrhea and more likely to develop the arthritis. Women may also find themselves suffering from pain in the abdomen and fever.

The typical patient with this disease is a young, sexually active person with signs and symptoms of venereal disease, so the doctor can often hone in on the diagnosis of gonococcal arthritis during the medical history and physical examination. He then checks for skin blisters and sends samples of various body fluids to the laboratory before making a definitive diagnosis.

Treatment with antibiotics is usually successful, although in recent years certain strains of gonorrhea have become resistant to both penicillin and tetracycline. Today, the disease is treated by a large number of new and potent antibiotics and, in most cases, vanishes without permanently damaging the joints

Surveying Psoriatic Arthritis

Psoriatic arthritis is an insult added to the injury of psoriasis, because it strikes those who are already suffering from this scaly skin condition. Fortunately, only about five percent of psoriasis sufferers develop the arthritis.

Summarizing the symptoms

In psoriatic arthritis, the joints of the fingers and toes become inflamed, swollen, and, in more severe cases, deformed. The spine, hips, and other joints may suffer as well.

Diagnosing and treating psoriatic arthritis

A specific test for psoriatic arthritis doesn't exist, so your doctor bases the diagnosis on your symptoms, and to some extent, your family medical history. (If you have psoriasis in your family, you're more likely to develop psoriatic arthritis.)

Treatment is important, because psoriatic arthritis can cause severe damage to your joints. Unfortunately, it has no cure. Your doctor can try to reduce your joint inflammation and keep your psoriasis under control through the use of NSAIDS. If the disease doesn't respond to NSAIDs or is aggressive, drugs such as methotrexate or sulfasalazine can be used. And certain biologic response modifiers (BRMs) have proven tremendously effective in fighting psoriatic arthritis: Enbrel has been FDA-approved for this purpose, and some doctors are also seeing good results with Remicade. Chapter 8 tells you more about these medications.

Considering Ankylosing Spondylitis

Ankylosing spondylitis (AS) attacks the cartilage, ligaments, and tendons of the spine, which become inflamed. The back becomes stiff, inflamed, and sore. As the disease progresses, the ligaments and tendons may become more like bone tissue, forming bony bridges between the vertebrae and locking them into place. In more severe cases, AS can turn the spine into an unbending rod, but the disease usually doesn't advance that far. Figure 4-2 shows the difference between a normal spine and one with AS.

A. Normal vertebra

Vertebra

B. Vertebrae with ankylosing spondylitis

Figure 4-2: Normal vertebrae compared to those with ankylosing spondylitis.

Intervertebral disc

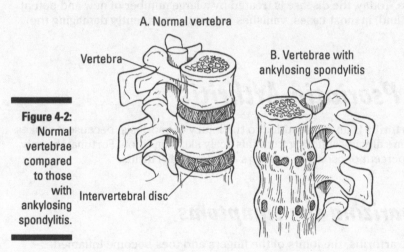

AS has attacked some 300,000 Americans. Men between the ages of 20 and 40 are the favorite targets. The disease has been linked to a certain gene and often runs in families. But having the gene doesn't guarantee that you'll get AS; it increases your susceptibility, but something else (perhaps an infection) must trigger the disease.

Summarizing the symptoms

AS generally comes on gradually. Pain or stiffness settles in the lower back or other joints. It may be worse at night or upon arising and then get better as the person begins to move around. AS can be fairly constant or it can come and go. Problems may also develop with the shoulders, hips, knees, and other joints.

A systemic disease, AS can cause skin and eye problems, loss of appetite, fatigue, and fever. There may also be difficulty in taking a deep breath, damage to the heart valves, and problems caused by pressure on the nerves.

Diagnosing and treating ankylosing spondylitis

No one test can detect ankylosing spondylitis, so doctors usually make the diagnosis on the basis of the patient's symptoms and family history, plus the physical examination. Your doctor will have you perform various bending exercises to test joint flexibility and will take an X-ray to look for characteristic bone damage. He will also order certain laboratory tests to rule out rheumatoid arthritis or other diseases.

Treatment is aimed at relieving pain and inflammation and preventing or correcting deformities of the spine and other problems. Your doctor typically prescribes NSAIDs and muscle relaxants. Although the damage that caused the spinal deformities can't be undone, exercises can help you remain as strong and flexible as possible. Physical therapy can be helpful as you work on coping with any deformities that arise. More extreme cases may require surgical replacement of a joint.

Though AS has no cure, most who have the disease suffer from mild to middling symptoms and do fairly well. One of the most exciting developments in rheumatology over the last few years is the effectiveness of BRMs in treating ankylosing spondylitis; they improve mobility while fighting progression of the disease. Also, Enbrel is FDA-approved as a treatment for AS.

Chapter 5

Exploring Other Conditions Linked to Arthritis

. . . .

In This Chapter

▶ Discovering the diseases that are linked to arthritis

▶ Understanding various disease processes

▶ Recognizing symptoms

▶ Finding out about diagnosis and treatment

▶ Knowing what you can do to help yourself

. . . .

Millions of people have been struck by symptoms ranging from joint stiffness to skin rashes to difficulty swallowing. Sometimes their conditions are diagnosed quickly. Other times, they're forced to endure myriad tests and bounce from doctor to doctor until they find out what's wrong. Along the way, they may be mistakenly told that their problems are caused by stress, lack of sleep, or depression, when in reality they're suffering from a condition related to arthritis. That is, arthritis is a major or minor part of the syndrome, although it's not the primary disease. Or arthritis may accompany another illness, while being a completely separate disease process.

These conditions that are somehow linked to arthritis can be categorized in one of three ways:

- Arthritis is a major player in the disease.

- Arthritis is a minor player in the disease.

- Arthritis is a companion condition to the disease.

Experiencing Arthritis as a Major Player

In ailments such as systemic lupus erythematosus and scleroderma, the joint problems that characterize arthritis are a major part of the syndrome. But even though arthritis is present — often in a big way — it isn't the primary disease process.

Systemic lupus erythematosus: The wolf disease

Systemic lupus erythematosus (commonly known as *lupus* or *SLE*) is a body-wide disease that often marks its victims with a red, wolf-like facial rash.

Lupus can attack the joints, heart, nervous and vascular systems, skin, lungs, and other parts of the body. The symptoms strike because the body produces large numbers of antibodies — called *autoantibodies* — that attack bodily tissue. No one knows exactly why this occurs. Those with lupus are at a higher risk of heart attacks, strokes, kidney failure, and osteoporosis than those without the disease.

Ninety percent of lupus patients are women, and most of them are in their childbearing years (ages 15 to 45). Perhaps as many as one million Americans suffer from the disease, which tends to favor African Americans (who are three times more likely to develop lupus than Caucasians). Hispanics, Asians, and Native Americans are also more likely than Caucasians to be struck by the disease.

Summarizing the symptoms

Symptoms can range from mild to deadly, with problems appearing in the joints, skin, organs, and/or elsewhere. Typical symptoms include fever, the blahs, joint pain and inflammation (in other words, arthritis), rash, hair loss, excessive sensitivity to sunlight, anemia, immune system weakness, problems with the kidneys and other organs, nervous system disorders, and depression.

Lupus settles in for the long haul but tends to hit and run, causing symptoms to flare up and then retreat. For many people, the "good" periods can last for weeks, months, or even years.

From wolves to butterflies

Today, we think the characteristic SLE rash looks more like a butterfly with its wings spread, but the French doctor who gave the disease its name back in the 1800s thought of a wolf when he saw the rash. The name *lupus,* which means *wolf* in classical Latin, has endured.

Diagnosing and treating lupus

Lupus can cause a bewildering variety of symptoms that may mirror those of other diseases, making the diagnosis difficult. Doctors sometimes follow a hunch, tying the fact that the patient is a young woman to one or more of her symptoms, and then ordering tests to confirm or rule out the diagnosis. Blood tests are used to look for antibody abnormalities, abnormal blood chemistries, problems with the immune system, kidney damage, and so on. Biopsies of the kidneys, lungs, and other tissues may be required, as well as X-rays, CT scans, MRIs, electrocardiograms, and more.

Treatment is as varied as the disease. In mild cases, the main thrust may center on relieving symptoms: non-steroidal anti-inflammatory drugs (NSAIDs) for arthritis symptoms and fever, aspirin or stronger blood thinners to prevent blood clots, other drugs for skin problems, and so on. More severe cases may require prednisone or other corticosteroids to bring down inflammation, immunosuppressants to keep the haywire immune system in check, and antimalarial medications for both skin and joint problems.

Fortunately, you can do several things to cope with lupus. You can't make the symptoms disappear, but you can certainly improve the quality of your life by doing the following:

- If you tire easily, cut back on your work or home duties.
- Look for ways to reduce stress. (See Chapter 15 for tips on coping with stress.)
- Protect yourself from the sun. (This is crucial, because excessive sun exposure leads to both worsening skin disease and disease flares. Complete sun avoidance is advisable, but for even short exposure, use of sun blocks *and* protective clothing is recommended.)
- Follow your doctor's dietary instructions carefully.

Discoid lupus erythematosus: A less dangerous form

A limited form of the disease, discoid lupus generally confines itself to the skin and usually doesn't venture into the body to attack the organs. The systemic form of lupus develops in approximately 5 percent of people with discoid lupus, and about one quarter of those with SLE demonstrate discoid disease at some time in their disease course.

Summarizing the symptoms

Like systemic lupus, discoid lupus tends to attack women and produces a characteristic skin rash. The rash begins with little, reddish, disclike patches, about as big around as the circumference of a drinking straw. Typically appearing on the face, scalp, and ears, they may also appear on the upper chest and back, the backs of the arms, and even the shins. Untreated, the rashes may begin to grow outward, and a scar may develop in the central area of each rash. Over time, there can be severe scarring and pitting of the skin, as well as hair loss.

The rash can come and go, or remain in place, and it may be accompanied by joint aches. A drop in the white blood cell count, indicating immune system depression, is also common.

Diagnosing and treating discoid lupus

Discoid lupus is difficult to diagnose because the primary symptom — the rash — can lead doctors to suspect other diagnoses such as psoriasis, actinic keratosis, seborrheic dermatitis, SLE (in fact, tests may confirm that it *is* SLE), or other diseases. Because there is no single, conclusive test for discoid lupus, much of the diagnostic workup is aimed at eliminating other diseases, then diagnosing discoid lupus by default. (A biopsy is often helpful in determining the diagnosis.)

Treatment usually consists of sun avoidance and the use of anti-malarial drugs to control the disease. If an active rash is present, topical or oral steroids are added to quiet things down. If the disease is detected and treated early, scarring can be kept to a minimum.

Scleroderma: When the skin hardens

Although it attacks various parts of the body, scleroderma is best known for its effects on the skin. In fact, the disease's name comes from the Greek words for *hard* and *skin*.

Technically speaking, scleroderma is a collagen vascular disease: collagen because an excessive deposit of collagen damages body tissue, and vascular because the blood vessels suffer.

No one knows why, but in the 50,000 to 100,000 Americans who have scleroderma, the body produces too much collagen. A fibrous material found in cartilage, skin, and bones, *collagen* is a structural material.

Unable to dispose of the excess collagen properly, the body starts storing it in body tissues in harmful ways. Too much collagen in the skin, for example, makes the skin tight and hard; too much in the organs makes it difficult — if not impossible — for them to work. To make matters worse, the cells in the lining of the blood vessels begin to grow abnormally. With these vital delivery and waste roads hampered, the body has even more difficulty operating effectively.

We don't know exactly why scleroderma develops. Immune system errors are a likely candidate. Hormonal upsets are also possible culprits, and this would explain why women are much more likely to get the disease than men.

Summarizing the symptoms

The symptoms of scleroderma vary from person to person. The disease often begins with joint pain, but sometimes the first symptom is difficulty swallowing. It may progress rapidly and fatally, or it may confine itself to the skin for years or decades before moving on to attack other parts of the body. Symptoms of scleroderma include:

- **Skin problems:** Thickening, hardening, roughness, and/or dryness of the skin on the fingers, arms, face, and elsewhere. There may also be "spider veins" on the face, tongue, chest, and fingers, as well as lumpy calcium deposits under the skin.

- **Joint pain, swelling, and locking:** Pain in the joints can make scleroderma appear to be rheumatoid arthritis. As the disease advances, the elbows, wrists, and fingers may become locked in a closed position.

- **Difficulty swallowing:** If collagen is deposited in the esophagus, you may experience trouble swallowing.

- **Shortness of breath:** Scleroderma can cause scar tissue to accumulate in the lungs. It may also cause changes in the blood vessels that service these vital organs.

- **Digestive difficulties:** If the intestines are strewn with collagen, you may have trouble digesting food and absorbing nutrients.

- **Raynaud's phenomenon:** Many scleroderma patients develop this extreme sensitivity to cold in the fingers and/or toes.

Scleroderma patients can also suffer from a host of other problems, depending upon which organs are overrun with collagen. If the heart is involved, for example, symptoms can range from irregular heartbeat to heart failure.

Diagnosing and treating scleroderma

Diagnosing scleroderma can be difficult in the early stages, especially if joint pain and tenderness are the only symptoms. After skin changes or difficulty swallowing become apparent, the identification process is much easier.

After a medical history and physical examination, the doctor calls for special X-rays to check the esophagus and gastrointestinal system, blood tests to assess lung function, a skin biopsy to search for excess collagen, and other tests to measure the extent of the problem.

There is no cure for scleroderma, but various drugs can weaken the symptoms, including NSAIDs for pain and inflammation, anti-hypertensives to lower elevated blood pressure, antacids or histamine-blockers for heartburn, and so on. Exercise and physical therapy can help strengthen muscles and "oil" the affected joints. Severe problems with swallowing may require placement of an artificial feeding tube.

Although no home cures for scleroderma exist, you can do several things to help relieve the problems it produces and improve the quality of your life:

- Help protect your skin by limiting yourself to short showers or baths, keeping it moist with creams and lotions, and avoiding strong soaps and household chemicals.

- Use a humidifier if indoor heaters are drying out your skin.

- Diligently perform the flexibility and strengthening exercises that your doctor or physical therapist prescribes. The exercises may be difficult to do, but they help you maintain joint function.

- If swallowing is difficult, chew your food well, avoid foods that are hard to swallow, and drink plenty of liquids with your meals.

- If nighttime heartburn is a problem, put blocks beneath the head of your bed or buy an adjustable bed so that you can elevate your head. You can get the same effect by placing blocks under the legs of the bed frame at the head of the bed. Also, try eating dinner earlier than usual or having a light meal so you have less in your stomach at bedtime.

The symptoms of scleroderma are daunting, and doctors have found no way to stop the overactive collagen "factories." Still, many people do well for years or even decades, and some patients have spontaneous remissions, especially when the disease first manifests in the joints and skin rather than in the organs.

Reactive arthritis: From a stomachache to arthritis

Like gonococcal arthritis, reactive arthritis can stem from a venereal infection. But it isn't necessarily the unhappy result of unprotected sex. It can also develop after an intestinal infection — and it sometimes seems to strike without an infectious prelude.

Summarizing the symptoms

Reactive arthritis has three classic groups of symptoms:

- **Arthritis** takes the form of mild to severe pain and inflammation, often in the feet, ankles, and knees. The wrists, fingers, and other joints may also be struck. The arthritis may vanish or return episodically for years.

- **Conjunctivitis** is an inflammation of the mucous membranes protecting the eyelid and eyeball, causing them to become red and swollen, to burn, itch, and water excessively.

- **Urethritis** is an inflammation of the urethra, the "pipe" that conducts urine from the bladder to the outside of the body.

In addition, patients may have thick, crusty rashes on the soles of the feet or the palms of the hands, sores in the mouth or vagina and on the tongue or penis, yellowish deposits under the fingernails and toenails, and problems with the heart. Men age 20 to 50 are the most likely group to be struck.

Young men are more likely to get reactive arthritis than any other form of arthritis. Three percent of all men who have a sexually transmitted disease are also struck by reactive arthritis.

Chlamydia trachomatis is the bacteria responsible for the largest number of reactive arthritis cases associated with sexual contact. As for reactive arthritis that is linked to gastrointestinal infections, the major culprits are campylobacter, salmonella, shigella, and yersinia.

Diagnosing and treating reactive arthritis

The diagnosis of reactive arthritis can be difficult and delayed, because doctors have no single symptom or definitive test to rely on. The presence of the three classic symptoms is an important clue, but they may not appear at the same time. Doctors generally send samples of a patient's joint fluid, plus samples swabbed from the urethra, to the laboratory for analysis.

Part of the diagnostic workup is designed to rule out other diseases such as lupus and rheumatoid arthritis, whereas other parts are designed to "rule in" reactive arthritis. For example, finding the HLA-B27 gene and the presence of an infectious agent such as Chlamydia increase the likelihood that reactive arthritis is the culprit. X-rays showing damage to the cartilage or bone, bony deposits where the bones and tendons meet, soft tissue swelling, and other signs also point to reactive arthritis syndrome.

Your doctor can prescribe antibiotics to treat the infection and NSAIDs for the arthritis symptoms. He may also prescribe stronger drugs, such as corticosteroids or immunosuppressives. The conjunctivitis usually isn't treated directly, although patients may be given eye drops or an ointment for symptomatic relief. Bed rest and exercise are also helpful.

The outlook is generally good for reactive arthritis patients. Many recover substantially within 5 or 6 months, although mild to moderate arthritis may linger. About a fifth of all patients wind up with chronic, generally mild arthritis, and only a small percentage suffer from severe, ongoing symptoms and joint deformity.

Lyme disease: When you're the bull's-eye

This new version of arthritis popped up during the 1970s in the town of Lyme, Connecticut. Local doctors were puzzled when individuals, groups of friends, and even entire families began developing a disease that looked a lot like arthritis but didn't fall into any of the known categories.

Fortunately, doctors realized that more people developed the disease during the summer than in any other time of the year, that many patients had developed a large, round bull's-eye rash, and that the town of Lyme was surrounded by wooded areas harboring deer and other wild animals. By putting these and other facts together, they discovered that they were looking at a new disease caused by bacteria called *borrelia burgdorferi,* which were carried by certain ticks hitching rides on deer in the nearby woods. When these ticks bit people, the bacteria passed into their bodies. (And you needn't go into the woods to contract Lyme disease — your dog or cat can bring the offending ticks into your home.)

Summarizing the symptoms

The first symptom of Lyme disease is likely a large red spot on your rear end, thigh, trunk, or armpit. The rash may have a "blank" spot area in the center, making it look like a bull's-eye. It may itch and be painful or hot.

About half of those with untreated Lyme disease develop recurrent attacks of arthritis, which manifest as swelling and pain in the knees and other joints, including the shoulders, elbows, wrists, and ankles. These arthritis attacks may last for several months. Unfortunately, up to 20 percent of those infected may go on to suffer from chronic arthritis.

Other common symptoms include fever, fatigue, chills, joint pain, muscle aches, headache, and stiff neck. Less common symptoms include sore throat, swollen lymph nodes, nausea, vomiting, backaches, and other problems. These early symptoms may come and go. There may also be nerve disorders, memory deficits and difficulty concentrating, heart and liver problems, skin disorders, and eye inflammation.

Diagnosing and treating Lyme disease

The diagnosis is made from a combination of the patient's personal history and the presence of the classic rash. If the diagnosis needs to be confirmed, blood tests can be performed. The patient's history is a very important part of the diagnostic procedure. Knowing that the patient went hiking in the woods and that the problems began in the summer, for example, are significant clues.

The key blood test looks for the presence of antibodies to *borrelia burgdorferi*. In patients that exhibit nervous system disorders, doctors may perform a spinal tap to look for the antibodies in the spinal fluid. Unfortunately, antibodies don't show up right away, so it may be a while before a definitive diagnosis can be made.

Arresting the spread of Lyme disease is often fairly easy if treatment is started early. Antibiotics, taken orally or given intravenously, can often halt the disease's progress and prevent the appearance of arthritis and other later-stage symptoms. More severe cases can require treatment with IV antibiotics for several weeks. In some people, years may pass before all the symptoms finally vanish.

The doctor may also prescribe NSAIDs for pain and swelling, as well as crutches or other specific treatments or aids, depending on the part of the body affected.

Staying in the clear(ing): Avoiding Lyme disease

The best way to keep clear of Lyme disease is to make your body a "tick-free zone." If you go into the woods or other areas where deer or other wild animals roam, you should remember the following precautions:

- Use insect repellent.

- Use your clothing as a shield over exposed areas of skin.

- Wear light-colored clothes so the dark-colored ticks stand out if they get on you.

- Walk on trails if possible, and stay in the center of the trails, giving a wide berth to ticks in the grass and brush.

- Admire any animals you come across from a distance.

- Afterward, carefully check yourself and your children for ticks. Pay special attention to the hairy areas of the body.

- If you live in a tick-infested area or near the woods, make sure your pets have flea and tick collars.

- Watch for the telltale bull's-eye spot on your trunk, rear end, thighs, or in your armpit. If you find one, see your doctor immediately.

- If a tick is found and a rash develops, bring the tick to your doctor, because only a certain species of tick carries the bacteria that cause Lyme.

Experiencing Arthritis as a Minor Player

In bursitis, polymyalgia rheumatica, and the other diseases in this category, arthritis is not the major disease process, but symptoms of arthritis (joint pain, inflammation, limitation of movement) are often present in varying degrees. The arthritis shows up as a symptom of the disease but doesn't cause the disease itself.

Bursitis: When the bursae become swollen

Bursae are little fluid-filled sacs strategically placed throughout the body. They're designed to help reduce the friction caused by movement in the joints. Unfortunately, a bursa can become inflamed if injured or overused. Infections or certain forms of arthritis, such as gout, can also prompt this inflammation.

Summarizing the symptoms

When one or more of the bursae become inflamed, you have bursitis. The normally flat sacs swell with excess fluid, producing pain and often limiting movement. The shoulders are common targets of bursitis; the elbows, joints of the foot, and other joints can also be struck. See Figure 5-1 for an example of where the bursae are located in the shoulder.

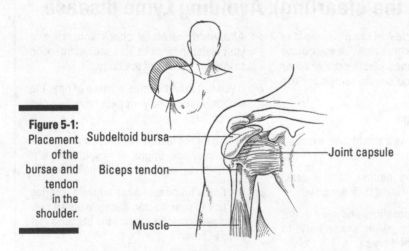

Figure 5-1: Placement of the bursae and tendon in the shoulder.

Subdeltoid bursa

Biceps tendon

Muscle

Joint capsule

The pain and resulting movement limitation can range from mild to severe. You may have a nagging little pain in one hip or such severe shoulder pain that dressing is difficult.

Diagnosing and treating bursitis

Ultrasound and MRIs are very good at identifying bursitis. Your doctor can also rely on your history and symptoms, as well as a physical examination of the affected areas, to make the diagnosis. Your doctor may also draw some fluid out of the bursae to try to determine the cause of the inflammation.

In many cases, treatment is limited to NSAIDs, rest, and perhaps joint immobilization. If this treatment doesn't work, corticosteroids may be injected into the bursa. If a bursa is infected, your doctor may drain it and give you antibiotics. Very rarely, in the case of chronic and severe bursitis, prednisone or another corticosteroid may be required. Exercise can help restore the range of motion and rebuild weakened muscles.

Tendonitis and tenosynovitis: Inflammation of the bone–muscle link

When certain muscles contract or relax, our bones move accordingly. But the bone-and-muscle, contract-and-relax-system depends on the connecting link: the tendons, which join muscle to bone.

Summarizing the symptoms

Tendons are the tough, fibrous extensions at the ends of the muscles that attach themselves to the bones. *Tendonitis* occurs when one or more of these tendons become inflamed. Most often associated with repetitive motions, impingements, strenuous activity, and advancing years, this ailment can leave tendons red, raw, and painful to the touch or upon movement.

The sheaths surrounding the tendons may also become inflamed, producing a condition known as *tenosynovitis*. If the sheaths dry out and rub against the tendon, they produce a grating sound or sensation. Various diseases, including scleroderma, gout, and gonorrhea can cause tenosynovitis.

Diagnosing and treating tendonitis and tenosynovitis

A diagnosis is based on your symptoms, medical history, and the physical examination. Your doctor may prescribe medications such as NSAIDs to counteract pain and inflammation. Corticosteroids or local anesthetics are sometimes injected right into the sheath surrounding the tendon. Chronic problems may require surgery to remove calcium deposits or release contracted tendons.

The outlook for those with tendonitis and tenosynovitis is good, and the problem often clears up on its own.

A few easy, inexpensive things can help alleviate the pain. You may want to try the following:

- ✔ Stop the activity that caused the inflammation.
- ✔ Rest.
- ✔ Apply hot or cold packs to the area.
- ✔ Immobilize the involved joints.

Raynaud's: A chilling problem

Raynaud's phenomenon involves changes to the small blood vessels in the hands and feet (or less commonly, the nose, lips, or ear lobes) when the patient gets cold.

Summarizing the symptoms

The hallmark of Raynaud's is discoloration in one or more fingers or toes, or the nose, lips, or ear lobes. The color changes can occur on their own or may be accompanied by tingling, burning, pain and/or numbness in the affected area. Although many people have cold hands and feet, the characteristic color changing (fingers or toes turning white or blue, followed by red) indicates Raynaud's.

Spasms of the small arteries that supply blood to these areas cause these symptoms by diminishing the blood supply. Brought on by cold temperatures and/or emotional stress, these spasms can last a few minutes or go on for hours. Chronic Raynaud's can lead to skin changes, as well as sores on the ends of the toes and fingers.

Raynaud's comes in two forms:

- ✔ **Raynaud's disease:** Also known as Primary Raynaud's, this is the more common form. Typically a milder version of the problem, it acts alone when it attacks.

- ✔ **Raynaud's phenomenon:** Also known as Secondary Raynaud's, this is less common. The more serious form of the ailment, it is brought on by another disease or condition, such as scleroderma or lupus.

Certain types of work increase a person's vulnerability to Raynaud's. Those who operate vibrating tools, who are exposed to vinyl chloride, and who type, play the piano, or otherwise subject their fingers to repetitive stress are more likely to develop this problem.

Diagnosing and treating Raynaud's

Diagnosing Raynaud's can be easy, but distinguishing one form from the other can be more problematic. Diagnosis and differentiation are made on the basis of the person's symptoms and laboratory tests, such as the antinuclear antibody test and erythrocyte sedimentation rate. Much of the laboratory testing is done to rule out other diseases. Treatment for Raynaud's may be as simple as teaching patients what they can do for themselves and monitoring the situation, or it may include administering powerful drugs. In very severe cases, nerves to the afflicted areas may be cut to provide temporary relief.

Your Raynaud's may be here to stay, but you needn't be a helpless victim. You can fight back in several ways:

- ✔ Stay warm all over. (Dress warmly, layer your clothing, and wear absorbent socks and underwear to draw perspiration away from your skin.)
- ✔ Immerse your fingers and toes in warm water to help keep them warm.
- ✔ If you smoke, stop. (Nicotine constricts blood vessels, a major problem with Raynaud's.)
- ✔ Speak to your doctor about the possibility of switching medicines if you are taking beta-blockers or other drugs that constrict blood vessels. (Decongestants like Sudafed are common offenders.)
- ✔ Work on controlling your reaction to stress.
- ✔ Exercise regularly.

Sjögren's syndrome: Dry mouth, eyes, and maybe more

No one knows what causes this disease, but the immune system is clearly involved. Sjögren's can occur alone or as a part of another autoimmune disease — most commonly in conjunction with RA. In fact, about 15 percent of RA patients go on to develop Sjögren's. Other disease associations include lupus, dermatomyositis, and scleroderma.

Summarizing the symptoms

The characteristic dryness in the mouth and eyes occurs when those mainstays of the immune system, the white blood cells, invade and damage the salivary and tear glands. The same problem can also cause dryness of the trachea, vagina, the lining of the gastrointestinal tract, and other parts of the body.

About one-third of Sjögren's sufferers develop an arthritis similar to, but usually less severe than, rheumatoid arthritis.

Those with Sjögren's are more than 40 times more likely to develop lymphoma than people who don't have Sjögren's.

Diagnosing and treating Sjögren's

The combination of dry mouth, dry eyes, and joint distress can make diagnosis a simple matter. Tests can confirm that the level of tears and saliva production is sub par. Further clues can be found in the abnormal blood tests. Antibody abnormalities and possibly anemia, fewer white blood cells, and an elevated erythrocyte sedimentation rate (ESR) may be found.

Sjögren's syndrome can't be cured, but many of the symptoms can be alleviated. By chewing sugar-free gum (it must be sugar free, because one of the most serious side effects in this disease is severe dental cavities), sipping fluid, and using a mouth rinse and artificial teardrops, you can help keep your eyes and mouth moist. Frequent dental visits are also necessary. A drug called pilocarpine and a new drug called cevimeline may be given to increase the production of saliva. Pain and swelling of the salivary glands and joints can be treated with painkillers, but stronger drugs may be needed to deal with any trouble arising from damage to the internal organs. For patients with severe joint or salivary symptoms, NSAIDs, anti-malarials, or steroids are sometimes used.

The outlook depends upon which parts of the body are affected. Most people manage reasonably well, but a small number succumb to kidney failure or other problems that arise when a key part of the body becomes too dry.

Polymyalgia rheumatica: The pain of many muscles

No one knows what causes *polymyalgia rheumatica*, which means *pain in many muscles*. It typically attacks people over the age of 50 and strikes more women than men. The older you are, the more likely you are to wake up one morning with the muscle pain and stiffness that are the hallmarks of this disease.

Summarizing the symptoms

Typically, a woman goes to bed at night feeling fine. But she wakes up the next morning with tremendous pain and stiffness in her neck, shoulders, upper arms, lower back, hips, and/or buttocks. She may say, "It feels like I worked out too much yesterday, like I really overdid it — but I didn't do anything!"

However, not everyone develops polymyalgia rheumatica overnight. Sometimes it comes on gradually. In addition to the pain and stiffness, fever, weight loss, and a general feeling of the blahs are common.

Navigating the road to the diagnosis

Arthritis and arthritis-related conditions may not be diagnosed right away. Many patients are mistakenly told that their problems are caused by stress, lack of sleep, or depression. Even when the disease is identified, the course may not be clear. Patients may spend money for one medicine after another or self-refer themselves to specialists outside their managed care or HMO programs, paying for the doctors themselves in the quest for relief.

The following examples illustrate the experiences of some people just like you:

✔ Recurring chest pain sent a frightened 25-year-old Kristen to her doctor.

✔ Stricken by severe pain on the right side of his "belly" that suggested appendicitis, Franklin found himself in the hospital, about to undergo exploratory surgery.

✔ Middle-aged Janice has felt weak and tired for the past several weeks.

✔ After drinking too much at a New Year's party, Rod woke early in the morning with excruciating pain in his big toe.

✔ Terry's fingers had a tendency to turn white, blue, and then red; they tingled, burned, and became numb.

✔ Fever, abdominal and joint pain sent 27-year-old Jennifer to her doctor's office.

What do these people, with such different and wide-ranging symptoms, have in common? They all have arthritis or an arthritis-related condition. Their pain is not all in their heads, and it's not due to depression or psychological problems. Their symptoms are absolutely real, and they need careful care.

Although the pain can be severe and may seem to resemble that of rheumatoid arthritis, the muscles involved don't show signs of inflammation, and the joints rarely show any signs of arthritis. However, inflammation of the joint linings may be present.

Diagnosing and treating polymyalgia rheumatica

With no characteristic joint damage, antibodies, skin rashes, or other obvious signs to look for, doctors must make the diagnosis of polymyalgia rheumatica by eliminating other causes of the pain and stiffness. The patient's age is one clue, with those over 50 most likely to be affected. Then there's the typically sudden onset of symptoms. People with the disease may also have anemia and a high erythrocyte sedimentation rate (ESR), but these are not definitive clues because they can be the result of many other health problems.

Sometimes the diagnosis is clinched by the patient's response to the standard treatment: low doses of prednisone or other corticosteroids. Almost all polymyalgia rheumatica patients respond well to low doses of these drugs.

This "pain of many muscles" often disappears on its own or improves dramatically with treatment. A significant number of patients do so well after a couple years that they can start cutting back on their medication.

Fifteen percent of those with polymyalgia rheumatica also have a life-threatening inflammation of the blood vessels called *giant cell arteritis* (GCA). Symptoms of GCA can include headaches, scalp tenderness, hearing problems, jaw pain, difficulty swallowing, and coughing. If you experience these symptoms, you should be evaluated by a medical professional immediately.

Paget's disease: Becoming too bony

Bones grow throughout life. They may not grow longer after a certain point, but they are constantly being broken down and restored, right up until the end of life.

With Paget's disease, the normal break down/rebuild system shifts into overdrive, causing excessive destruction of the bone and poor-quality bone repair. As a result, bones may become bulkier, softer, and weaker, with a greater tendency to fracture.

Summarizing the symptoms

Many people with Paget's have no idea anything is wrong, whereas others suffer from gradual joint stiffness and fatigue. Sometimes the bones become enlarged, deformed, and painful. And there can be secondary damage, such as pain, osteoarthritis, loss of height, and bowleggedness.

Diagnosing and treating Paget's disease

Making the diagnosis of Paget's is fairly simple: X-rays of the bones show the abnormal areas of growth, and a laboratory test detects elevated blood levels of alkaline phosphatase, an enzyme necessary for bone formation.

Treatment depends upon the symptoms — if you don't have symptoms, perhaps nothing may be done. Surgery may be needed if nerves are being pinched or if a joint is no longer functioning properly. In more severe cases, your doctor may prescribe drugs that slow the disease, such as alendronate and calcitonin, or drugs used to strengthen bones, such as alendronate sodium.

Experiencing Arthritis as a Companion Condition

In these conditions, the disease is centered in the structures that surround the joint (muscles, tendons, ligaments, and nerves) instead of in the joints themselves. Although the joints are painful, these maladies don't begin in the joints and aren't classified as "true" arthritis.

Carpal tunnel syndrome: Nerve compression

You may have seen office workers or supermarket checkers wearing splints on their hands and lower arms to immobilize their wrists. Or perhaps you've noticed people rubbing and shaking their hands, complaining of pain and tingling in their thumbs and fingers.

They may be suffering from carpal tunnel syndrome, a problem caused by compression of the nerve and tendons that pass through the *carpal tunnel* (a corridor between the ligaments and bones in the wrist). This syndrome causes pain, numbness, decreased sensation, and tingling in the thumb, index, and middle fingers that can sometimes spread all the way up to the arm and shoulder. If left untreated, carpal tunnel syndrome can cause the muscles on the thumb side of the hand to waste away, making it difficult to make a fist or grasp objects.

Your doctor bases the diagnosis on your symptoms, medical history, and physical examination and looks for weakness and decreased sensation in your hand. An X-ray may provide helpful information, and nerve tests can confirm the diagnosis.

Treatment often begins with a splint, followed by medication to reduce pain and inflammation. Corticosteroid injections into the afflicted nerve can be temporarily helpful. If the problem is related to water gain, you may be given diuretics to help rid your body of excess fluid. More advanced cases may by helped by surgery.

 In addition to these medical measures, look for ways to cut back on — or completely eliminate — any repetitive motion that may bring on the pain. Also, look for ways to relieve joint stress. For example, if you type a lot, consider getting an ergonomically designed keyboard.

The outlook for those with carpal tunnel syndrome is generally good. Most recover, and only a very small percentage of those treated develop permanent nerve injury.

Fibromyalgia: The pain no one can find

It's an odd situation: You hurt, perhaps all over, but the doctor can't find any inflammation or damage to explain the pain. He may even suggest, "It's all in your head" and say that you're stressed, depressed, or need more sleep.

Pain and stiffness in the muscles, ligaments, and tendons are the primary signs of fibromyalgia. The pain and stiffness generally occur throughout the body, although they can begin in one area and spread (see Figure 5-2). Fatigue is also a major problem; as many as 90 percent of fibromyalgia sufferers also experience moderate to severe fatigue.

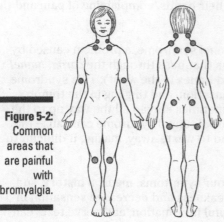

Figure 5-2: Common areas that are painful with fibromyalgia.

Symptoms may come and go and are often associated with sleep disturbances; sufferers may also experience mood changes, numbness and tingling in the extremities, and headaches. No one knows what causes the disorder, but it is often triggered by stress, injury, lack of sleep, infections, and other diseases. Although fibromyalgia can be painful, it is not life threatening or otherwise dangerous. For some people, however, the symptoms can become so severe that work is impossible.

The Arthritis Foundation estimates that 3.5 million Americans suffer from fibromyalgia. Women are seven times more likely than men to suffer from this condition, especially those in their childbearing years.

The diagnosis can be difficult to make, because the symptoms of fibromyalgia may be similar to those of other diseases. Finding the location and pattern of your pain helps your doctor make the diagnosis.

Increasing physical activity improves symptoms and is possibly the most important component of therapy. Treatment may include medicines to kill pain, local anesthetics injected directly into painful areas, and antidepressants to aid in sleep. Your doctor may also prescribe massage therapy, along with application of heat to the affected areas. Relaxation techniques and education to help you manage your pain may also be prescribed.

Fibromyalgia is not all in your head; it's not a hysterical response to stress or a cry for help. It's a real disease that happens to have an important psychological component. That's good news, in a sense, because it means you can begin doing something right now to help relieve your symptoms by controlling stress. (See Chapter 14 for methods of dealing with stress.)

For immediate relief, try taking a warm bath or applying compresses to your sore muscles. And you may have a little more luck sleeping with a different mattress, a white noise machine to block disturbing sounds, blackout curtains, and a more comfortable pillow. (See Chapter 15 for the basics of good sleep.) Overall, the outlook for fibromyalgia patients is good. It causes no long-term damage to the joints or the rest of the body and can be eased with medicine and stress reduction. Check out *Fibromyalgia For Dummies* (Wiley) to find out more.

Polymyositis: A rare sapping of strength

An uncommon disease affecting less than one tenth of 1 percent of the population, polymyositis is an inflammation of the muscles that saps the victim's strength.

Summarizing the symptoms

In severe cases, those with polymyositis may have trouble just lifting themselves out of a chair or brushing their teeth. The larger muscles closest to the torso — the muscles of the shoulders, upper arms, thighs, and hips — are usually the ones that suffer. But the neck muscles may also be stricken, as well as those used to breathe and swallow. Patients may also experience fever, weight loss, pain in the joints, Raynaud's phenomenon, and the blahs.

Polymyositis can strike at any age but usually hits adults between 30 and 60 years of age and children aged 5 to 15. And the disease prefers women to men, striking women about twice as often. No one knows what causes polymyositis. Infections and immune system disorders are suspected, whereas genetics are not.

Diagnosing and treating polymyositis

Lacking a quick-and-easy test that can provide a definitive diagnosis, doctors look for identifying signs and symptoms. These include unexplained muscle weakness, certain microscopic changes in the structure of the muscle tissue, and changes in the levels of certain enzymes in the blood.

A corticosteroid called prednisone, given to strengthen the muscles and quell the inflammation, is a standard medication for this disease. But although some people respond quickly and dramatically to this medicine, others don't.

Ironically, when used over time, prednisone can cause muscle weakness and a host of other unpleasant side effects. So your doctor may eventually prescribe other immunosuppressants, while gradually tapering off your steroid dosages.

Although many children stricken with the disease can stop their medication after a year or so, most adult patients continue taking their drugs for many years — or indefinitely. Some adults suffer from progressively more severe symptoms and eventually die from respiratory failure, pneumonia, or other problems, but most are able to keep the disease under control and live fairly normal lives.

Dermatomyositis: Polymyositis plus

With dermatomyositis, one suffers of all the symptoms of polymyositis, plus rashes and other skin problems.

Summarizing the symptoms

There may be a reddish rash on the face, reddish-purple swelling about the eyes, and a rash elsewhere on the body. Typically appearing on the knuckles, the rash may be raised, smooth, or scaly. With time, the rash fades but may leave behind areas with brownish pigmentation or no pigmentation at all, as well as scarred or shriveled skin.

Diagnosing and treating dermatomyositis

Dermatomyositis is diagnosed and treated in much the same way as polymyositis. Doctors look for unexplained muscle weakness, certain microscopic changes in muscle tissue structure, and changes in the levels of certain blood enzymes.

To treat dermatomyositis, prednisone or other corticosteroids are used to decrease the inflammation and suppress autoimmune responses that are believed to cause the disease. Topical medicines (creams, ointments, gels, solutions, sprays, or foams) can also be applied to the skin to bring some relief.

Part II

Tests and Treatments: What to Expect from Your Doctor

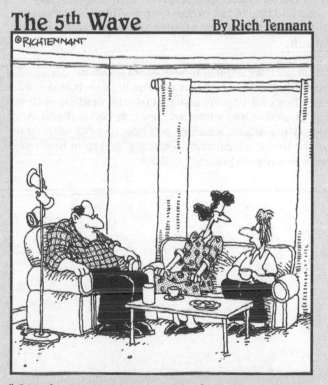

The 5th Wave   By Rich Tennant

@RICHTENNANT

"Stan's taken salmon pills for years for his arthritis. Other than an urge to swim upstream each fall, he hasn't experienced any side effects."

In this part . . .

*1*t would be great if a single test could tell you whether you had arthritis, which type, and which treatment is appropriate for your condition. Unfortunately, such a test doesn't exist. Diagnosis can be quick and easy, a long and drawn-out process, or anything in between. And making the treatment decisions can sometimes be difficult.

In this part, we explain how doctors go about diagnosing the many forms of arthritis and the high-tech and low-tech tests they may use. We also discuss the medicines they may prescribe and surgeries they may recommend. And, equally important, we show you how to work with your doctor to make treatment decisions, and then how to manage any pain you may suffer.

Chapter 6

Your Doctor and You: Allies Against Arthritis

. . . .

In This Chapter

▶ Deciding what you need from treatment

▶ Finding and interviewing a reputable doctor

▶ Communicating effectively with your doctor

▶ Deciding if and when it's time to switch doctors

. . . .

*I*n the old days — well, just 15 or 20 years ago — the doctor said, "Jump," and the patient answered, "How high?" In other words, the doctor was completely in charge, ordering tests as she saw fit, deciding how aggressively or conservatively to attack the disease, pushing patients toward surgery or drugs, taking a dim view of alternative approaches, and so on.

Fortunately, a new approach to health care exists today: Doctor and patient work together as a team with you, the patient, staying in charge. Research has shown that patients who play active roles in their treatment tend to fare better than those who are stuck in a passive role. So selecting your doctor carefully, helping draw up the treatment program, and then following that program to the letter is important. Your odds of recovery improve if you believe in your treatment and pitch in with your recovery efforts, doing everything you can to get well.

Positioning Yourself for Treatment Success

Doctors are experts who are well-trained in diagnosis and treatment. They'd better be, because we put our health (and our lives) into their hands. Still, doctors are only human, which makes them subject to limitations and foibles just like the rest of us. To make sure you get the best treatment, follow these three cardinal rules:

✔ **Select your doctor carefully.** Find someone who is not only thoroughly familiar with and experienced in treating your kind of arthritis, but who is also up on the latest research and treatments. You don't want to miss out on an effective therapy because your doctor is uninformed. The following section, "Choosing a Good Doctor," tells you how to find the right person for the job.

✔ **Research all you can about your condition.** How can you gauge whether your doctor is following correct procedure and doing everything possible to treat your condition unless you know something about the topic? Plenty of information about every type of arthritis, its symptoms, treatments, alternative healing methods, and so on is available from the Arthritis Foundation (phone 800-283-7800; Web site www.arthritis.org) and similar organizations. Appendix B gives you more information.

✔ **Be a team player with your doctor.** After you've decided on a doctor, regard him as the expert — your trusted advisor. Unless something feels wrong about the advice you're getting, follow it to the letter. Get behind your treatment and do all you can to make it successful. Only then can you get the best possible results.

Choosing a Good Doctor

How do you find a good doctor? Ideally, you begin by getting recommendations from doctors or other people in the medical field, including your own general practitioner or internist (if you're searching for a specialist), or perhaps a highly regarded nearby hospital or medical center. You can also ask friends for their recommendations. You then need to check the candidates' credentials on the Internet or call the local chapter of the American Medical Association to narrow the field. Finally, you personally interview those left on your now-shorter list and select the doctor who seems to suit you best. However, in real life, you may not have the opportunity to select your doctors quite so freely — you may be restricted to the ones on the list that your insurance company or HMO provides.

Luckily, you have a good chance of finding an excellent doctor through your HMO or on your insurance-approved list. After all, the overwhelming majority of doctors are well-qualified to help. But some are undoubtedly a better match for you than others. Assuming that you have some choice, looking around for the physician best suited to your needs is worth your while.

Determining whether the doctor is knowledgeable

Almost every doctor has an office wall covered with diplomas and certificates, and although you may find them interesting to look at, most of these fancy, framed pieces of paper can't offer you much useful information. Not even a diploma from Harvard Medical School, you ask? Isn't a diploma from a super-prestigious school better than one from Tiny Town Med? Not necessarily. Plenty of brilliant doctors have graduated from little-known medical colleges.

What about the official-looking paper that the state issues proclaiming that the doctor is licensed to practice medicine? Remember that every practicing physician *has* to have one of those to treat patients. (Think of it as a driver's license for doctors.)

As for membership in the American Medical Association, the AMA is primarily a trade association. If Dr. Smith can pay the dues, he can join the AMA, but that doesn't necessarily mean he's better than a non-AMA doctor.

And what about the certificates indicating that the doctor is a member of various medical societies? Again, these documents guarantee nothing. A doctor can belong to an organization that offers wonderful seminars and educational materials without ever taking advantage of them. On the other hand, a doctor who doesn't belong to a medical organization may spend hours studying medical journals and swapping tips with colleagues. What if the doctor is a diplomate in a medical society? Sometimes this title can mean something. Certain medical societies require that their members pass rigorous written tests before allowing the doctors to call themselves diplomates. On the other hand, some societies offer diplomate tests that aren't so difficult.

The one thing that *does* mean something is board certification. *Board certified* means that the doctor has passed difficult written and/or oral tests in his or her field. Certification is generally considered an impressive credential, because it isn't required to practice. Being board certified is an extra stamp of validation that not every doctor receives.

Sharing the same treatment philosophy

Many people think of medicine as a science, but it's often just as much an art. For example, doctors frequently follow hunches during their diagnostic workups. And although standard approaches to treating most diseases exist, doctors know that everybody responds a little differently. Therefore, most treatment programs must be individualized and then changed as time goes on — anywhere from slightly tweaked to radically altered.

Because everyone responds to treatment differently, physicians have some leeway when diagnosing and treating patients — some wiggle room that also allows for the expression of personality. Some doctors are more aggressive than others; some like the idea of alternative approaches, and others are determined to stick strictly to Western medical techniques. Some doctors want to tell you exactly what to do, but others are more willing to involve you in the decision-making process.

Although no diploma hanging on the wall is going to let you in on a doctor's treatment philosophy, these framed documents *can* offer you some clues. Framed certificates of membership in medical or nonmedical organizations dedicated to nutrition or exercise, for example, suggest that the doctor is open to alternative therapies, as do certificates stating that the doctor has attended lectures in chiropractic or herbal medicine. But the best way, by far, to figure out a doctor's philosophy about diagnosis and treatment is simply to ask.

Interviewing a prospective doctor

When you're ready to interview those on your "short list" of prospective doctors, call and make an appointment with each one, explaining that you simply want to talk about the possibility of becoming a patient. Yes, it will cost whatever the doctor wants to charge — which can be hefty. And no, your insurance company probably won't pay for it. But it can mean the difference between finding a doctor who's just right for you or getting stuck with one who isn't right. Your future health is worth the investment.

Your primary goal for the interview is to get a feel for what the doctor is like, how he responds to you and your questions, and what makes up his or her general treatment philosophy.

You may want to bring a list of questions, such as the following:

✔ What is your background and training in arthritis treatment?

✔ Which kinds of cases (osteoarthritis, rheumatoid arthritis, and so on) do you typically treat?

✔ Do you like to work as part of a team (rheumatologist, physical therapist, chiropractor, massage therapist, and so on) or do you prefer to handle the treatment alone?

✔ If you do like to work as a team, who is in charge of the treatment?

✔ Do you think medication is always, or almost always, the best treatment for arthritis?

✔ How valuable are diet, exercise, and stress reduction in treating arthritis?

✔ Do you favor the use of vitamins, herbs, and other supplements as adjuncts to treatment? If so, which ones?

✔ How do you feel about using other alternative therapies (chiropractic, massage, homeopathy, magnets, acupuncture, and so on) in conjunction with standard treatment? Which do you feel are best?

No right answers to these questions exist. Look for a doctor whose attitude dovetails with yours.

Considering compatibility

After you're sure that your prospective physician is qualified, you must try to predict whether the two of you can work together. Don't automatically assume that the answer is *yes*. You, the patient, should be considered a member of the treatment team — the most important member — rather than a passive pincushion who acquiesces to whatever medicines and surgeries your doctor deems necessary. How can you find out if your prospective doctor seems like a team player?

After you visit with a doctor for either an interview or an appointment, think carefully about what went on during your time together. Did the doctor:

- Try to rush you through the interview?

- Keep looking at her watch?

- Solicit your opinions?

- Give you ample time to express your thoughts, wishes, concerns, and fears?

- Listen carefully?

- Give you thoughtful, complete responses in plain English (instead of confusing medical speak)?

- Invite you to ask questions?

- Ask about your preferred approach to treatment? (For example, whether you wish to begin treatment with strong painkillers or prefer to give exercise and a back brace a chance before moving on to medication?)

- Push you to pursue much more aggressive or conservative treatment than you prefer?

- Brush aside your concerns by saying, "Trust me," or, "I know what's best"?

- Focus on drugs and surgery for treatment and downplay your desire to work with a physical therapist, chiropractor, or other alternative healer?

You can gather a lot of information by asking questions, listening carefully, and observing the doctor's behavior. If you aren't comfortable, find another doctor.

Working with Your Doctor

Nothing can be quite as educating, enlightening and reassuring as a long talk with your doctor about your condition. But for many people, the time actually spent with the doctor seems all too short. Certain things you wanted to report

General practitioner versus rheumatologist

Whether you need a specialist depends upon the kind of arthritis you have. If you have osteo-arthritis (see Chapter 2), you may do well under the care of a general practitioner or internist. But if you have a more complicated kind of arthritis, one that involves entire body systems (such as rheumatoid arthritis — check out Chapter 3), you probably need to see a rheumatologist.

Rheumatologists specialize in diseases of the joints, muscles, and bones. They treat arthritis, musculoskeletal pain disorders, osteoporosis, and various autoimmune diseases. An important part of the rheumatologist's job is proper diagnosis of the disease, because symptoms can point to many different conditions. After the rheumatologist pinpoints the disease, proper treatment can begin, so early and accurate diagnosis is crucial. If you don't have a clear-cut case of osteoarthritis, or if your family physician or internist seems baffled by your symptoms, consult a rheumatologist.

can slip your mind, and you might miss the opportunity to ask important questions or clarify confusing explanations. But you can make the most of your appointments by doing a little advance planning.

Before your first appointment, gather the information your doctor will need and come prepared. Bring the following information along with you to your appointment:

- ✔ Medical records from other doctors, chiropractors, or health professionals: Have them forwarded to your doctor's office.

- ✔ A log of your arthritis symptoms: Describe how each symptom feels, the intensity of the pain, when it occurs, and what you were doing when you noticed it.

- ✔ A list of all prescription and non-prescription medications you're currently taking, plus all herbs, vitamins, minerals and other supplements.

- ✔ A list of all the treatments you've used (including home remedies) to ease arthritis symptoms.

- ✔ Questions that you'd like your doctor to answer. For example:

  - How did you determine that I have this particular kind of arthritis?

  - What's causing my arthritis?

  - Do I have any joint deformity?

  - What kinds of treatment do you recommend?

  - What outcome can I expect?

  - Which non-medication kinds of treatment do you recommend?

  - Will physical therapy help? Which kinds?

- Will I need surgery? If so, how long can I wait before I have it?

- What will happen if I do nothing?

- What will my treatment cost?

✔ A notepad: Take notes so that you can review your doctor's answers at home when you have no distractions.

 If, when you get home and review your notes, you find that you don't understand an answer or that you've forgotten to ask a question, don't be afraid to call the doctor's office and ask for a phone consultation. The more you know, the better prepared you'll be to tackle your condition head-on.

Speaking Your Doctor's Language

Although you're not expected to know everything (any more than an orchestra conductor has to play every instrument proficiently), you do need to know enough to communicate with your doctor(s) and the other members of your medical team. Doing so requires a certain amount of education. You needn't become an expert, and you don't have to stay up all night mastering arcane medical terms and memorizing medical books. However, you should read all you can about the type of arthritis you have, as well as the medications that have been prescribed, to become informed about your disease. Some good information sources include the following:

✔ *The Merck Manual of Medical Information, Home Edition* (Pocket Books). This is the layman's version of the technical manual that doctors use.

✔ *The PDR Pocket Guide to Prescription Drugs* (Pocket Books). This is a slimmed-down and simplified version of the *PDR (Physician's Desk Reference),* the doctor's reference guide to medications. In regular, nonmedical English, *The PDR Pocket Guide* spells out important issues concerning each medication, such as:

   - Why it's prescribed

   - The most important facts about the drug

   - Tips on how you should take the medication

   - Side effects

   - Tips for when you shouldn't use the drug

   - Clues concerning how the drug may interact with foods and other drugs

✔ **Arthritis support groups.** Consider joining an arthritis support group. The other members understand what you're going through, so they listen sympathetically, and they've been in your situation, so they can give you helpful advice. Likewise, if you join the group, at some point you become a regular, which gives you the great satisfaction of helping others. You can find support groups by asking your doctors, nurses, or the community support staff at your hospital.

You can also find arthritis support groups through the Arthritis Foundation. Call the foundation at 800-283-7800 or check out its Web site at www.arthritis.org. If you go to the Web site, click **Communities** and then click **Local Offices** in the left-hand column to find the Arthritis Foundation office nearest you. Call to ask for the location and meeting time of a support group in your area.

✔ **The Internet.** Three great places to begin your search are the Arthritis Foundation (www.arthritis.org), the National Institute of Arthritis and Musculoskeletal and Skin Diseases (www.nih.gov/niams), and the American College of Rheumatology (www.rheumatology.org). You can find more Web sites in Appendix B of this book.

The Internet is a great place to find information. Unfortunately, you can't treat everything you find there as gospel. Before accepting what you read, ask yourself who is offering the material, who wrote the material, and why and when it was written. If the information is offered by well-known, reputable organizations, such as the Arthritis Foundation, the National Institute of Arthritis and Musculoskeletal Diseases, or the American College of Rheumatology, it's undoubtedly good information. However, if an organization devoted to selling products mentioned in the literature prepares and posts the information you find, take what you read with a grain of salt.

No matter where you find information, ask yourself who wrote it: A physician or other health professional? A respected nonmedical educator? Some guy off the street? Is the author qualified to present information or give advice? Ask yourself whether the article is offered to provide information or to sell a product. There's nothing wrong with selling products, and some pieces that are written with the idea of selling are packed with unbiased, useful information. However, others aren't. Be sure to check the date that the information was posted. Even a well-researched article may contain erroneous information if it hasn't been updated in several years.

Figuring Out When You Should Find a New Doctor

Not every marriage is made in heaven, and not every patient/doctor partnership works out for the best. If you're wondering whether you ought to switch to a different doctor, take a look at the following list (adapted from the article "Red Flags" by Doyt Conn, MD) and see if the situations ring any bells for you:

✔ **Feeling the progress of your treatment is too slow.** It may take a while before your doctor finds the right treatment for you, and complete relief of your symptoms isn't always possible. If your doctor is still trying to adjust your treatment, you may want to stick it out a little longer. If not, find someone else.

✔ **Noticing that your treatment consists of medication only.** Treatment of arthritis is multifaceted and should include nondrug therapies, such as exercise, diet, joint protection techniques, rest, and so on.

✔ **Realizing that your doctor relies solely on NSAIDs.** At one time, NSAIDs (see Chapter 8) were the treatment-of-choice for arthritis and are better at relieving the pain of hip and knee OA than acetaminophen. But it may be a better choice to start with acetaminophen and then escalate to NSAIDs, if necessary, because NSAIDs are notorious for causing stomach problems. As for RA, treatment may require the use of more aggressive drugs, such as methotrexate or sulfasalazine, in addition to NSAIDs. In some cases, waiting too long to use these drugs can allow affected joints to become irreparably damaged.

✔ **Finding that your doctor gives you too many "cortisone" injections.** Injecting corticosteroids into an inflamed joint is a fast way of stopping an RA flare or decreasing the pain associated with OA. But overuse of injectable steroids (most experts recommend no more than four injections per joint per year) can have serious side effects, including tendon rupture, destruction of the joint, and, occasionally, high blood pressure, diabetes, cataracts, and osteoporosis. As long as the injections aren't performed too frequently and are used in combination with other therapies, they can be safe and effective.

Generally, the best advice is to go with your gut feeling. If something feels wrong or you and your doctor don't seem to click, find someone with whom you do feel comfortable. Having confidence in the type and quality of medical care that you receive can make a positive difference in your recovery.

Chapter 7

Judging Joint Health with Low- and High-Tech Tests

. . . .

In This Chapter

▶ Discovering what a good doctor does to diagnose arthritis

▶ Introducing common tests for the various forms of arthritis

▶ Looking at biopsies and blood tests

▶ Finding additional tests that are used to help pin down your diagnosis

. . . .

iagnosing arthritis can be as easy as 1-2-3. Or it may take months or even years of following up on clues and running endless tests. With osteoarthritis, the diagnosis is usually pretty clear: The patient is typically over 40, has pain in a single joint but no swelling, and an X-ray shows the narrowing of the joint space. But with other forms of arthritis, such as infectious arthritis, the symptoms can be much vaguer: fatigue, chills, fever, rash, inflammation of the heart, meningitis, and joint aches that may come and go for years. However, doctors have many tests available to narrow the long list of possibilities and pinpoint a diagnosis.

Checking In for a Check-Up

No one test can determine for sure whether you have arthritis. Instead, your doctor has to go through several procedures, such as taking a thorough medical history, examining you carefully, and performing a series of tests. Together, these clues should provide a pretty accurate picture of what's going on in your body.

Presenting the past: Your medical history

Your doctor needs to assemble a great deal of information about your overall health, as well as your specific complaints. The medical history includes that questionnaire you answer in your doctor's waiting room and questions your

Tracing arthritis from dinosaur to tick

200,000,000 B.C.: A dinosaur was struck by osteoarthritis. We know this is true because examination of dinosaur bones shows evidence of the disease.

2,000,000 B.C.: An otherwise unknown prehistoric man developed chronic arthritis of the spine. He may not have been the first human to do so, but he's the oldest of those whose arthritic bones have been found.

8,000 B.C.: An Egyptian important enough to be mummified had the evidence of his arthritis wrapped up with him.

440 B.C.: Hippocrates, the father of Western medicine, offered the first known description of arthritis. He described gout as a "violent attack on the joints."

Circa 300 A.D.: Arthritis was so endemic in the Roman Empire that the Emperor Diocletian gave a tax break to the citizens who were most afflicted with the disease. One reason the disease was so widespread may have been that the ancient Romans used lead to clarify their red wines — lead poisoning in adults can produce arthritic symptoms.

Circa 400 A.D.: Colchicum, from which the drug colchicine is derived today, was introduced as a treatment for gout.

Circa 1600 A.D.: Guilaurne de Bailou introduced the term *rheumatism* and suggested that it was a type of arthritis different from gout.

1907: X-rays were added to doctors' diagnostic arsenal, allowing them to further distinguish one type of arthritis from another.

1949: The rheumatoid factor, which plays a role in rheumatoid arthritis, was discovered. In the same year, cortisone was introduced as a treatment for this disease.

1951: Drugs to suppress an errant immune system and modify the course of rheumatoid arthritis were first used.

1960: Surgeons began performing total joint replacement.

Early 1960s: The urate crystals that cause gout were identified, and new drugs to control the disease were introduced.

1963: The introduction of indomethacin, a new non-steroidal anti-inflammatory drug that blocks the action of the enzyme cyclooxygenase, takes the control of arthritic inflammation one step further.

1977: Lyme disease was recognized and named.

1998: A new class of drugs, the biological response modifiers (BRMs), takes arthritis treatment in a new direction by inhibiting or shoring up certain components of the immune system, called cytokines, to ease stubborn cases of joint inflammation.

doctor asks you in person. Medical histories commonly include general information, such as your age, sex, and occupation, as well as specific information about

- ✔ Any accidents or injuries that you've sustained
- ✔ Diseases that run in your family
- ✔ Illnesses you've had (especially recently)

✔ Other problems, including recent weight loss, depression, sleep disturbances, aches and pain, skin changes, and fatigue

The doctor also reviews your activities at work and at home. Knowing that you type eight hours a day may help the doctor connect your hand pain and tingling to carpal tunnel syndrome, and likewise, knowing that you drink a lot of alcohol may point him to the possibility of gout. You may help guide your doctor to the diagnosis of Lyme disease by revealing that you went camping in the woods and discovered a rash on your back shortly before your joints began hurting. And of course, you should tell the doctor about any and all of your symptoms.

Don't hold back information because you think it's not important. You may not mention that you've had some difficulty in swallowing, because you don't think it's related to your joint and muscle pain. But if you have scleroderma or polymyositis (see Chapter 5 for information on both of these conditions), it very well may be.

From head to toe: The physical exam

Even if you have pain in just a single joint, you should be examined from head to toe. Your primary physician (internist or family practitioner) is the doctor most likely to do perform this examination. If you see a rheumatologist or other specialist, she probably won't look you over from stem to stern, but she *should* carefully examine all affected and related areas.

How important is the head-to-toe examination? Well, urinary difficulties in men can be due to reactive arthritis, gonococcal arthritis, or something totally different, such as an enlarged prostate gland. Without a thorough examination, the proper diagnosis may be missed.

At some point, the examination focuses on your painful joint(s). Your doctor is particularly interested in the following key symptoms:

✔ How many joints are affected?

✔ Does the pain affect the same joints on both sides of the body?

✔ Do redness, swelling, and warmth surround the joint, and is it tender to the touch?

The doctor may ask you to bend and straighten your affected joint(s) several times as he determines the range of motion. He will manipulate your joints(s) for you, checking for joint crackling and pain upon bending and flexing. Your doctor will also examine any related areas and check your reflexes and muscle strength.

The doctor may ask you to walk, sit, rise from a chair, bend, and do other movements so she can assess the way you use your joints. You may be asked to reach for something or make a fist around a pencil so the doctor can estimate the impact of your condition on your ability to perform daily activities.

You and your doctor need to discuss in detail the kind and amount of pain you're experiencing, and you need to answer questions that are specifically geared to the pain itself. You may want to pay special attention to these issues before you see your doctor so that you can have your answers ready. The following is a pain checklist you can use to check off symptoms, write in your own comments, and take with you to your doctor's appointment.

❑ Is it an ache, a burn, a throb, or a stabbing pain?

❑ Does it come and go, or is it constant?

❑ What activities or movements make the pain worse?

❑ What makes the pain recede?

❑ Are you stiff in the morning?

❑ Do your joints lock up?

❑ Is the pain more intense at a certain time of day?

❑ How does your condition affect your work and home life?

You may also be asked to rate your pain on a scale of one to ten, with ten indicating intolerable pain.

 If you keep a pain diary or a symptom diary for several days or weeks before visiting your doctor, you can paint a more accurate picture of your pain and other problems.

Explaining X-Rays and Scans

In order to understand what's making your knee hurt, your hip ache, or your finger swell, your doctor needs to take a peek inside the affected joint. Luckily, looking inside your joint is painless; your doctor has sophisticated equipment designed to do just that via X-rays and scans, while you relax on a table.

Exposing the benefits of an X-ray

An X-ray is usually one of the first tools that a doctor uses when gathering information to make a diagnosis. X-rays are useful in distinguishing between two of the most common forms of arthritis, osteoarthritis (Chapter 2) and rheumatoid arthritis (Chapter 3), and are also used to diagnose gout (Chapter 4), reactive arthritis (Chapter 5), and ankylosing spondylitis (Chapter 4).

X-rays are particularly helpful in confirming that cartilage and/or joint damage does exist and in distinguishing between osteoarthritis and rheumatoid arthritis. Ankylosing spondylitis and similar conditions can also be confirmed with an X-ray.

In osteoarthritis, roughened bone ends, cartilage deterioration, uneven narrowing of the joint space, bone spurs, and thickened bone-ends can be seen clearly in an X-ray. A joint afflicted with RA shows tissue swelling, decreased bone density, narrowing of the joint space in an even manner, and, possibly, bone erosion. In ankylosing spondylitis, X-rays can reveal inflammation, small bone growths, and changes in the sacroiliac joints.

X-rays are very helpful in detecting rheumatoid arthritis, osteoarthritis, and reactive arthritis, but aren't so useful in diagnosing Raynaud's phenomenon or bursitis.

Seeing more with a scan

Sometimes a standard X-ray can't tell the doctor what he or she needs to know, because X-rays can't produce images of soft tissue or give the doctor a three-dimensional view. That's where CT scans and MRIs come in handy.

✔ **MRI scans:** MRI stands for magnetic resonance imaging (MRI). Magnetism, radio waves, and a computer are used to create detailed images of body structures. MRIs are especially helpful in diagnosing ailments that affect soft tissues and may detect OA even before symptoms are present. Some experts use MRI scans when they suspect a case of early RA, to detect erosions in the joints that are too subtle to be seen on X-rays.

For a traditional MRI scan, you lie on a narrow table that is wheeled inside a tunnel-like scanner. Unfortunately, you must lie perfectly still, you can feel claustrophobic while squeezed inside the tunnel, and the machine makes a great deal of noise. Plus the scan can go on for as long as an hour and a half! The new open-MRI scanner is more comfortable, less noisy, and less likely to cause claustrophobia because it's similar to a tanning bed that's open on all sides.

✔ **CT scans:** The CT scan (which stands for computerized axial tomography) is a marriage of X-rays and computer technology in which a series of X-rays of one area are taken from different angles. The computer builds these images into three-dimensional pictures, which can be helpful for examining organs, such as the lung or GI tract that can be affected by diseases like lupus. Unlike MRIs, CT scans are completed in 15 to 30 minutes, make minimal noise, and, because the machine isn't tunnel-shaped (CT machines are shaped more like doughnuts), they don't cause claustrophobia.

Backing Up a Diagnosis with Biopsies and Blood Tests

Sometimes the best way to figure out what's going on inside the body is to take samples of blood or tissue for an up-close look. Doctors do this with blood tests and biopsies.

Taking tissue for a biopsy

A *biopsy* is when a doctor takes a sample of tissue from a diseased area of the body and gets it analyzed by a lab to determine what might be causing the problems. A joint biopsy, which involves taking a sample of the joint lining or synovial membrane, is done to determine why a joint is swollen or painful. It is used to help diagnose gout, pseudogout, bacterial infections, lupus, reactive arthritis, and rheumatoid arthritis.

Diagnoses of some forms of arthritis may require samples of the skin, muscle, kidneys, liver, arteries, or nerves. For example, a muscle biopsy can help in the diagnosis of polymyositis, or a skin biopsy may be necessary to confirm diagnoses of psoriatic arthritis, lupus, or scleroderma.

Testing the blood

Blood tests can help confirm a tentative diagnosis or rule out other causes of joint pain. Certain substances found in the blood can indicate inflammation, infections, muscle damage, or other signs of a particular type of arthritis. For example, the presence of RA factor suggests rheumatoid arthritis; certain antibody abnormalities can suggest lupus; and the presence of antibodies to

Borrelia burgdorferi indicate Lyme disease. However, blood abnormalities can point to many different diseases, so these tests are usually used to supply diagnostic clues only.

Common blood tests for the various kinds of arthritis include:

- **Fluorescent antinuclear antibody (FANA):** More than 95 percent of lupus patients have antinuclear antibodies (ANA) that attack and take over the nuclei of healthy cells. The fluorescent dye used in the FANA test can show these antibodies clinging to the cell nuclei. Because this test requires the utmost skill in the laboratory to ensure correct results, it may have to be repeated. Besides those with lupus, up to 40 percent of patients with RA and even some healthy patients test positive for ANA.

- **Anti-DNA and anti-Sm:** If the FANA test is positive, your doctor confirms the results by testing for antibodies to DNA (the cell's genetic material) and Sm, another substance found in the nucleus of the cell. Antibodies to either or both of these are commonly found in those with lupus. Because these antibodies are rarely present in the blood of people who don't have lupus, this test is a reliable diagnostic tool. If the FANA test was negative, these tests are unnecessary.

- **Blood chemistries:** Abnormal amounts of various chemical substances can indicate the possibility of certain forms of arthritis. A high level of uric acid, for example, can be a sign of gout. High levels of creatinine indicate disturbed kidney function, which may point to lupus or another disease of the connective tissue.

- **Complement:** A group of blood proteins that are activated as part of the immune process, the *complement system* releases substances that kill bacteria and send white blood cells rushing to fight off invaders. A low complement level suggests that your immune system is working in overdrive and that you may have a disease, perhaps lupus.

- **Complete blood count (CBC):** Although the presence of arthritis can't be confirmed by a CBC, it can be indicated. For example, a low red blood cell count (anemia) can be a sign of chronic inflammation, which is found in rheumatoid arthritis, Sjögren's syndrome, and polymyalgia rheumatica. A high white cell count may signal some kind of infectious arthritis, such as Lyme disease or gonococcal arthritis. Low levels of blood platelets may be an indication of lupus.

- **Erythrocyte sedimentation rate (ESR):** During inflammation, the red blood cells (*erythrocytes*) clump together, becoming heavier than normal. When left to stand in a test tube, these heavy red blood cells fall faster than normal. The rate at which your red blood cells settle in a one-hour period is called the *erythrocyte sedimentation rate* or *ESR*. A high ESR indicates inflammation.

✓ **Rheumatoid factor (RF):** About 80 percent of patients with rheumatoid arthritis have an antibody called *rheumatoid factor (RF)* in their blood. No one is quite sure whether RF causes the disease or is the result of the immune system's reaction to the disease. Although the factor is a pretty good indicator of rheumatoid arthritis, some people with RA don't have it, and some who do have the factor don't have RA. Like most blood tests, this one must be factored in with other symptoms before an accurate diagnosis can be made.

These are not the only blood tests that your doctor may order, and the examples given are not the only reasons for using them. They are, however, common among the tests doctors use.

Taking Other Tests on the Road to Diagnosis

Doctors often have a good idea of what may be wrong after listening to you describe your symptoms, examining you, and considering your medical history. With many forms of arthritis, they may need nothing more than an X-ray or scan, a blood test or a biopsy to confirm the diagnosis. However, sometimes more testing is necessary. If, for example, your doctor suspects you have gout, she may draw a sample of joint fluid to be examined in the laboratory. If ankylosing spondylitis is likely, genetic testing may be required.

Joint aspiration

Your doctor may want to insert a needle into one or more of your affected joints to withdraw a small amount of fluid for examination under a microscope. He can draw out additional fluid to help relieve pain and pressure inside of your joint, if the swelling is intense.

Called *joint aspiration* or *tapping a joint,* the process consists of the doctor sterilizing the area, using a local anesthetic, and inserting a needle to pull out a small amount of fluid (as little as a couple of drops or as much as a tablespoon or two). She then sends the joint fluid to a laboratory for analysis.

Healthy joints contain clear fluid; anything else probably indicates a problem. Blood in the fluid may be the result of a substantial injury to the joint. Cloudy fluid or the presence of large numbers of white blood cells can indicate either infectious or inflammatory arthritis. Crystals in the fluid are probably due to gout or pseudogout. Bits of cartilage or bone that are present in otherwise clear fluid usually indicate osteoarthritis.

Arthroscopy

An *arthroscope* (a fiberoptic camera about as big around as a straw) is inserted into your joint through a small incision, allowing the doctor to check out your joint's insides in all their glory. The doctor may use this as a diagnostic tool or even as a way to perform surgery inside your joint by repairing torn cartilage, cutting away inflamed or diseased tissues, removing bits of bone or cartilage, or reconstructing ligaments. Only orthopedic surgeons perform arthroscopy.

Recent studies have stirred up controversy by showing that arthroscopy as a surgery compared with sham surgery (the patient had arthroscopic tools inserted into the joint but no corrections were made) had similar effects in pain relief and joint function. That is, neither seemed to do much for the patients. So although it's still used for diagnostic and surgical purposes, the role of arthroscopy has yet to be defined.

Genetic testing

Scientists have discovered that certain genes may be associated with certain types of arthritis. The genetic marker HLA-B27, for example, is often found in those with ankylosing spondylitis. HLA-DR4 occurs in 80 percent of adults with RA. Doctors can't rely solely on genetic testing, because many people who have these genes do not get arthritis, and many who do have arthritis don't have these genes. But these tests may show an inclination toward developing a particular kind of arthritis.

Urine testing

In this test, your urine is examined for protein, red blood cells, or other abnormal substances. Protein or red blood cells in the urine may be an indication of kidney disease, which is often seen in lupus. Protein in the urine may also be due to toxicity caused by certain medications used to treat arthritis, including gold therapy and penicillamine.

Chapter 8

From Aspirin to Steroids: Medicines for Arthritis

● ●

In This Chapter

▶ Discussing medications with your doctor

▶ Looking at the major types of arthritis medication

▶ Treating different forms of arthritis with typically prescribed medicines

● ●

Many of the medicines that doctors prescribe for arthritis are briefly described in this chapter. Naturally, whether any of these medications may be right for you is a decision that you and your doctor should make together.

Talking to Your Doctor

Your doctor's job is to diagnose and treat you, but this important task can't be done without your help. In order to diagnose and treat your condition properly, your doctor must be thoroughly familiar with all of your symptoms — and you're the only one who can supply that information. He needs to ask a lot of questions to build a "knowledge database," but the doctor probably won't think of everything. If you haven't already been asked, be sure to give this information to your doctor:

✔ List everything that's bothering you. You should relate every little symptom and problem, whether physical, mental, or emotional.

✔ Tell her about all of your allergies and any allergic reactions you've had to any medications over the years.

✔ List every prescription and nonprescription medicine you're taking, as well as any vitamins, minerals, amino acids, herbs, other supplements, weight loss products, muscle builders, and so on.

✔ List every medicinal cream or ointment you're using.

Generic name, brand name, generic equivalent: I'm so confused!

A *generic name* is a medication's official moniker, bestowed upon it by the United States Adopted Names Council. A *brand name,* on the other hand, is a proprietary name given to the medication by the pharmaceutical company that owns it. Generic names often tell you something about the drug's structure or chemical formula. As far as lay people are concerned, generic names tend to be dull and unpronounceable. But brand names are often chosen with an eye toward "sales sizzle." For example, the drug with the generic name of methotrexate is sold under the brand name Rheumatrex.

You can quickly distinguish generic from brand names by looking at how they're written: Generic names begin with lowercase letters; brand names start with capitals. (This rule doesn't apply when the drug name appears at the beginning of a sentence, of course, where it is always capitalized.)

A *generic equivalent* is a drug whose active ingredients are chemically identical to the drug your doctor prescribes under its brand name, but the inactive ingredients (binders, fillers, etc.) may not be the same.

- ✔ If you're pregnant, planning to become pregnant, or are nursing, be sure to mention this to your doctor.
- ✔ Inform the doctor if you're on hormone replacement therapy.
- ✔ List the foods that you like to eat. (Grapefruit, for example, can interfere with the workings of some medicines.)
- ✔ Tell the doctor what chemicals, liquids, or fumes you're exposed to at work and at home.
- ✔ Explain the tasks you handle at work and home, and tell your doctor about your hobbies and recreational activities.

In short, tell your doctor all about yourself, your job, your habits, and everything you're ingesting. Tell her about your previous experience with medicines, even if it was good. (Knowing that you tolerated a certain drug well may help your doctor choose a new medicine for you, or it may persuade him to stick with the same one.) The more your doctor knows about you, the better off you are. If you're not asked for the information, volunteer it.

The following questions are good ones to ask your doctor concerning any medications prescribed for you:

- ✔ How do I take this drug, exactly? (With or without food, in the morning, with fluid, after shaking the bottle, and so on.)
- ✔ What activities are unsafe while I'm taking this medication? (For example, can I drive? Take other medicines? Take my vitamins?)

✔ Are there any drugs, supplements, foods, or anything else that I should avoid while I'm taking this medicine?

✔ What is my pill or capsule going to look like? Get a picture from the *PDR (Physician's Drug Reference), Pocket Guide to Prescription Drugs,* or a similar book. Compare what the doctor or pharmacist gives you to the description or picture of the drug to make sure you have the right thing.

 Doctors love to use big words, especially when talking about drugs. When you talk to your doctor, you're likely to hear words like *analgesic, antimalarials, NSAIDs,* and *immunosuppressants* tossed around. If your doctor uses any word that you don't understand, ask for a definition. You may also want to ask your doctor to spell it for you.

Exploring the Five Classes of Drugs for Arthritis

Before deciding exactly which drug to prescribe, doctors first consider which class of medication is best. Doctors can choose from five primary classes to prescribe: nonsteroidal anti-inflammatory drugs (NSAIDs), analgesics, corticosteroids, disease modifying antirheumatic drugs (DMARDs), and biologic response modifiers (BRMs).

Nonsteroidal anti-inflammatory drugs (NSAIDs)

NSAIDs (pronounced EN-seds) help relieve pain and reduce inflammation by interfering with an enzyme called COX (cyclooxygenase). Widely used for many forms of arthritis, NSAIDs come in prescription and nonprescription (over-the-counter) variations, ranging from ibuprofen to Naproxen, and from Anacin to Vioxx. The over-the-counter variations that you can buy in supermarkets and drug stores have lower dosages and are generally well-tolerated. The more powerful prescription forms, on the other hand, can trigger numerous side effects, often centered in the stomach. As you can see in the review of medicines later in this chapter, some of these side effects are potentially dangerous.

Aspirin, perhaps the best known of the NSAIDs, is available under several brand names and also as plain old aspirin. It works by interfering with the body's manufacture of the inflammation products that cause swelling, pain, and other problems. Aspirin's side effects are similar to those seen with the other NSAIDs, and it has a few more all its own.

When traditional NSAIDs cause stomach upsets, doctors often prescribe a newer version that falls into the class of cyclooxygenase-2 (COX-2) inhibitors. COX-2 inhibitors (Bextra, Celebrex, and Vioxx) seem to be just as effective at relieving pain and inflammation as traditional NSAIDs but are less damaging to the stomach. But they're very expensive, so your doctor probably won't prescribe them unless you develop a real problem with traditional NSAIDs.

Analgesics

If you have arthritis pain without inflammation (as is often the case with osteoarthritis or fibromyalgia), your doctor may recommend an analgesic. Analgesics fight pain but do nothing to interfere with the inflammation process, making them easier on the stomach than the NSAIDs. The best-known and most commonly used analgesic is acetaminophen, often recommended as a first-line treatment for osteoarthritis pain. Brand names for acetaminophen-containing analgesics include

- Tylenol
- Excedrin's "Tension headache" formula
- Aspirin-free Excedrin

Prescription varieties include the following, all of which contain opiates:

- Vicodin
- Percocet
- Darvon
- Codeine

A combination of acetaminophen plus a prescription analgesic, like codeine, may be used for more intense pain. If you still hurt after taking an analgesic or NSAID alone, your doctor may prescribe a combination of the two, which may be more effective.

Although opiate-containing analgesics are potentially addicting, when properly prescribed and taken by those with no tendency toward substance abuse, the risk for addiction is very small.

Corticosteroids

Corticosteroids are man-made versions of certain natural hormones that your body produces. And just like the "real thing," they can be quite powerful in both good and bad ways. The corticosteroids, including prednisone, hydrocortisone, and methylprednisolone, are powerful anti-inflammatories that can quickly reduce damaging inflammation of the joints or organs. Unfortunately, they also have significant side effects, including increasing your risk of infections, diabetes, high blood pressure, skin thinning, easy bruising, increased weight, loss of muscle, osteoporosis, and glaucoma. Because of these side effects, doctors look for the lowest effective dose when prescribing these medicines. Corticosteroids may be used to treat rheumatoid arthritis, lupus, polymyositis, and other forms of arthritis.

Disease-modifying antirheumatic drugs (DMARDs)

DMARDs are generally reserved for serious forms of arthritis — such as rheumatoid arthritis, psoriatic arthritis, and ankylosing spondylitis — that aren't helped by other medicines. But because these diseases can be so destructive, many doctors prescribe DMARDs early on to try to prevent inflammation-related joint damage. DMARDs work by altering the way the immune system works and slowing or halting its disastrous attack on the body. DMARDs take time to work — in some cases, months — so they may be prescribed along with an NSAID or a corticosteroid to ease inflammation in the meantime. Methotrexate, sulfasalazine, and anti-malarials are a few examples of DMARDs.

Biologic response modifiers (BRMs)

For those who don't respond to DMARDs, a new class of drugs, the BRMs, may be the answer. First introduced in 1998, the BRMs help ease stubborn cases of inflammation by inhibiting or shoring up certain components of the immune system, called cytokines. The cytokines play a part in the inflammation seen in rheumatoid arthritis, ankylosing spondylitis, and psoriatic arthritis, and BRMs inhibit their inflammatory action. Enbrel, Humira, and Remicade are three of the four BRMs currently approved for treatment of rheumatoid arthritis, and they work to suppress a cytokine called tumor necrosis factor (TNF), and the fourth, Kineret, blocks a cytokine called interleukin-1.

The BRMs are either injected or infused, and are quite expensive, although researchers are working on less expensive versions that can be taken by mouth.

Possible side effects include redness, pain, swelling, itching, or bruising at the injection site, and infections of the upper respiratory tract. Some BRMs may increase your risk of developing serious infections, such as tuberculosis or pneumonia. Tell your doctor if you have tuberculosis, pneumonia, a current infection, a history of serious infections, or asthma.

Uncovering Specific Medicines for Specific Types of Arthritis

In addition to NSAIDs, analgesics, corticosteroids, DMARDs, and BRMs, doctors may prescribe muscle relaxants, sleeping pills, anti-anxiety drugs, or opiates. And when treating certain forms of arthritis and related conditions, they may prescribe drugs that deal with problems extending beyond the joints. For example, people with Raynaud's phenomenon are often treated with drugs normally thought of as heart medications, such as *vasodilators,* to open up (dilate) the blood vessels and increase circulation to the extremities. Unfortunately, some drugs may also be necessary to counteract or ameliorate the side effects of arthritis medicines.

No matter what medication you take, remember that you must always get complete instructions from your doctor and follow those instructions carefully. If anything seems amiss or if you have any questions, ask your doctor!

Following is a list of some of the drugs that a doctor may prescribe for arthritis and arthritis-related conditions. In most cases, we have listed them under their brand names, with their generic names included in the discussion that follows.

Actonel

Actonel (generic name, risedronate) is used to prevent and treat osteoporosis and belongs to a class of drugs called bisphosphonates. Those who have Paget's disease or those who take medications that can cause osteoporosis (such as prednisone) may take Actonel to inhibit bone breakdown.

Possible side effects include upset stomach, flatulence, constipation, diarrhea, heartburn, and bone or joint pain, among others. Actonel must be taken while sitting upright and with a full glass of plain water at least 30 minutes before eating or drinking anything else.

Amoxil

Amoxil (generic name, amoxicillin) is an antibiotic used to treat a wide variety of bacterial infections including Lyme disease. It's available under the brand names Trimox and Wymox.

Some possible side effects include agitation, anxiety, confusion, diarrhea, hives, hyperactivity, insomnia, rash, nausea, and vomiting.

It's not just gulp and swallow

Medicines are tricky. Some are best absorbed on an empty stomach, so you must be sure to take them between meals. Others can irritate the stomach, so you should take them with food. You take some long-lasting medicines once a day; others only work for a brief period of time and must be taken several times a day. Sometimes, it's necessary to have a constant level of the drug in your body, so you need to take it according to a rigid schedule. Other drugs may be taken whenever you feel they're necessary. Some medicines mix well with others, and some don't.

The point is that there's more to taking medicines than gulp and swallow. Ask your doctor for precise instructions on taking all your medicines: when, how (for example, with or without food), how often, and so on. Ask what to do if you forget to take a dose. Ask what side effects you can expect, which of them are dangerous, and which are not.

If your doctor doesn't tell you all about the medicine(s), don't be afraid to ask!

You should not take this medication if you're allergic to penicillin or cephalosporin antibiotics (for instance, Ceclor). If you've had asthma, hives, hay fever, or other allergies, make sure your doctor knows this before you take this drug.

Anaprox

Anaprox (generic name, naproxen sodium), also available as Naprelan and Aleve, is an NSAID used for osteoarthritis, rheumatoid arthritis, tendonitis, bursitis, gout, juvenile rheumatoid arthritis, ankylosing spondylitis, and others. It reduces joint pain, swelling, inflammation, and stiffness.

Some possible side effects include abdominal pain, diarrhea or constipation, indigestion, breathing difficulties, headache, dizziness, sweating, and fluid retention. See your doctor regularly to monitor for possible internal bleeding or ulcers.

Ansaid

Ansaid (generic name, flurbiprofen) is an NSAID used for osteoarthritis and rheumatoid arthritis. It reduces joint pain, swelling, inflammation, and stiffness.

Some possible side effects include headache, swelling, infection of the urinary tract, gastrointestinal upset, the blahs, anxiety, and an altered sense of smell. See your doctor regularly to monitor for possible internal bleeding and stomach ulcers.

Arava

Arava (generic name, leflunomide) is a DMARD that attempts to reduce the symptoms and tissue damage seen in rheumatoid arthritis by slowing the growth and reproduction of white blood cells. By interfering with white blood cells, which are involved in the inflammation process, Arava may help relieve joint pain and swelling and can slow the progression of tissue damage.

The first new DMARD to be approved by the government in a decade or more, Arava produces the same kind of relief seen with methotrexate, an effective drug treatment for rheumatoid arthritis. Arava may work for people who haven't been helped by methotrexate or other medications, who can't tolerate methotrexate's side effects, or who have pre-existing kidney failure.

Some possible side effects include liver problems, thinning or loss of hair, and stomach and digestive problems. It may also cause birth defects and should be used with caution by women in their childbearing years. Careful monitoring is required in those who have elevated blood pressure, problems with the immune system, or kidney disease.

Arava doesn't cure rheumatoid arthritis, but it can help relieve symptoms and reduce the rate at which the disease progresses.

Arthrotec

Arthrotec, a combination of the NSAID diclofenac sodium plus the anti-ulcer medication misoprostol, is used for people with arthritis who are likely to develop an ulcer. Arthrotec helps relieve the pain and inflammation seen in rheumatoid arthritis, osteoarthritis, ankylosing spondylitis, and juvenile rheumatoid arthritis, and protects the stomach against the severe irritation and ulcers often seen with NSAID use.

Some possible side effects include abdominal pain, diarrhea, edema (swelling of the feet), dizziness, heartburn, or indigestion. Arthrotec may also reduce fertility.

Aspirin

Aspirin (generic name) is an NSAID used for various types of arthritis. It reduces pain, inflammation, and fever. It's available under various brand names, such as Bayer, Empirin, and Ecotrin.

Some possible side effects include bleeding stomach ulcers, stomach pain, upset stomach, and heartburn. Aspirin may also cause complications during pregnancy.

Azulfidine

Azulfidine (generic name, sulfasalazine), a DMARD, is an anti-inflammatory and antibiotic used to treat rheumatoid arthritis and ankylosing spondylitis in adults and children whose disease has not responded well to other medications. Rheumatoid arthritis patients usually take this medication in its time-release form, azulfidine EN-tabs.

Azulfidine should not be taken if you are allergic to sulfa drugs, PABA-containing sunscreens, or local anesthetics. It may cause increased sensitivity to the sun or to bright light. Use sunscreen and wear sunglasses and protective clothing.

Some possible side effects include hives, nausea, vomiting, loss of appetite, and headaches.

Bextra

Bextra (generic name, valdecoxib) is an NSAID of the COX-2-inhibitor variety. COX-2 drugs have been shown to relieve arthritis pain and inflammation as well as traditional NSAIDs do but with less stomach damage.

Some possible side effects include abdominal pain, diarrhea, edema (swelling of the feet), dizziness, heartburn, or indigestion. Tell your doctor if you're allergic to sulfonamides, a kind of sulfa drug. Bextra is also significantly more expensive than standard NSAIDs. And because it's relatively new, the sum total of its effects, both good and bad, is not yet known.

Celebrex

Celebrex (generic name, celecoxib) is an NSAID and a COX-2 inhibitor. It's used to relieve the pain, inflammation, and stiffness of osteoarthritis and rheumatoid arthritis with fewer of the gastrointestinal side effects seen with standard NSAIDs.

Although designed to have fewer side effects, Celebrex may cause diarrhea, abdominal pain, indigestion, ulceration, bleeding, perforation of the stomach or intestines, and other problems. It may also be dangerous to use Celebrex while you're on other medications or if you have liver or kidney disease, asthma, allergies to sulfa drugs, or you're pregnant.

Celebrex is also much more expensive than standard NSAIDs, and its long-term effects are yet to be seen.

Clinoril

Clinoril (generic name, sulindac) is an NSAID used for osteoarthritis, rheumatoid arthritis, bursitis, tendonitis, gout, and ankylosing spondylitis. It reduces joint pain, swelling, inflammation, and stiffness.

Some possible side effects include headache, nervousness, ringing in the ears, swelling, and many stomach problems including pain, diarrhea, constipation, nausea, and loss of appetite. See your doctor regularly to monitor for possible internal bleeding or stomach ulcers.

ColBenemid

ColBenemid (generic name, probenecid-colchicine) is an antigout medicine. It contains both colchicine, an antigout medicine that slows the movement of white blood cells to the joints, and probenecid, which removes extra uric acid from the body. It doesn't cure gout but can prevent gout attacks. However, relief lasts only as long as you take it.

Some possible side effects include muscle weakness, nausea, vomiting, diarrhea, and blood and kidney problems. Probenecid can trigger dizziness, headaches, fever, and blood problems.

Cytoxan

Cytoxan (generic name, cyclophosphamide), a DMARD, is an anticancer drug used for serious cases of rheumatoid arthritis and lupus. It apparently kills some of the white blood cells that bring on arthritis symptoms.

Some possible side effects include severe nausea and vomiting, damage to the bladder or bleeding from the bladder, loss of appetite, hair loss, mouth ulcers, darkening of skin and fingernails, low blood counts, and abdominal pain.

Daypro

Daypro (generic name, oxaprozin) is an NSAID used for osteoarthritis and rheumatoid arthritis to reduce joint pain, swelling, inflammation, and stiffness.

Some possible side effects include rashes, depression, confusion, indigestion, nausea, and constipation. See your doctor regularly to monitor for possible internal bleeding or stomach ulcers.

Decadron

Decadron (generic name, dexamethasone) is a corticosteroid used to treat rheumatoid arthritis and lupus by reducing inflammation.

Some possible side effects include increased infections, diabetes, high blood pressure, skin thinning, easy bruising, increased weight, loss of muscle, osteoporosis, and glaucoma.

This drug can increase your susceptibility to infections and make them harder to treat. It can also "hide" the presence of infections, making it difficult for your doctor to diagnose the problem.

Deltasone

Deltasone (generic name, prednisone) is a corticosteroid used to reduce inflammation in rheumatoid arthritis, lupus, and many other conditions.

Some possible side effects include increased infections, diabetes, high blood pressure, skin thinning, easy bruising, increased weight, loss of muscle, osteoporosis, and glaucoma.

This drug can increase your susceptibility to infections and make them harder to treat. It can also "hide" the presence of infections, making it difficult for your doctor to diagnose the problem.

Didronel

Didronel (generic name, etidronate) is an anti-hypercalcemic used to treat Paget's disease. It inhibits the breakdown and release of calcium from bone. Also available as EHDP, Didronel helps regulate bone development. Be aware that it takes at least a month of treatment with Didronel before you see improvement in Paget's disease.

Some possible side effects include bone pain, nausea, diarrhea, and swelling of various parts of the body.

Disalcid

Disalcid (generic name, salsalate) is an NSAID used for osteoarthritis, rheumatoid arthritis, and others to relieve pain and inflammation.

Some possible side effects include nausea, rashes, ringing in the ears, and hearing problems. Disalcid contains salicylate, which has been linked to Reye's syndrome in children.

Doryx

Doryx (generic name, doxycycline) is a tetracycline antibiotic used to treat gonococcal infections and Lyme disease. It works by inhibiting the growth and multiplication of bacteria. It's also available as Vibramycin and Vibra-Tabs.

Some possible side effects include serious allergic reactions causing swelling of the face, difficulty swallowing, inflamed tongue, and pain in the chest. Other side effects include serious sun sensitivity and abdominal discomfort.

Enbrel

Enbrel (generic name, etanercept) is a biologic response modifier (BRM) used to reduce the pain and swelling seen in rheumatoid arthritis, juvenile rheuma- toid arthritis, psoriatic arthritis, and ankylosing spondylitis. Enbrel works by blocking the activity of tumor necrosis factor (TNF), a substance that causes arthritis-related swelling and joint damage. Enbrel is given — usually twice a week — in the form of injections in the thigh, stomach, or upper arm.

Some possible side effects include redness, pain, swelling, itching, or bruising at the injection site, and infections of the upper respiratory tract. Enbrel may also increase your risk of developing a serious infection, including tuberculosis. Tell your doctor if you have or have ever had tuberculosis, recurrent infections, a nervous system disorder, or a neurologic disorder, such as multiple sclerosis or a seizure disorder. Though rare, symptoms of lupus have occurred with treatment with Enbrel.

Feldene

Feldene (generic name, piroxicam) is an NSAID used to reduce the joint pain, swelling, inflammation, and stiffness seen in osteoarthritis and rheumatoid arthritis.

Some possible side effects include abdominal pain, anemia, dizziness, nose- bleed, elevated blood pressure, sweating, stomach ulceration, the blahs, headache, itching, and nausea. See your doctor regularly to monitor for possible internal bleeding or stomach ulcers.

Fentanyl

Fentanyl (generic name), an opiate analgesic that comes in the form of a patch applied to the skin, is used to relieve chronic pain. The medication, which is sold under the brand names of Astramorph, Demerol, Ultiva and others, is slowly and continuously released into the body via the patch. Each patch is designed to last for 72 hours before being removed and replaced by another. It may take a day or so before the effects of the first patch are felt.

Some possible side effects include abdominal or stomach pain; breathing problems, confusion, constipation, diarrhea, dizziness, drowsiness, headache, indigestion, loss of appetite, nausea or vomiting, nervousness, sweating; or weakness.

Fosamax

Fosamax (generic name, alendronate sodium) is used to treat Paget's disease and postmenopausal osteoporosis (thinning of the bones). It prevents or slows down the weakening of the bone and helps maintain bone integrity. Fosamax (which comes in tablet form) must be taken with a full glass of water 30 minutes before a meal. During that time, you should stand or sit upright to reduce the risk of developing heartburn or injuring your esophagus.

Some possible side effects include bloating, diarrhea, constipation, stomach irritation, muscle or bone pain, difficulty swallowing, and ulcers in the esophagus. Be sure to get enough calcium and vitamin D while taking this drug.

Humira

Humira (generic name, adalimumab) is a biologic response modifier (BRM) used either by itself or with other medications (such as methotrexate) to reduce the pain, swelling, and difficulty in moving seen in rheumatoid arthritis. Humira works by blocking the activity of tumor necrosis factor (TNF), a substance that causes arthritis-related swelling and joint damage. Humira is given in the form of injections, usually every other week, and is only given to those who have not been helped by other rheumatoid arthritis medications.

Some possible side effects include redness, pain, swelling, itching, or bruising at the injection site, and infections of the upper respiratory tract. Humira may also increase your risk of developing a serious infection, including tuberculosis. Tell your doctor if you have or have ever had tuberculosis, recurrent infections, a nervous system disorder, or a neurologic disorder, such as multiple sclerosis or a seizure disorder. Rarely, symptoms of lupus have occurred with treatment with Humira.

Ibuprofen

Ibuprofen (generic name) is an NSAID used to relieve the pain and swelling seen in osteoarthritis, rheumatoid arthritis, juvenile rheumatoid arthritis, and carpal tunnel syndrome. It's available under several brand names, including Advil, Motrin, and Nuprin.

Some possible side effects include headache, itching, nervousness, ringing in the ears, and abdominal problems, including pain, bloating, constipation, diarrhea, and flatulence.

Motrin and Advil are available over-the-counter without a prescription. See your doctor regularly to monitor for possible internal bleeding and ulcers.

Imuran

Imuran (generic name, azathioprine) is a DMARD used for rheumatoid arthritis and lupus. It decreases the body's response to infections and interferes with the action of the white blood cells, which worsen the symptoms of rheumatoid arthritis and lupus. Imuran is also used with other medications to prevent the rejection of kidney transplants.

Some possible side effects include infection, suppression of the bone marrow, loss of appetite, liver damage, hair loss, skin rashes, diarrhea, nausea, and vomiting.

Indocin

Indocin (generic name, indomethacin) is an NSAID used to reduce the joint pain, swelling, inflammation, and stiffness seen in osteoarthritis, rheumatoid arthritis, bursitis, ankylosing spondylitis, gout, and tendonitis.

Some possible side effects include hair loss, hepatitis, vaginal bleeding, depression, fatigue, dizziness, indigestion, nausea, stomach pain and upset, and vertigo. See your doctor regularly to monitor for possible internal bleeding or stomach ulcers.

Keflex

Keflex (generic name, cephalexin hydrochloride) is an antibiotic used for bacterial infections, including those found in infectious arthritis. If you have an infected joint, your doctor may give you an intravenous form of Keflex

(Cefazolin) as a first-line treatment. After two weeks of this treatment, your doctor may switch to the oral form of Keflex. (Other brand names include Biocef and Keftab.)

Some possible side effects include upset stomach, diarrhea, vomiting, mild skin rash, colitis, yeast infections, fatigue, fever, hallucinations, joint pain, and joint inflammation.

Kineret

Kineret (generic name, anakinra) is a biologic response modifier (BRM) used either by itself or with other medications to reduce the pain, swelling, and joint stiffness seen in rheumatoid arthritis. Kineret works by blocking the activity of interleukin-1, a substance that causes arthritis-related swelling and joint damage. Kineret is given in the form of daily injections and is only given to those who haven't been helped by other rheumatoid arthritis medications.

Some possible side effects include redness, pain, swelling, itching, or bruising at the injection site, and infections of the upper respiratory tract. Kineret may also increase your risk of developing a serious infection, including pneumonia. Tell your doctor if you have pneumonia, a current infection, a history of serious infections, or asthma.

Lodine

Lodine (generic name, etodolac) is an NSAID used to reduce the joint pain, swelling, inflammation, and stiffness seen in osteoarthritis and rheumatoid arthritis.

Some possible side effects include blurred vision, chills, pain or difficulty upon urinating, more frequent urination, asthma, fever, black stools (a sign of stomach bleeding), rapid heart beat, and congestive heart failure.

See your doctor regularly to monitor for possible internal bleeding or stomach ulcers.

Medrol

Medrol (generic name, methylprednisolone) is a corticosteroid used to reduce the inflammation seen in rheumatoid arthritis, gout, and lupus.

Some possible side effects include increased infections, diabetes, high blood pressure, skin thinning and easy bruising, increased weight, loss of muscle, osteoporosis, and glaucoma. This drug can increase your susceptibility to infections and make them harder to treat. It can also "hide" the presence of infections, making it difficult for your doctor to diagnose the problem.

Miacalcin

Miacalcin (generic name, calcitonin-salmon) is a synthetic hormone used for Paget's disease and osteoporosis (thinning and weakening of the bones). Also available as Calcimar, it helps regulate calcium levels in bone and blood. It is given as an injection (either into the muscle or directly beneath the skin) or can be used as a nasal spray. Those using Miacalcin as a treatment for osteoporosis should also take a calcium and a vitamin D supplement.

Some possible side effects include diarrhea, upset stomach, flu-like symptoms, muscle aches, and fatigue.

Naprosyn

Naprosyn (generic name, naproxen) is an NSAID used to treat the joint pain, swelling, inflammation, and stiffness seen in osteoarthritis, rheumatoid arthritis, juvenile rheumatoid arthritis, bursitis, tendonitis, gout, and ankylosing spondylitis. It's also available as EC-Naprosyn.

Some possible side effects include difficulty breathing, drowsiness, skin eruptions, bleeding in general, stomach ulcers, itching, abdominal pain, bruising, and constipation. See your doctor regularly to monitor for possible internal bleeding, ulcers, and stomach ulcers.

Orudis

Orudis (generic name, ketoprofen) is an NSAID used to treat the joint pain, swelling, inflammation, and stiffness seen in osteoarthritis and rheumatoid arthritis. It's also available as Oruvail (an extended-release form used for long-term treatment of osteoarthritis and rheumatoid arthritis), as well as the nonprescription, over-the-counter drugs Actron and Orudis KT.

Some possible side effects include kidney damage, insomnia, nervousness, fluid retention, belching, loosening of the fingernails, impotence, flatulence, headache, and nausea. See your doctor regularly to monitor for possible internal bleeding and stomach ulcers.

Pediapred

Pediapred (generic name, prednisolone sodium phosphate) is a corticosteroid used to reduce the inflammation seen in rheumatoid arthritis, gout, lupus, and others. Some possible side effects include increased infections, diabetes, high blood pressure, skin thinning and easy bruising, increased weight, loss of muscle, osteoporosis, and glaucoma. This drug can increase your susceptibility to infections and make them harder to treat. It can also "hide" the presence of infections, making it difficult for your doctor to diagnose the problem.

Penicillamine

Penicillamine, also available as Cuprimine and Depen, is used to treat rheumatoid arthritis. We don't know exactly how penicillamine helps. It may interfere with the action of certain white blood cells that inadvertently damage joints.

Penicillamine is a slow-acting drug that may take two to three months to bring about beneficial effects. If and when it works, it reduces joint pain, swelling, and tenderness.

Some possible side effects include lack of appetite, swollen lymph glands, diarrhea, and skin rashes.

Penicillin

Penicillin is an antibiotic used to treat bacterial infections including Lyme disease. It's available in a variety of generic and brand names, including Bicillin, Duracillin, Pentids, Pen Vee, and Pipracil.

Some possible side effects include allergic reactions, such as rashes, tongue swelling, itching, nausea, diarrhea, and acute kidney failure.

Plaquenil

Plaquenil (generic name, hydroxychloroquine sulfate) is an anti-malarial drug used to treat the joint pain, swelling, inflammation, and stiffness seen in rheumatoid arthritis and lupus.

Some possible side effects include changes in eye pigmentation, blind spots, difficulty focusing the eyes and other eye problems, decreased muscle coordination, hair loss, and changes in skin and hair coloration. Plaquenil is a slow-acting drug that may take several weeks to bring about beneficial effects.

Prosorba

Although Prosorba isn't a drug, it may be an effective treatment for rheumatoid arthritis. The Prosorba column is a therapeutic device that cleans the blood in a process similar to kidney dialysis. The goal is to filter out certain antibodies in an attempt to calm an immune system that has turned on the body.

Designed for patients with severe rheumatoid arthritis who have not been helped by standard medications, Prosorba therapy requires 12 once-a-week sessions, each lasting about two hours. During the sessions, blood is taken from the arm, the fluid (plasma) and blood cells are separated, and the fluid is passed through a Prosorba cylinder. Inside the cylinder, the blood is filtered to remove the offending antibodies. Then the fluid and blood are combined before being returned to the body, via the other arm.

Not all patients are helped by Prosorba therapy, although 20 percent of those in clinical trials enjoyed good results, and some experienced remissions that lasted a year or longer. One thing is certain: It takes a while to see results. On average it takes 9 to 12 weeks, and some people don't respond until they've undergone 16 to 20 weeks of treatment.

Unfortunately, Prosorba treatment is quite expensive, with each of the 9 to 20 sessions costing well over $1,000. And side effects are possible, including nausea, muscle and joint pain, chills, fever, a temporary drop in blood pressure, and fatigue.

Overall, the role of this therapy is still unclear. It's an expensive alternative with many serious side effects, though it may have a role in treating patients who haven't found relief from other therapies.

Relafen

Relafen (generic name, nabumetone) is an NSAID used to reduce the joint pain, swelling, inflammation, and stiffness seen in osteoarthritis and rheumatoid arthritis. Some possible side effects include itching, insomnia, nervousness, constipation, diarrhea, dizziness, ringing in the ears, and stomach inflammation. See your doctor regularly to monitor for possible internal bleeding and stomach ulcers.

Remicade

Remicade (generic name, infliximab) is a BRM used to treat rheumatoid arthritis. It's also often used to treat psoriatic arthritis, ankylosing spondylitis, and juvenile rheumatoid arthritis, although it has not yet been FDA-approved for these purposes. It helps slow the progression of joint damage, relieve pain and stiffness, and improve joint function. Remicade is infused intravenously every two months and is often used in conjunction with the drug methotrexate.

Side effects can include reactions that occur during or just after infusion, such as abdominal pain, cough, rash, muscle pain, unusual fatigue, or shortness of breath, among others. Infections have been reported during treatment with this drug, so it should not be used if serious infections are present. Discontinue if a serious infection develops.

Rheumatrex

Rheumatrex (generic name, methotrexate) is an anticancer drug used for rheumatoid arthritis when drugs such as NSAIDs haven't worked. It helps slow immune system reactions that cause many of the problems seen in rheumatoid arthritis. But in the process, methotrexate may lower your body's overall resistance, so a chance for infection exists. You should avoid getting any live vaccines while on Rheumatrex, because you may contract the disease you're trying to avoid. It's important to note that methotrexate is taken once a *week,* not once a day.

Besides a greater susceptibility to infections, some possible side effects include liver toxicity, lung toxicity, bone marrow suppression, mouth ulcers, the blahs, dizziness, fatigue, abdominal pain and distress, impotence, and diabetes. It's important to get blood tests to check your liver and blood counts every two months and get immediate medical attention if a cough or shortness of breath develop.

Sandimmune

Sandimmune (generic name, cyclosporine) is a BRM that is used to treat severe cases of rheumatoid arthritis and lupus by suppressing the immune system.

Some possible side effects include elevated blood pressure, kidney damage, growth of the gums, tremor, convulsions, coughing, acne, tumor of the lymph system, difficulty breathing, and joint or muscle pain. Because Sandimmune suppresses the immune system, you may be more likely to develop other diseases, including cancer.

The amount of cyclosporine absorbed from Sandimmune varies from person to person, so your doctor needs to check the levels in your blood regularly.

Sulfinpyrazone

Sulfinpyrazone (generic name) is an antigout medication available under brand names such as Antazone, Anturan, Anturane, and Novopyrazone. It works by lowering uric acid levels.

Some possible side effects include itching, redness, rash or other signs of skin irritation, difficulty urinating, nausea, and lower back pain.

Tetracycline

Tetracycline (generic name) is an antibiotic used to treat bacterial infections, including Lyme disease. Many generic and brand name tetracyclines exist, including Doryx, doxycycline, methacycline, minocycline, Sumycin, and Vibramycin.

Some possible side effects include allergic reactions, sore mouth, nausea, vomiting, vaginal discharge, dark tongue, faintness, anemia, and skin sensitivity to sunlight.

Tolectin

Tolectin (generic name, tolmetin sodium) is an NSAID used to reduce the joint pain, swelling, inflammation, and stiffness seen in osteoarthritis, rheumatoid arthritis, and juvenile rheumatoid arthritis.

Some possible side effects include weight changes, weakness, elevated blood pressure, hives, kidney failure, painful urination, and dizziness.

Tolectin is used for both short-term and long-term treatments. It can damage the liver, kidney, and eyes, and increase bleeding. See your doctor regularly to monitor for these problems, as well as for possible internal bleeding and stomach ulcers.

Trilisate

Trilisate (generic name, choline magnesium trisalicylate) is an NSAID used to treat the joint pain, swelling, inflammation, and stiffness seen in osteoarthritis, rheumatoid arthritis, and juvenile rheumatoid arthritis.

Some possible side effects include stomach pain, heartburn, vomiting, constipation, and diarrhea.

Trilisate may be linked to Reye's syndrome, a serious ailment. See your doctor regularly to monitor for this problem, as well as for possible internal bleeding and stomach ulcers.

Tylenol

Tylenol (generic name, acetaminophen) is a fever- and pain-relieving medication used to treat aching joints and muscles. It is also available as Aspirin-Free Anacin and Panadol. It should not be used for more than ten days to relieve pain or three days to relieve fever.

Some rare but possible side effects include indications of an allergic reaction, such as hives, swelling, and difficulty breathing. Liver damage is possible when large amounts of Tylenol and alcohol are combined.

Vioxx

Vioxx (generic name, rofecoxib) is a COX-2 inhibitor, designed to relieve osteoarthritis pain and inflammation, as well as menstrual pain and acute pain, with fewer side effects than the standard NSAIDs. Yet Vioxx can cause bleeding in the intestines, kidney problems, nausea, and itching. There may also be flu-like symptoms, headache, dizziness, diarrhea, heartburn, swelling of the legs and/or feet, fatigue, kidney failure, vomiting, and other problems.

Certain conditions make it dangerous to take Vioxx, including pregnancy, asthma, swelling of the throat and face or other allergic reactions. It can also be dangerous to take Vioxx if you have liver disease, kidney disease, heart failure, high blood pressure, or certain other ailments. A drawback to Vioxx is that it's significantly more expensive than standard NSAIDs, costing between $90 and $120 per month.

Voltaren

Voltaren (generic name, diclofenac sodium) is an NSAID used to treat the joint pain, swelling, inflammation, and stiffness seen in osteoarthritis, rheumatoid arthritis, and ankylosing spondylitis. It's also available as Voltaren-XR and Cataflam (diclofenac potassium).

Some possible side effects include diarrhea, itching, cramps, constipation, ringing in the ears, and rash. Voltaren-XR is used for long-term treatment.

Tell your doctor if you have kidney or heart problems or elevated blood pressure, and see your doctor regularly to monitor for these and other problems, including internal bleeding and stomach ulcers.

Zyloprim

Zyloprim (generic name, allopurinol) is used to treat gout by reducing the production of uric acid. It's also available as Lopurin. Zyloprim does not stop gout attacks that have already begun; in fact, it can worsen acute attacks of gout. Instead, it's used after an acute attack has subsided as a long-term treatment to prevent future attacks.

Some possible side effects include chills, fever, diarrhea, rash, itch, stomach pain and other problems, and headache. The most serious side effect is a life-threatening allergic reaction, which, although very rare, requires immediate medical attention because it is fatal about 25 percent of the time. Its symptoms include a skin rash, fever, and liver and kidney failure.

Chapter 9

Cuts That Cure: Surgeries for Arthritis

The idea of having surgery is always a scary one. Any time you allow a surgeon to ply his trade on your body, you're taking certain risks, some great, and others small. But under the right conditions, surgery performed on a diseased joint can bring results that are nothing short of spectacular. Pain can be reduced or eliminated, range of motion restored, deformities corrected, and joint function vastly improved. Still, surgery isn't for everybody. Whether it's right for you depends on many factors.

If you're considering surgical treatment for your arthritis, you need to consult with an *orthopedic surgeon* or *orthopedist* (the kind of doctor who specializes in treating diseases of the muscles, bones, and joints). An orthopedic surgeon is trained in both surgical and nonsurgical methods. *Nonsurgical treatments* consist of casting, splinting, and joint injections. *Surgical treatments* include removal of the joint lining, cutting and resetting of the bone, bone fusion, and joint reconstruction. *Arthroscopic surgery*, a special technique that has gained great popularity in recent years, is one of many techniques in the orthopedic surgeon's repertoire.

Your family physician or internist may be able to refer you to a competent orthopedic surgeon, but don't automatically assume that this person is the right choice for you. Review the suggestions in Chapter 6 for finding a doctor and apply them in your current search.

Finding out if you're (mentally) prepped for surgery

Although your doctor can tell you all about what goes on inside your body, only you know what's going on inside your head. Do a little soul-searching to determine whether you really want and need the surgery by asking yourself the following questions:

✔ Is the pain interfering with my ability to lead a productive and satisfying life?

✔ Do I rely on pain relievers taken at the maximum allowable dosage to get through the day?

✔ Have I tried all other pain-relieving methods (physical therapy, exercise, pain management strategies, and so on) without success?

✔ Are my expectations of the surgery results realistic?

✔ Will I participate fully in my post-surgery rehabilitation?

If you can answer "yes" to all of these questions, you may be mentally and emotionally ready to undergo joint surgery.

Knowing What to Ask Your Doctor Before Undergoing Surgery

Because surgery is a drastic and (at least somewhat) risky option, you shouldn't consider it until all other measures have been exhausted. First, you and your doctor should thoroughly investigate and make use of the any non-surgical options, such as medication, diet, physical therapy, pain management strategies, exercise, and alternative methods. The truth of the matter is that most people don't need surgery to manage their arthritis.

In some cases, though, surgery can be a godsend. When rheumatic finger joints render your hands nearly useless, or when a painful, osteoarthritic hip makes walking out to the mailbox a major feat, certain surgical procedures may be able to give you a new lease on life.

Whether a surgery succeeds depends on two things: the condition itself and the body in question. Some disease states respond wonderfully to surgery, whereas others show little or no improvement. People are like that, too. One person may come through a surgical procedure with flying colors, zip through recovery, and be thrilled with the results. Another person, equally affected and undergoing an identical surgery, may become trapped in a long, drawn-out recovery period that garners less-than-optimal results. Putting it simply, surgery is a highly individual matter and may or may not be best for you. To find out, begin by asking your orthopedic surgeon the following questions:

✔ **Do my symptoms and my test results go hand-in-hand?** In other words, can your doctor confirm your diagnosis? You certainly don't want to undergo surgery for a problem that may not exist.

✔ **Does my kind of arthritis respond well to surgery?** Surgery is most often performed on those with rheumatoid arthritis (Chapter 3) or incapacitating osteoarthritis (Chapter 2); on the other hand, surgery is rarely the treatment-of-choice for gout (Chapter 4), scleroderma (Chapter 5), or lupus (Chapter 5). Those with ankylosing spondylitis (Chapter 4) are "iffy" candidates for surgery; Sometimes surgery is used to straighten their spines or replace joints, but excessive bone growth can complicate the recovery process.

✔ **How do I know if I need surgery?** In most cases, surgery for arthritis is not an emergency — it doesn't absolutely have to be done at a certain time. The decision to undergo surgery and the timing of the operation is usually dictated by pain, your overall health status, and your degree of disability. Although a few arthritis-related problems need surgery right away (for example, a ruptured tendon), most can wait. But delaying an "optional" surgery (for example a hip replacement) for too long can be a bad idea, leading to a poor surgical outcome, the irreversible contraction of certain muscles supporting the joint, and increased postoperative pain. Ask your doctor about the possibility of irreversible damage or disability brought about by waiting too long.

✔ **What results can I expect from this surgery?** In other words, what is the surgery going to do for you? How may it affect your pain, your range of motion, and the stability of your joint(s)? What kind of activities will you be able to participate in after you recover? What limitations will you have?

✔ **What risks are involved?** Make sure the doctor explains all the complications that can result from the surgery (for example, infection, nerve damage, and so on), as well as the risks involved in undergoing the surgery itself (such as cardiac arrest).

✔ **What is involved in the post-surgery rehabilitation?** Rehabilitation can be a long, sometimes painful process that usually requires your utmost dedication and hard work. Be sure you know what lies ahead before you consent to surgery. If you're not willing to do the work, the outcome of your surgery may be compromised.

✔ **Am I physically able to withstand the surgery?** It is common practice to have a physical examination before surgery to make sure that you and your body are up to the procedure. The condition of your heart, respiratory system, blood, and overall health are taken into account when assessing whether you can withstand the rigors of surgery.

✔ **What does the future hold if I don't have surgery?** If you are already in great pain, finding out that it may get worse unless you have the surgery could tip the scales for you in favor of the procedure. In some cases, arthritis surgery can be put off indefinitely without compromising its effectiveness. But sometimes waiting too long can result in muscle wasting, a decline in joint function, or permanent deformities, all of which can make future surgeries less successful.

Looking At Different Kinds of Joint Surgery

Because the joint is an intricate piece of "machinery," and many different things can go wrong with it, joint surgery is complex and wide-ranging. It can involve flushing the joint with water, resurfacing rough bone ends or cartilage, cutting away inflamed membranes, growing bone where it otherwise wouldn't be, and even taking the whole joint out and starting from scratch with a new one.

Synovectomy: Removing a diseased joint lining

People who have rheumatoid arthritis may benefit from having a *synovectomy*, in which the surgeon removes an inflamed, overgrown joint lining *(synovium)*.

In rheumatoid arthritis, the inflamed, thickened synovium can overgrow to the point that it invades the joint's supporting structures — the bones, cartilage, muscles, and ligaments. This growth can cause damage to the joint over time. At the same time, the synovium releases enzymes that cause bone and cartilage to break down. Removing the offending lining stops the synovial invasion and reduces the amount of destructive enzymes released.

The surgeon may make a large incision that exposes the entire joint. Or, in the case of arthroscopic surgery, tiny incisions may be made that are just large enough to accommodate the insertion of an arthroscope. The *arthroscope* is a flexible tube about the diameter of a pencil that has a camera on the end. It's used for diagnostic and surgical purposes. In either procedure, the joint lining is cut away, leaving just enough behind to produce lubricating fluid. This type of surgery isn't a permanent cure, as the synovium eventually grows back. Pain relief and protection against joint destruction can last for a couple of years, so more radical treatments, such as joint replacement, can be postponed.

Osteotomy: Cutting and resetting the bone

To perform an *osteotomy*, the surgeon removes a section of bone to correct joint alignment. (*Osteo* is the Greek word for *bone; tomy* means *to cut.*) Those suffering from osteoarthritis (especially of the knee) (Chapter 2) and ankylosing spondylitis (Chapter 4) can benefit from this surgery. It's also helpful for joints that are wearing improperly but still have a healthy area.

Taking a look at the total hip replacement procedure

The total hip replacement surgery gives you a good idea of how joint replacement (arthroplasty) surgeries are performed. A ball-and-socket joint, the hip must provide a secure anchor between the pelvis and thigh bone (femur) to do its job properly. In a total hip replacement, the ball and the socket are separated, removed, and then replaced with artificial structures. The surgery is completed in several stages:

✔ The tendons and ligaments that are connected to the femur's ball-shaped end are carefully detached.

✔ The hip joint is dislocated, in order to separate the pelvis and femur.

✔ The ball-shaped end is cut away from the femur.

✔ A special tool is used to hollow out the socket to make it large enough to hold the new socket, a cup-like structure made of polyethylene plastic.

✔ The plastic socket is cemented into place using joint compound.

✔ A shaft is cut down the center of the femur. A metal ball with a rod attached (it looks like a door knob with a root) is inserted in the shaft and cemented into place.

✔ The metal ball is inserted into the plastic socket, the ligaments and tendons repaired, and the wound is closed.

Recovery from a total hip replacement can take time. Patients usually stay in the hospital for 4 to 5 days after surgery and may use a cane, a walker, or crutches for the first 6 weeks. After that, most normal activities can be resumed — walking, bicycling, driving, golfing, and so on. Some doctors estimate that 80 percent of a patient's recovery occurs within the first 10 to 12 weeks after surgery, and the last 20 percent occurs during the following 3 to 6 months.

A misaligned joint can cause uneven wearing on the bones and cartilage as well as general joint pain. After proper alignment is restored, the force exerted on the joint is distributed more evenly. Excess pressure is released from cartilage and bone, "worn spots" have the chance to repair themselves, and pain is reduced.

If the patient is suffering from osteoarthritis, a slice or wedge of bone is surgically removed, allowing the joint to realign. The "raw edges" of the bone are connected with screws and eventually grow together again. If the patient has ankylosing spondylitis (the spinal disease), the damaged tissue and bone that lock the spine into its unnatural, bent-over position are removed so that the spine can return to its natural, upright position.

Pain relief, improved joint function, increased range of motion, and greater joint stability are the benefits of this type of surgery.

Recovery may take anywhere from 6 to 12 months, but the possibility exists that joint function may not improve. Alterations in joint alignment can make future joint replacements difficult. For many, the benefits last only a few years.

Arthrodesis: Fusing the bone

Folks who suffer from rheumatoid arthritis may benefit from having certain bones fused. The surgeon positions the joint into its most functional alignment and then "locks" it in place permanently.

This surgery helps to stabilize and relieve pain in highly unsteady and painful joints. Arthrodesis is primarily performed on the spine but also can be used on the thumb, hip, knee, and wrist when replacement is either not feasible or has already proved unsuccessful. Fusion of the hip joint may be required for those who need a total hip replacement but can't have one, either because their bones aren't healthy enough or because they're too young or too active. (Hip replacements typically last only about 10 to 15 years, and second replacements often don't work as well.) Fusion of the thumb joint can make grasping possible. Fusion of the knee is sometimes performed when a knee replacement becomes infected and won't "take." The wrist may be fused, because it's a highly unstable joint and very difficult to replace.

The surgeon removes cartilage from the opposing bone ends and also removes a surface layer of bone. The joint is positioned in the way in which it can be of greatest use, and then the bone ends are joined using pins, rods, or screws. Splinting or casting helps keep the joint stable, while new bone growth fuses it permanently into place.

The surgery helps to relieve pain and can increase the ability to use the joint (in a limited way). Although joint motion is forfeited with arthrodesis, joint function improves. A person with a fused hip, for example, *can* walk, even if it is with a limp, which may be progress for one who is otherwise wheelchair-bound. Recovery from this surgery can take several months.

Arthroplasty: Replacing the joint

Sometimes a joint degenerates to the point where the pain is severe or constant and function is seriously impaired. By surgically removing the old, diseased parts and replacing them with new, man-made ones, the pain is usually relieved, and mobility is restored. This procedure is called *arthroplasty,* or joint replacement surgery, and it has revolutionized the treatment of hip and knee arthritis.

Hip and knee arthritis routinely sidelined people in the past (especially the elderly), but today replacing old worn-out joints with artificial parts can offer relief from excruciating pain, loss of mobility, and disability.

Surgery can help to stabilize a wobbly joint, realign a joint to improve function, and in some cases even make cosmetic improvements. Many people undergoing hip or knee replacements feel that they've gotten a new lease on life — suddenly they can walk, hike, cycle and just move around without pain! Hoping to get similar benefits, and encouraged by the surgery's high rate of success (joint replacement surgery is successful in 9 out of 10 cases), approximately 440,000 Americans undergo joint replacement surgery every year. The hip and knee are the most commonly replaced joints (200,000 and 300,000 per year, respectively), but ankles, shoulders, elbows, and knuckles are also done routinely and successfully.

A better idea may be to get the surgery earlier, instead of waiting. A study of 222 OA patients undergoing total hip or knee replacement surgery found that those who delayed their surgeries until joint function had severely declined and pain was severe had the worst surgical outcomes and were most likely to need assistance with bathing, dressing, and other daily tasks. (For the latest on joint replacement surgery techniques, see Chapter 23.)

With cement or without?

Over time, the cement used in hip replacements can crack and break into little pieces, causing the prosthesis to loosen. These wayward little pieces of cement can take fragments of bone with them as they fall away, weakening and degrading the overall bone structure. Some people opt for cementless hip replacements to avoid this problem. The ball-and-stem part of the cementless prosthesis has a rough, bumpy outer skin, like a horned toad, that causes bone to grow into the spaces between the bumps, securing the real bone to the artificial part.

Advantages of cementless replacements:

✔ This type of replacement may last longer, because you don't have any cement to crack and break away.

✔ Revision surgery can be easier.

Disadvantages of cementless replacements:

✔ Recovery can take a long time, with activity limited for as much as three months while bone "grows into" the replacement part.

✔ Soft or porous bones may not be able to bond tightly enough to the prosethesis to allow a successful cementless hip replacement.

✔ It's hard to get a perfect fit — 10 to 20 percent of patients experience pain in the thigh that is sometimes severe.

Those with the best outcomes are usually older, have arthritis-related pain, loss of movement, or stiffness that hasn't responded to other forms of treatment, and are otherwise in good health. In addition, they're highly motivated to help themselves and willing and able to participate in an exercise regimen once they've received their new joint.

TIP

You have a much better chance of enjoying a successful hip or knee replacement if you exercise, stay away from high-impact sports and activities, and maintain your ideal body weight.

Joint replacement surgery involves the use of artificial parts as well as some of the existing natural tissues. With the patient under anesthesia, the surgeon opens the joint and detaches the tendons and ligaments from the bone. He dislocates the joint, and cuts away the diseased or weakened parts of the bone. The surgeon uses plastic and/or metal prostheses to replace the missing parts of the joint and may cement them into place. He then fits the joint parts together, reattaches ligaments and tendons, and closes the incision. (See Figure 9-1 and the sidebar "Taking a look at the total hip replacement procedure" precedng this section.)

Figure 9-1:
The hip socket is replaced with a polyethylene cup, and the head of the femur is replaced with a metal ball.

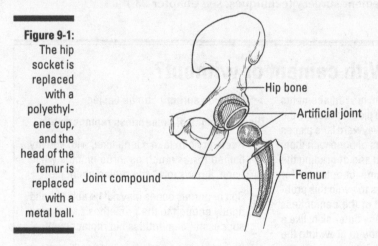

Hip bone

Artificial joint

Joint compound

Femur

MEDICAL SPEAK

Although we call it "joint replacement surgery," a more accurate description is "joint rebuilding surgery." The surgeon tries to maintain the integrity of your natural joint as much as possible. He may simply resurface certain areas and cut away diseased tissue. He may replace just part of the joint, for example the "socket" of the ball-and-socket joint in the hip, while leaving the "ball" intact. Or he may reconstruct the entire joint using artificial parts.

In the majority of cases, joint replacements provide pain relief, restored mobility, and improved joint stability. In the case of the weight-bearing joints, such as the hip or knee, this improved function can restore not only a patient's independence but also his or her overall outlook on life. Complications exist, however. Infection at the site of the surgery may require removal of the implant, the prosthesis can loosen, or the joint may dislocate. Replacements of weight-bearing joints can wear out — hips last only 10 to 15 years, but knees may last as long as 20 — and when joint replacements wear out, the surgery must be repeated. (A shoulder replacement, however, can last for life.) Other complications of joint replacement include blood clots (especially in the leg), damage to the nerves surrounding the replacement, and legs that are unequal in length.

Until recently, total joint replacement was thought of as a last resort, because replacement parts (implants) tended to wear out or loosen with the passage of time. Those who might benefit from this kind of surgery were asked to hold out as long as possible, because most implants had to be replaced within 10 to 20 years. So if you were 40, you didn't want to have joint replacement surgery unless you were absolutely desperate, because you'd probably have to have another surgery by the time you were 60, if not sooner!

But recent advances in the durability of implant materials (things like prepared polyethylene and metal or ceramic surfaces) have made it more likely that a joint replacement will last longer. That means that earlier total joint replacement surgery is now an option. Great news for baby boomers or young adults with arthritic knees and hips! And joint replacement surgery doesn't seem to have a cutoff age: A study released by the Mayo Clinic found that even those 90 years old and up can undergo safe and effective hip replacements.

If you're planning to have a knee replacement, you may think it's a good idea to replace both knees at once and save yourself some time and money. But studies show that those undergoing double knee replacements are more likely to suffer from serious complications (dislocation, inflammation, nerve damage, and so on) than those who take it one step (or one knee) at a time. Healing is also easier when you have one "good" leg to put your weight on, while allowing your newly-replaced knee to heal.

Although the risk of developing an infection in a joint replacement is relatively rare (1 in 100), it's a complication that can require more surgery and the removal of joint replacement parts. Any infection in your body can spread to your joint replacement, so be scrupulous about taking antibiotics as prescribed both before and after surgery. Also, during the months or even years after surgery (infection can occur years later) you should take antibiotics if you develop a skin or bladder infection, undergo a dental treatment that's more than just a simple procedure, or if you undergo another surgery. These are all high-risk times for bacteria to enter the bloodstream and travel to the site of your joint replacement, where they can settle in and cause an infection.

Autologous chondrocyte implantation: Transplanting cartilage

Osteoarthritis sufferers (especially those under 40 years old who have experienced trauma to the joint) benefit from this procedure.

For this procedure, the surgeon takes healthy cartilage cells from one part of the body and transplants them into a joint with damaged cartilage. These transplanted cells continue to grow, producing a new, healthier cartilage that eventually replaces the old.

When a joint suffers trauma, the *chondrocytes* (cartilage-producing cells) can change the way they act. They may make smaller amounts of certain cartilage components (*proteoglycans* and *collagen*), while churning out more of the enzymes that break down the cartilage. This decrease in the building up of cartilage, plus an increase in cartilage destruction, adds up to damaged, poor-quality tissue. But if the old chondrocytes can be replaced with new chondrocytes that work properly, production and maintenance of healthy cartilage may be restored.

The surgeon harvests healthy cartilage cells from another area in the body (not the damaged joint) and mixes them together with a special solution that includes some fluid taken from the patient. The cells are carefully cultured in a laboratory for a few weeks, where they grow and multiply. Then these cells are injected into the patient's damaged joint, where they take hold and begin to grow new cartilage. Because the cells and fluid come from the patient's own body, less chance of rejection exists.

The surgery helps relieve pain and restores mobility through a relatively non-invasive method.

The cost of the surgery is very high (as much as $40,000), and few insurance companies pay for the procedure. Because this is a new approach, no one knows how long the new cartilage will last.

Getting Ready for Surgery

If you decide to undergo surgery, you need to do a little planning for the event, starting by taking excellent care of your health. Your doctor should review the medications, vitamins, minerals, herbs, and other supplements that you're currently taking and tell you which ones to stop taking prior to surgery. (Certain drugs and supplements can thin the blood and increase the risk of bleeding.) You may also want to donate some of your own blood so that you can receive it during or after surgery, if necessary. Making careful plans for your postoperative care, figuring out the financial and insurance angles, and arranging for someone to handle your daily responsibilities ensures that you can relax while convalescing and lets you concentrate on getting well!

Getting yourself into the best possible physical shape

Prepare for your surgery as if you were an athlete training for a competition. Eat highly nutritious meals, exercise regularly (if you're up to it), get plenty of sleep, and stay away from alcohol or unnecessary drugs. Surgery is done carefully, utilizing every precaution, but it is still a major assault on the body. The better your health is going in, the better your body can withstand the trauma and the faster you recover.

Your doctor will undoubtedly give you several presurgical instructions. You may be asked to wash with a special soap or take a course of antibiotics. Most certainly, you need to avoid taking certain drugs that can thin the blood and increase bleeding time.

Arranging adequate postoperative care

You need someone to take you home from the hospital, someone who can take care of you for the next several days, and someone who can help around the house for at least a week or two, depending on the extent of your surgery. You may have an angel in your life who can play all three roles, or you may have to call on a variety of friends and family members. One thing is sure: You can't recover alone.

Finding someone who can handle your responsibilities

If you are undergoing major surgery on a weight-bearing joint, you may be at least partially out of commission for months. Driving, shopping, taking care of children, doing housework, or going to work may be impossible for quite some time. You must have a solid support system in place. The last thing you need is to be forced into doing things that are beyond your capabilities.

Resolving financial and insurance matters

Before your surgery, find out exactly what your insurance company covers and how much of the tab you have to pick up. The stress of unexpected medical expenses is extremely disruptive mentally and emotionally and can be a major hindrance to your recovery.

Making a recovery plan with your doctor

Although no one can predict exactly when you'll pass certain milestones on the road to recovery, it may ease your mind and give you something to look forward to if you have a list of the progressive steps of healing. Ask your doctor to help you construct a recovery plan that maps out these steps. Studies show that people recover better and faster if they have a good idea of what to expect both during and after surgery.

Your recovery begins while you're still in the hospital, where you'll undergo physical therapy beginning the day after surgery. If you're doing well after four to five days, you'll go home. But if you need more help, you may go to a rehabilitation center for a short time to get more in-depth therapy.

After you're home, your doctor will set up an at-home therapy program for the first four to six weeks, during which time you'll be visited by a physical therapist. Often your physical therapist will visit you only a few times and then set up a home exercise program for you to do on your own. (This will depend upon your insurance program.)

After about six weeks, if all is going well, you'll begin an outpatient therapy program. The success of your joint replacement will depend heavily on your doing the required exercises and following the treatment plan. It's a lot of work, but your health is worth it.

Chapter 10

Overcoming the Ouch: Strategies for Pain Management

. . . .

In This Chapter

▶ Understanding the causes of arthritis pain

▶ Knowing the difference between acute and chronic pain

▶ Breaking the pain cycle

▶ Exploring noninvasive ways to control pain

. . . .

It's hard to be happy when you hurt. Pain has a way of enveloping your mind, hijacking your brain, and making it difficult to concentrate on work, family, hobbies, or anything else. You desperately want to be fully involved in life, but the pain distracts, worries, irritates, and depresses you to the point where you can think of little else. The things that you used to do with ease can suddenly become difficult or even impossible to accomplish. Living with long-standing chronic pain can wear you down, exhaust you, depress you, and make you feel that life isn't worth living. Fortunately, plenty of strategies (both physical and mental) can help you cope with pain. So even if your pain isn't completely banished, you can release its stranglehold on your life.

In this chapter, we focus on physical strategies for managing the pain. (See Chapter 14 for mental pain-management strategies.)

Understanding Arthritis Pain

Arthritis pain comes in many forms: stabbing, aching, twisting, burning, pressing, stretching, and crushing. Some people describe it as "killing," "a fire," "a knife that someone keeps jabbing into me," "a bowling ball knocking the pins down over and over," "a continual car wreck," and "something I wouldn't even wish on my worst enemy."

Several things can cause the pain of arthritis. For example, it may result from something about the disease process itself:

- ✔ **Inflammation:** Swollen, hot, inflamed joint tissues
- ✔ **Joint damage:** Bones grinding against each other, tendons that have slipped, joint misalignment or loosening, invasion of the bone by the synovium (joint lining), and so on

Your arthritis pain may also be related to your body's response to the disease:

- ✔ **Muscle tension:** Tensing up as a reaction to your pain can spread pain to the muscles and make everything feel worse.
- ✔ **Strained muscles and supporting tissues:** When overcompensating for an injured area, you can unintentionally put excessive stress on a different area.
- ✔ **Fatigue:** Feeling dragged out due to illness can make your pain even more intense and difficult to cope with.

Of course, when you're hurting, it doesn't matter much whether your pain is caused by or related to the arthritis. You just want it to stop! But for many people, the pain just seems to go on and on — and on.

Differentiating Between Acute Pain and Chronic Pain

The kind of pain you feel when you touch a hot stove, called *acute pain,* is absolutely vital to your well-being. Acute pain is a warning that you've injured yourself and need to do something about it — now! Acute pain is episodic, meaning that it comes on quickly, builds rapidly to a crescendo, then tapers off and disappears. Suppose, for example, that you fall down and skin your knee: It really hurts! But, by the time you wash, disinfect, and bandage the area, your pain is already receding and soon disappears entirely. The acute pain has served its purpose — it got you to remove the source of the pain and attend to the damage that it caused. Although acute pain can be excruciating, at least it has a purpose and an end.

Chronic pain, however, is another story. Like a barrage of telegrams repeating the same message over and over, chronic pain is not a useful warning, but an agonizing, debilitating tirade. More resistant to medical treatment than acute pain, chronic pain can become the constantly tormenting drumbeat underlying your every activity, day and night. Bam! Bam! Bam! It won't let up. You may not be surprised to hear that the number one cause of chronic pain is arthritis.

Breaking the pain cycle

Many arthritis sufferers become extremely frustrated and depressed by pain and the decline in their physical abilities. Unfortunately, stress and depression can, and do, make pain worse. The physical pain from arthritis causes stress and upset about the lost physical abilities. This stress, in turn, can trigger muscle tension that worsens the pain and further limits physical activities, causing even more stress and depression; thus, the cycle continues.

Happily, you can do many great things to break the pain cycle and live more comfortably, even if your pain is chronic. The key is to block the pain signals moving through your nerves and spinal cord so they can't register in your brain. The medicines discussed in Chapter 8 can eliminate a little or a lot of your hurting.

With medication and the pain management methods that we describe in this chapter and the next, you should be able to block many of these signals and manage your arthritis pain. The key word here is *manage*. Managing chronic pain means reducing its severity and decreasing it to the point where you can get on with your life, not eradicating it completely.

Dealing with chronic pain

You usually don't have to worry much about dealing with acute pain. It certainly hurts, but it often responds well to medicine and doesn't wear out its welcome. Getting rid of acute pain is typically your doctor's job. Dealing with chronic pain, however, is a different matter.

The goal in chronic pain management is to block pain messages before they reach the brain. You can try several natural things, apart from using drugs:

- Exercise that's appropriate to your condition
- Hot or cold treatments
- Water therapy
- Massage
- Magnets
- Topical pain relievers
- Relaxation
- TENS (transcutaneous electrical nerve stimulation)

On the other hand, several "natural" things can make your pain even worse, all of which we discuss in Chapter 14:

- ✔ Anxiety
- ✔ Depression
- ✔ Fatigue
- ✔ Focusing on your pain
- ✔ Physical overexertion
- ✔ Progression of the disease
- ✔ Stress

Assembling your treatment team

Chronic pain is a complex phenomenon that involves the original or ongoing disease process, the way your body deals with the problem mechanically, and your mental and emotional responses. A team of professionals, each with her own expertise, best handles this multifaceted problem. Your treatment team may include the following people:

- ✔ **Your doctor** guides your treatment and prescribes medication, if necessary.
- ✔ **A physical therapist** helps you build strength and restore range of motion. (See the sidebar "What does a physical therapist do?" later in this chapter.)
- ✔ **An occupational therapist** teaches you how to place less strain on your joints when performing daily activities, overcome limitations, and prevent further damage.
- ✔ **An exercise physiologist** helps you devise an exercise program that increases strength, flexibility, and endurance without putting undue strain on your joints. (This is also a function of the physical therapist, whose services may be paid for by insurance.)
- ✔ **A psychologist, psychiatrist, or other mental health professional** helps you cope with depression, anger, and/or other emotional issues.
- ✔ **A pharmacist** offers advice on the proper use of medication.
- ✔ **A social worker** recommends support groups or other special services.

You can also visit pain management clinics that have such teams already assembled for you. Although some of these clinics specialize in treating specific types of pain, others treat all types. (Insurance coverage varies according to plan, and you may need a referral from your doctor.) For a pain clinic in your area, contact one of the organizations listed under "Pain management" in Appendix B of this book.

MEDICAL SPEAK

Controlling pain the natural way

Your body makes certain substances that can decrease or even block pain sensations, as well as others that can increase your pain. The pain blockers include *endorphins* and *enkephalins,* substances that can slow or stop nerve cells from firing and sending pain messages to the brain. These chemicals are so powerful that their effects are often compared to those of morphine. Naturally, you want to produce more endorphins and enkephalins when you're in pain. You also want to have plenty of the brain hormone serotonin and other substances that play a role in manufacturing and releasing these internal painkillers.

Natural irritants — substances that increase the neurons' sensitivity to pain — are the flip side of

the body's natural pain blockers. These irritants include *lactic acid, potassium ions, substance P,* and the stress hormones *noradrenaline* and *norepinephrine.* Most of the pain-control process revolves around increasing the production of the pain blockers while decreasing the production of the pain intensifiers. For example, massage can increase the production of endorphins while helping the body dispense with excessive amounts of lactic acid. Meditation, deep breathing, and a good belly laugh also can do much to increase endorphin levels, and transcutaneous electrical nerve stimulation (TENS – which is described later in this chapter) can decrease substance P.

Relieving Pain with Noninvasive Therapies

Remember getting sick when you were a child? Your mother probably had a whole bag of tricks that could make you feel better: a cool cloth on your forehead, a warm bath, letting you lie in her bed to watch television, chamomile tea, and so on. Her methods were just simple little things, but they really *did* make you feel better.

Mom's methods were *noninvasive,* which means they didn't intrude on or cause harm to the body. Noninvasive methods may be physical or psychological, and they are the least traumatic approaches to pain management.

We discuss several noninvasive physical treatments in this section. Other techniques include psychotherapy, self-hypnosis, deep breathing, progressive relaxation, creative imagery, and biofeedback. (See Chapter 14 for more on these mental strategies for pain relief.)

At best, noninvasive approaches to pain management are very helpful; at worst, they're probably harmless. With no side effects, incisions, blood loss, addiction potential, or other hazards, these techniques should be thoroughly explored by you and your doctor before you move on to the harsher, more dangerous methods of pain relief.

You may be surprised at how much relief you can get from your arthritis pain by adopting the following simple physical strategies. Although these techniques don't *cure* your arthritis (the relief is temporary), any respite from the pain is welcome! So, next time your arthritis pain flares, try some of the following methods.

Applying heat

Warmth encourages the blood vessels to expand, bringing more blood to the painful area and stimulating the healing process. It also helps your muscles relax, which may be just what you need if the pain you experience makes you tighten up. You can use hot packs, heating pads, heat lamps with infrared bulbs, electric blankets, or hot paraffin wax treatments to rev up your circulation, encourage overall relaxation, and make you feel better.

Another way to apply heat is to wrap yourself in a flannel sheet or a throw blanket that you've just popped into the clothes dryer for a few minutes. Although the heat won't last long, it's very cozy!

Ultrasound is a more high-tech way of accomplishing the same thing, and it can penetrate more deeply into the muscles and joints. High-frequency sound waves are aimed at the affected area, producing deep tissue heat, which increases circulation and promotes muscle relaxation. Ultrasound is typically performed in your doctor's office or at a rehab center, although your physical therapist can bring along a portable machine for at-home visits. Ultrasound machines also are available for sale on the Internet, but they're pretty expensive.

Be careful not to damage your skin when applying heat. Follow these rules to protect yourself:

- ✔ Limit heat applications to no longer than 30 minutes in one area.

- ✔ Wrap the hot pack or heating pad in towels to insulate it; don't place the source of heat directly on your skin.

- ✔ To avoid steam burns or skin reactions, make sure that your skin is dry and that you haven't applied lotion or cream to it (particularly deep-heating creams).

- ✔ Inspect the area every five minutes for purplish-red skin, hives, or blisters, which are signs of skin damage.

- ✔ Allow your skin temperature to return to normal before reapplying heat.

Heat may make some conditions worse. Check with your doctor in advance to see if heat treatments are appropriate for you.

Applying cold

Cold packs are used to reduce inflammation, ease muscle spasms, and block pain signals by numbing the affected area. Although blood flow to the chilled area is temporarily reduced, cold applications eventually *increase* circulation, acting much like hot packs (perhaps because the body senses the need to warm up the area). Ice is the usual medium used to numb painful areas, but you may find it more convenient to use cold packs containing chemical mixtures that thaw slowly and don't drip.

A bag of frozen peas makes a good cold pack, because you can mold it around any shape, unlike a block of ice or bulky cubes. But make sure that you put the bag inside an airtight plastic bag and wrap it in a towel, because it does drip.

Protect your skin and other tissues when using cold packs by following these steps:

- ✔ Limit treatment to no longer than 20 minutes.
- ✔ Remove the cold pack after the area is numb.
- ✔ Be on the lookout for skin damage — redness, white patches, and so on.
- ✔ Avoid cold packs if you have Raynaud's, poor circulation, sensitivity to cold, nerve damage, a lack of sensation, or heart problems.

In general, if inflammation is present, use cold; if not, use hot, although many doctors recommend that you use whatever feels good to you. The best advice is to consult your doctor before using either method.

Hot paraffin wax treatments

Hot paraffin wax treatments are a nice, comfortable way to warm up painful joints in your hands and feet. These treatments sustain their warmth because they use wax as insulation. A physical therapist usually applies hot paraffin wax treatments, but you can also do it yourself at home.

How do hot paraffin wax treatments work? Your painful hand or foot is repeatedly dipped into a blend of melted wax and mineral oil and allowed to cool in between immersions so that the wax can harden. When the build-up is thick enough,

your hand/foot is wrapped in plastic and covered with towels to preserve the heat. The locked-in warmth can be very soothing to your stiff, painful fingers or toes. After 20 minutes or so, the wrapping comes off, and the wax is peeled away.

As if pain relief weren't enough, hot paraffin wax treatments leave your skin wonderfully soft!

Don't use this treatment if your hand or foot shows any signs of skin damage (excessive redness, blisters, and so on).

Washing away pain with water therapy

Ah, what feels better than easing your stiff, sore body into a nice warm bath? The ancient Romans evidently agreed, building several health resorts throughout their wide-ranging empire for the express purpose of bathing. Most notable was their bath in the town of Bath, England, where people with arthritis came from far and wide to "take the waters."

Warm showers, baths, and whirlpools can help ease your stiffness and make you feel better. Warm-water therapy is also a good way to warm up your muscles before an exercise session, relaxing them and making movement easier.

Cool water can also help, especially when inflammation is present. Immersing a painful, swollen joint in cool water or using cool compresses is a milder, less jolting version of applying an ice pack.

Pool exercises are another extremely effective form of water therapy. Because water supports your body, exercising in a pool is like exercising in a weightless environment. With the tiresome pull of gravity greatly reduced in water, your joints can rest, even as your muscles are put through a real workout. Because water provides resistance, your muscles have to work harder to perform a movement in water than they do on land. This combination adds up to more effective exercise, with less wear and tear on your joints. (See Chapter 12 for more on water exercise.)

Whether warm or cool, water can be used in a variety of ways to help ease your pain:

✔ Cool hand or foot baths

✔ Cool moist compresses

✔ Drinking warm tea

✔ Warm full-body baths

✔ Warm hand or foot baths

✔ Warm, moist compresses

✔ Warm showers

✔ Whirlpool baths

Trying topical pain relievers

Many topical creams, lotions, rubs, and sprays can help with chronic arthritis pain. They typically contain one or more of the following ingredients:

- **Capsaicin** is a substance derived from chili peppers that decreases the nerves' concentration of substance P in the painful area, thus reducing pain. See the sidebar "Controlling pain the natural way" for more on substance P.

- **Irritants** include menthol, camphor, and other substances that produce feelings of heat, cold, or itching. These distract you from the sensation of pain.

- **Salicylates** are aspirin-like compounds that desensitize nerve endings.

Topical pain relievers are usually safe and at least somewhat effective. If you decide to use them, make sure you don't apply them to broken skin, and watch for signs of skin irritation.

Manipulating the joints

Joint manipulation is also known as *passive movement,* because something other than your own energy is moving your joints for you. That "something" is usually a physical therapist. During joint manipulation, the physical therapist uses his hands to move your joints through their range of motion. Then, by applying pressure (stretching) or simply moving the joint back and forth or around and around (depending upon the joint type), the therapist can help loosen up your joints. Joint manipulation must be done carefully, however, and never overdone. Otherwise, your joints can become even more irritated and painful.

If you don't move your joints, you may lose the ability to do so. In most cases some joint movement is *absolutely necessary.* People with arthritis have a tendency to guard their stiff, sore joints by moving them as little as possible. Unfortunately, this can be the worst thing for them. When the joints are held still, they aren't being lubricated or nourished, their supporting muscles become weaker, circulation decreases, and ligaments and tendons tighten up, losing their resilience. Over time, an immobile joint can actually become frozen into position. That's why you must keep moving your joints, whether they hurt or not. Even splinted joints should be moved, at least a little, every day.

Helping the joints with splints and supports

Splints are designed to support and immobilize an injured or inflamed joint. A molded piece of metal or plastic is strapped to the affected area and then wrapped with elastic bandages. You can find splints for the wrists, fingers, hands, ankles, knees, back, and neck. Splints are widely available in off-the-rack varieties or can be custom-made by taking an impression of your joint and then molding heat-sensitive material to replicate the shape. Splints help by doing the following:

- ✔ Providing support, stability, protection, and rest for injured or inflamed joints

- ✔ Immobilizing a joint after surgical fusion (arthrodesis) and allowing healing

- ✔ Easing pain during arthritis flares, although they're only temporary measures

- ✔ Keeping inflammation under control

- ✔ Correcting or preventing deformities (in certain cases) by correctly positioning the joint

Supports (sometimes called *braces*) are strong, elasticized wraps designed to fit certain body parts (your wrist, knee, ankle, and so on). Their tight fit lends stability to the joint, and their elasticity allows movement and blood circulation.

Supports are used two ways: to support and stabilize an injured joint or to protect a weakened joint from becoming injured in the first place. You should use supports in conjunction with a good exercise program, so the muscles and supporting structures themselves become strengthened and don't rely solely on the wrap to do the trick.

Magnetizing the pain

Magnets seem to be everywhere these days. You can buy them at the local pharmacy, at medical-supply stores, via mail-order houses, and even at the grocery store! Magnets used for pain relief are generally embedded within a belt or wrap designed to fit a specific body part (your neck, knee, ankle, wrist, and so on). You can also purchase them in sets that you can tape wherever the pain settles.

The magnets used for pain relief are much like the horseshoe-shaped toy you used to play with as a child, except they're small, flat discs. Just like your old toy, they exert a pull — a magnetic field that can attract or repel certain elements in the environment. A few researchers propose that this magnetic field can produce a calming effect on the body and help normalize bodily function. More important, the magnetic field helps block pain signals to the brain, causing a release of endorphins (the body's natural morphine). Finally, like many of the other pain-relieving techniques that we discuss in this chapter, magnets may help increase blood flow to the painful area.

Therapeutic magnets are measured in the hundreds or thousands of gauss. (By way of comparison, the earth's natural magnetic field is approximately .05 gauss, and refrigerator magnets weigh in with about 60 gauss.) The actual amount of gauss delivered to the skin is much less than the amount listed on the magnet's packaging, however. For example, a 6,000-gauss magnet may transmit only 1,800 gauss to the skin. And, the more wrapping or distance between the magnet and the skin, the weaker the magnetic effect. If possible, find a physical therapist or other health professional well-versed in magnetic therapy to advise you.

The beneficial effects of magnets are still largely unproven, so mainstream medicine has yet to fully embrace their use as a valid therapy. Still, they appear to be safe for most people, and some have found that they help to relieve pain. If you'd like to try magnetic therapy, consult with your doctor first. If you're pregnant or have a pacemaker or other electronic implant, you may not be a candidate for this treatment.

Transmitting a tingle with TENS

Transcutaneous electrical nerve stimulation (TENS) is a mild electrical buzz that overrides pain signals in tender areas. The process may sound scary, but it really isn't, and it's easy to apply. Electrodes are affixed to your skin with a small amount of gel, and then a very mild shock (from a battery-powered unit connected to the electrodes) is transmitted to the pained area. As a result of these shocks, the production of endorphins is supposed to increase. The physiologic basis for TENS is the Gate Theory of Pain (discussed in Chapter 14). TENS helps to "close the gates," thus inhibiting pain impulses.

TENS is usually used to treat back and spine problems that don't respond to other treatments. It offers welcome temporary relief for many people, but isn't a cure.

You can purchase your own TENS unit and give yourself treatments at home, but only with a doctor's prescription. (If you decide to do your own treatments, knowing how to operate the TENS unit properly is important. Some people don't benefit from TENS simply because they use the equipment incorrectly.) Because the units are very expensive, you want to try TENS at your doctor's office several times before purchasing your own unit. Consider renting one before committing yourself to a purchase.

What does a physical therapist do?

Described as a combination of buddy, drill sergeant, cheerleader, and workout partner, the physical therapist works with you to help increase your range of motion, reduce your pain, build strength, and decrease disability.

"The hardest part is getting the patients to do exercises that remind them that they can't move like they used to," Kari, a physical therapist in San Diego, California, told us. "That seems to make them angrier and more depressed than feeling the pain does. But my job is to keep pushing, because that's the only way anybody gets better."

A physical therapist takes you through a series of exercises designed to get your joints lubed and stretch your range of movement. Joint manipulation and massage are also important parts of the physical therapy session. Perhaps most importantly, the physical therapist helps you stamp out procrastination and get to work!

Part II: Tests and Treatments: What to Expect from Your Doctor

Don't use TENS if you have a pacemaker or are pregnant. Also, don't use it on open wounds or sensitive parts of the body, such as the eyes.

Taking Pain Relief to the Next Level

When noninvasive techniques don't work and your pain is interfering with your ability to live a comfortable and productive life, it may be time to look into medications or, in more serious cases, surgery.

Medicating the pain away

From mild aspirin to powerful DMARDS (see Chapter 8), medicines can be beneficial but risky. The most commonly prescribed painkillers for most forms of arthritis are NSAIDs (non-steroidal anti-inflammatory drugs, like aspirin or ibuprofen) and analgesics (drugs that reduce pain without reducing consciousness, like acetaminophen).

If a joint is particularly painful and not responding to painkillers, the doctor may recommend injecting substances like corticosteroids (high-powered anti-inflammatory agents) right into the afflicted area. DMARDs (disease modifying antirheumatic drugs, like methotrexate) alter the way the immune system works and are reserved for serious forms of arthritis — rheumatoid arthritis, psoriatic arthritis and ankylosing spondylitis. And BRMs (biological response modifiers, like etanercept and infliximab) also target the immune system, and are used for those with aggressive, debilitating arthritis who have not been helped by one or more of the DMARDS.

All medications, from aspirin to joint injections have side effects. Although they can be helpful initially, their long-term use can cause problems ranging from stomach upsets to drug dependence. And, over time, their effectiveness can wane. So it's important to take medication exactly as prescribed and to see your doctor regularly to monitor its effects on your body.

Undergoing surgery

Surgery, which involves making incisions and manipulating the inner workings of the body, is always a risky and traumatic procedure.

Undergoing surgery to relieve pain can produce dramatic results in some cases, but it always carries serious risks and side effects, ranging from infection to death. Consider surgery only as a last resort. (See Chapter 9 for a complete discussion of the surgeries for arthritis.)

Part III
The Arthritis Lifestyle Strategy

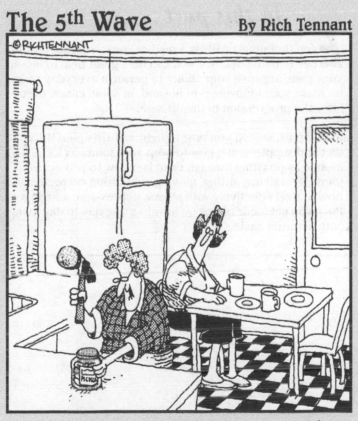

The 5th Wave   By Rich Tennant

©RICHTENNANT

"I've learned a few tricks for dealing with my
arthritis. One is to invest in a good
jar opener."

In this part . . .

*E*ven though arthritis is a medical problem that continues to baffle doctors, you can do a great deal to lessen your pain, improve your ability to perform everyday tasks, increase your enjoyment of life and, in some cases, even slow the progression of the disease.

In this part, we tell you how to fight arthritis pain through diet and supplements; how to keep your joints as loose and mobile as possible through exercise; how to protect your joints by walking, sitting, moving, and lifting correctly; and how to deal effectively with stress, depression, and anger. Plus, you get loads of tips on how to make day-to-day living with arthritis easier.

Chapter 11

Fighting the Pain with Foods and Supplements

The idea that food can cause or relieve arthritis isn't new. More than two hundred years ago, English doctors prescribed cod-liver oil to treat gout and rheumatism. More recently, some health writers have insisted that arthritics should eat or not eat specific foods. The debate is in full swing. Do certain foods cause arthritis? Is there an "Arthritis Begone" diet? All the evidence isn't yet in, but thanks to the studies currently available, more and more physicians are convinced that diet plays a valuable role in arthritis treatment plans.

And what about supplements? Can they eliminate arthritis pain, unlock "frozen" joints, or prevent the immune system errors that lead to rheumatoid arthritis (RA)? Researchers have not yet come up with definitive answers, but more and more scientific evidence suggests that supplements can be helpful aids in the battle against arthritis. So get ready to discover more about some of the foods, "food parts," and supplements that can help — and a few that might best be avoided.

Reviewing in detail all of the supplements that people take for various forms of arthritis is beyond the scope of this book, but this brief account will give you enough information to start a discussion with your doctor.

Discuss *everything* you plan to take with your physician. There are subtle and sometimes hidden reactions caused by the combination of body chemistry, supplements, medications, and disease processes that may make your condition worse.

Finding Foods That Heal

Way back in the 1920s, researchers looked into treating osteoarthritis (OA) with the mineral sulfur. In 1963, a letter to the editor in the prestigious medical journal called *Lancet* described the use of a B vitamin called pantothenic acid in treating osteoarthritis. The idea that foods and the vitamins, minerals, and other substances they contain can aid in the battle against arthritis isn't new. What is new is that researchers are finding out why certain foods can be helpful — exactly *why* an apple a day may keep the doctor away.

Which fruits, vegetables, meat, or fish should you eat? There are no absolute rules, but the results of studies and case histories suggest that these foods may be helpful:

- **Anchovies:** Three-and-a-half ounces of anchovies contain almost a gram and a half of omega-3 fatty acids. The omega-3 fatty acids help regulate the prostaglandins, which play a role in inflammation and, hence, pain. Anchovies are extremely high in sodium, however, so if sodium-sensitivity or water retention is a problem for you, choose a different kind of fish. Because anchovies also are high in purines (nitrogen-containing compounds), you should probably avoid them if you have gout.

- **Apples:** Not only can an apple a day keep the doctor away, but it may also help to hold your arthritis at bay. Apples contain boron, a mineral that appears to reduce the risk of developing osteoarthritis. And when boron is given to people who have osteoarthritis, it helps relieve pain.

- **Broccoli:** This popular vegetable contains a powerful antioxidant and detoxifying agent called glutathione. New studies indicate that people with low amounts of glutathione are more likely to have arthritis. Other foods rich in glutathione include avocados, cabbage, cauliflower, grapefruit, oranges, potatoes, and tomatoes.

- **Cantaloupe:** This sweet fruit contains large amounts of vitamin C and *beta-carotene,* the plant form of vitamin A. These two powerful vitamins help to control the oxidative and free radical damage that may contribute to arthritis. (For more on oxidative and free radical damage, see "Saving Your Joints with Supplements" in this chapter.)

- **Curry:** A combination of spices that often includes turmeric, garlic, cumin, cinnamon, and so on, curry contains powerful antioxidants that may help relieve inflammation and reduce pain.

✔ **Fish:** The omega-3 fatty acids in Norwegian sardines, Atlantic mackerel, sablefish, rainbow trout, striped bass, and other fish may help reduce inflammation and pain. (See "Using omega-3s and omega-6s to fight arthritis pain and inflammation" in this chapter.)

✔ **Garlic:** An ancient treatment for tuberculosis, lung problems, and other diseases, garlic also appears to relieve some forms of arthritis pain. Although never tested in large-scale, double-blind studies, garlic has been found helpful in many case reports. These helpful benefits may be due to the fact that garlic contains sulfur, which has been known for many years to help relieve certain arthritis symptoms.

✔ **Grapefruit and other citrus fruits:** The skin, peel, and outer layers of citrus fruits are rich sources of bioflavonoids like quercetin, hesperidin, and rutin. Among other things, bioflavonoids help increase capillary strength and permeability, fight inflammation, inhibit viruses, and strengthen the collagen that's so important to joint health.

✔ **Grapes:** This sweet, bite-sized fruit is a good source of the mineral boron, which is important for strong bones. The skin of the grape also contains resveratrol, a compound that can block the inflammation that causes arthritis pain.

✔ **Mango:** A sweet treat, mangoes are packed with three powerful antioxidants. One medium mango provides 90 percent of vitamin C, 100 percent of beta-carotene, and about 25 percent of vitamin E that you need in an entire day.

✔ **Nuts:** Almonds, peanuts, and hazelnuts are good sources of boron, a mineral that helps keep bones strong, and certain arthritis symptoms at bay.

✔ **Oysters:** Oysters are an excellent source of zinc: Six medium-sized oysters offer just about 125 milligrams of the mineral, which is well over the RDA. RA patients often have low blood levels of zinc, and depleted zinc supplies have been associated with the joint pain and stiffness of arthritis, in general.

Stay away from raw oysters, which are notorious for their high bacteria levels and are especially unhealthy for those who have compromised immune systems or liver disease. Either eat them well-cooked, or not at all.

✔ **Papaya:** Long used as a folk medicine for diarrhea, hay fever, and other problems, a single papaya contains three times the RDA for the antioxidant vitamin C, plus more than half the daily allotment of beta-carotene.

✔ **Spinach and other leafy greens:** Unfortunately, eating spinach won't dispatch arthritis as quickly as Popeye does Brutus, but the vitamin E found in this vegetable can help reduce the pain of RA, inhibit the prostaglandins that help "stir up" inflammation, ease certain symptoms of fibromyalgia, and improve or stabilize lupus lesions.

✔ **Water:** Drinking eight glasses of water per day can help prevent kidney stones in some people who have gout. Eight glasses is also the amount most health experts recommend to keep your body well-hydrated and healthy.

✔ **Whole grains:** Whole grains such as wheat, rye, and barley are good sources of the B vitamins, which can be helpful in relieving some of the symptoms of arthritis. For example, vitamin B12 has reportedly helped reduce the pain of both chronic and acute bursitis. Niacin can help improve joint mobility in osteoarthritis patients and may help lessen the skin lesions seen in lupus. Vitamin B6 reduced pain and improved performance in a study of patients with carpal tunnel syndrome. Because whole grains are an excellent source of B vitamins, eating plenty of servings on a daily basis may help you battle arthritis.

Managing RA Mediterranean-style

Fat is considered a boogeyman. It causes heart disease, and it contributes to obesity, cancer, and a host of other ills. You're told to cut the fat off of your meat and out of your diet. But at least one diet that is high in fat, the Mediterranean diet, is actually good for you — and may help ease rheumatoid arthritis (RA).

The Mediterranean diet was first studied over 50 years ago, when researchers noticed that the people living on the Greek island of Crete had low rates of heart disease and certain types of cancer, plus a long life expectancy, even though they ate plenty of fat. Countless studies since that time found the same results in other areas of the Mediterranean region — Greece itself, Italy, southern France, and parts of Spain, Portugal, North Africa, and the Middle East. What are these people doing that the rest of us aren't? Part of the answer has to do with the kind of fat they eat.

Olive oil, which has long been linked to heart health, is the main fat used in the Mediterranean diet, replacing other oils, butter, and margarine. Olive oil can actually help lower harmful LDL cholesterol, and it contains antioxidants that discourage artery clogging and chronic diseases, including cancer. But it's only one part of this super-healthy style of eating. The bulk of the Mediterranean diet is made up of plenty of plant foods (vegetables, fruits, whole-grain breads, pasta and cereal, nuts, and legumes), eaten as fresh and as close to their natural state as possible. Cheese and yogurt are eaten every day, and small-to-moderate amounts of fish, poultry, and eggs are eaten a few times a week. Red meat is included just a few times a month, while a glass or two of red wine (it's loaded with antioxidants!) is taken just about every day, with meals. Sweets are limited, and fresh fruit is a favorite dessert. (See Figure 11-1 for the Mediterranean diet food pyramid.)

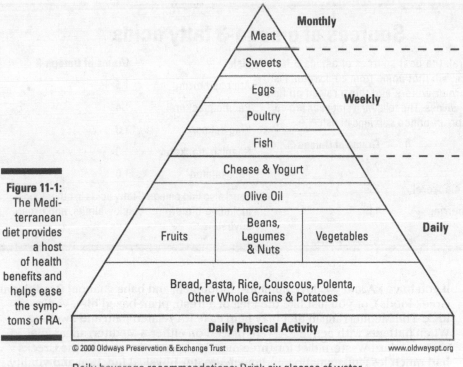

Figure 11-1:
The Medi-
terranean
diet provides
a host
of health
benefits and
helps ease
the symp-
toms of RA.

Daily beverage recommendations: Drink six glasses of water.
If you drink wine, do so in moderation.

What does "omega" mean?

A fatty acid is built around a line of carbon atoms. There may be a few, 6, 10, 12, or more carbons lined up, one behind the other, like a line of school children. Each of the carbons has a "left hand" and a "right hand," and can "hold" one hydrogen atom in each hand, off to either side. If each of the carbons in the line is holding two hydrogens, one in each hand, the fatty acid is saturated. Like a sponge that's full of water (saturated), the fatty acid can't possibly hold any more.

Often times, however, some of the carbons in the line "let go" of one of their hydrogens. Now

they're each holding only one. When that happens, the fatty acid is either unsaturated or poly-unsaturated (depending on how many carbons have let go of a hydrogen).

If the first carbon holding only one hydrogen happens to be the third in line, the fatty acid is called an omega-3 fatty acid. If the first carbon holding only a single hydrogen is sixth in line, it's called an omega-6 fatty acid, and so on. They're called "omega" this or "omega" that because the counting starts at the side of the fatty acid called the omega side.

Sources of omega-3 fatty acids

In general, the best sources of omega-3 fatty acids are fish that come from cold water. Fish from warmer waters and those raised on fish farms have less. The following statistics are calculated on 3½-ounce servings of fish.

Fish	Grams of Omega-3
Roe	2.3
Atlantic mackerel	2.3
Pacific herring	1.6

Fish	Grams of Omega-3
Atlantic herring	1.5
Pacific mackerel	1.4
King salmon	1.3
Spanish mackerel	1.3
Pink salmon	1.0

You'll also find omega-3 fatty acids in other foods, including butternuts, black walnuts, and green soybeans.

If you have RA and you love hummus, tabbouleh, and baba ghanouj (traditional Greek foods), or you just like the idea of a fresh, plant-based diet, you're in luck: The Mediterranean diet may help ease RA-related pain and swelling. When patients with active RA were placed on either a Mediterranean diet or a standard Western diet for three months, those who ate like the Greeks had much less inflammation and much greater physical function and vitality. Researchers concluded that the Mediterranean diet seemed to suppress the activity of RA, at least for the short term.

Using omega-3s and omega-6s to fight arthritis pain and inflammation

Two other kinds of fat, the omega-3 and the omega-6 fatty acids, can also help fight arthritis. Omega-3s can be converted to natural anti-inflammatory substances called *prostaglandins* that help decrease the inflammation and pain that plague so many arthritis sufferers. And a certain type of omega-6 fatty acid (gamma linoleic acid, or GLA) can help lessen pain by calling off the disease-related invasion of white blood cells that trigger the joint swelling and tenderness seen in rheumatoid arthritis.

Omega-3 fatty acids

Studies have shown that the omega-3 fatty acids, which are found primarily in certain fish, can help reduce the pain of osteoarthritis, as well as the joint stiffness and tenderness seen in rheumatoid arthritis. The omega-3 fatty acids are believed to help fight arthritis by "dampening" the inflammation response, thus reducing joint pain and tenderness. In one study, women with rheumatoid arthritis were compared to women of the same age who did not have the disease. The researchers found that women who ate more than one serving of grilled or baked fish (other than tuna) per week had less risk of developing rheumatoid arthritis than those who did not. Another study found that those who already had RA could ease pain and inflammation and reduce their use of NSAIDs (pain relievers such as aspirin and ibuprofen) just by eating a diet rich in antioxidants and omega-3s.

Don't deep-fry your fish. Doing so destroys the omega-3s.

The Arthritis Foundation agrees that omega-3s can help in the battle against arthritis, especially rheumatoid arthritis, and to some extent Raynaud's syndrome and lupus. Good fish sources of omega-3 fatty acids include mackerel (Atlantic, Pacific, and Spanish), herring (Atlantic and Pacific), salmon (king, Chinook, and pink), and roe. Check out the sidebar "Sources of omega-3 fatty acids" for more. In general, the best sources of omega-3 fatty acids are fish that come from cold water. Fish from warmer waters and those raised on fish farms have smaller amounts. Some nonfish foods also contain omega-3 fatty acids, such as green soybeans, black walnuts, and flaxseed oil.

Omega-3 fatty acids have some long, complicated names such as *alpha-linoleic acid, DHA (docosahexaenoic acid),* and *EPA (eicosapentaenoic acid).* But they're often referred to as omega-3s or *fish oil* (because that's where you typically find them in their most concentrated form), for short.

You can also get omega-3s through supplements. If you use a supplement, make sure that it clearly lists the amount of DHA and EPA per capsule. There is no RDA for fish oil: Some authorities suggest taking 3 grams of DHA and/or EPA per day.

Take supplements only after discussing them with your physician. And make sure your doctor always knows what supplements you're taking, for they may interfere with certain aspects of treatment.

Taking fish oil thins the blood, which can be dangerous if pushed too far. Overly thin blood may not clot properly, causing bleeding to increase to dangerous levels. Consult a physician before taking fish oil supplements if you take blood-thinning medication, NSAIDs, supplements that contain ginger, or anything else that thins the blood.

The good omega-6 fatty acid — GLA

Although most of the omega-6s are best avoided (see the section "Avoiding Foods That May Be Trouble," later in the chapter), one of them gives hope to arthritis patients: gamma-linoleic acid, or GLA for short. Your body converts GLA from another omega-6 fatty acid, linoleic acid, and oddly enough, although linoleic acid *promotes* inflammation, GLA actually helps *calm* it. Some studies have shown that GLA helps reduce the number of tender joints, pain, and inflammation in RA patients. In a study of 56 patients with active RA, taking 2.8 grams of GLA for six months significantly improved joint pain, stiffness, and grip strength.

An often-suggested dose of GLA in supplement form is 1.8 to 2 grams per day. If you decide to take a supplement, make sure that it lists the GLA content on the label so you know exactly how many capsules or spoonfuls you need to take to get the desired dose. To get 1.8 grams of GLA, you need to take a lot of borage or black currant oil, and even more evening primrose oil.

Getting a grip on arthritis with green tea

Green tea, that delicious drink sometimes referred to as a "cup of steaming medicine," has been linked to prevention of heart disease, strokes, and certain kinds of cancer. It also appears to protect against the cartilage breakdown seen in OA. That's because the unfermented green tea leaves contain large amounts of some potent health promoters called *catechins,* which are powerful antioxidants and disease fighters. Two of the most potent catechins, EGCG and ECG, may actually block cartilage-destroying enzymes. So when you drink green tea, your precious cartilage is better able to stave off the breakdown process and stay intact. It may not work if your joints are already severely damaged, but if you start drinking green tea early enough, you may be able to keep OA at least somewhat in check. (Tell your kids!)

Green tea's EGCG can also put a damper on the inflammatory response. And green tea may help boost bone density through certain compounds like fluoride, flavonoids, and phytoestrogens.

For best results, look for the higher grades of green tea, use flow-through tea bags, allow the tea to steep in just-boiled water for 3 minutes, and drink at least 3 cups of tea per day. Also, be sure to keep your tea bags in an airtight container because exposure to air or dampness lessens both the polyphenol content and the flavor.

Avoiding Foods That May Be Trouble

No foods actually *cause* arthritis. At worst, a food may exacerbate a preexisting condition. For example, alcohol can trigger gout, but only in certain people. However, some foods are known to give some people trouble, so you may want to consider cutting back or avoiding intake of the following:

✔ **Nightshades:** Peppers, potatoes, eggplant, and tomatoes are some of the members of the nightshade family of vegetables. Some people feel that eating nightshades aggravates their rheumatoid arthritis and other forms of the disease. Although it hasn't been proven, if you feel that eating nightshades worsens your symptoms, avoid them.

✔ **Organ meats:** Liver, kidney, sweet bread, and other organ meats contain the purines that can trigger gout. If you have gout, avoid organ meat and other foods high in purines, including sardines, anchovies, and meat gravies.

✔ **Processed meat:** Cold cuts, hot dogs, bacon, and other processed meats contain various chemicals that may trigger allergic reactions, bringing about arthritis-like symptoms. Or, they may cause flares of existing arthritis conditions. It's not clear whether these substances actually trigger arthritis and allergies, or whether they tend to replace the vegetables, fruits, and whole grains that provide nutrients needed to hold arthritis at bay.

✔ **Foods containing linoleic/arachidonic acid:** The omega-3 fatty acids help reduce inflammation, but linoleic acid, an omega-6 fatty acid, does the opposite. Linoleic acid is found in salad or cooking oils, such as corn, safflower, and sunflower. It's used to make many kinds of fast food, and large amounts of it are fed to the cattle that eventually end up in the meat department of your grocery store. Linoleic acid is converted into arachidonic acid, which the body uses to build the substances that trigger inflammation and arthritic pain. Naturally, the less linoleic acid you consume, the better for your arthritis! To avoid linoleic acid, switch to olive, flaxseed, or canola oil for cooking, eat less meat and poultry, and avoid fast foods. At the same time, increase your consumption of the fish and other foods that contain the helpful omega-3 fatty acids (see "Omega-3 fatty acids," earlier in this chapter).

Watch for food allergies

If you've noticed that a food tends to make your arthritis worse, try eliminating it from your diet for a while. Reports (including some published in prestigious medical journals) abound of arthritis cases being "cured" when the sufferer stopped eating certain foods, including cheese, corn, milk, and various members of the nightshade vegetable family. Most likely, their arthritis-like symptoms were the result of simple food allergies. This diagnosis may not be true for you, but it can't hurt you to check it out.

To test for a food allergy, eliminate all foods that contain the suspected culprit for at least two weeks and keep a diary so that you can write down everything you eat and drink, plus your symptoms — especially any reactions or changes in the way you feel. After the two-week period, if you've noticed no difference, gradually add the foods back into your diet, one at a time, in small amounts, once again recording your diet, symptoms, and any changes. Remember: This test is not a true, scientifically valid elimination diet. Only a health professional can conduct a scientifically valid elimination diet.

Saving Your Joints with Supplements

Various studies have linked poor nutrition to rheumatoid arthritis, juvenile arthritis, and other forms of arthritis. However, the connection between nutrition and arthritis isn't yet fully understood. For example, researchers can't say that eating too few apples will cause arthritis or that drinking too much beer *always* triggers gout. However, good nutrition *is* an important part of the battle against arthritis. Evidence also suggests that careful use of supplements can be very helpful. And not just the omega-3 and omega-6 fatty acids can help you out. Antioxidants and free radical scavengers, plus some regular vitamins and minerals, can also have beneficial effects.

Take *all* supplements with care, because even helpful ones can interact with medicines or herbs that you're taking and cause trouble. Supplements can increase the effect of blood-thinning medications (which makes you more likely to bleed unnecessarily), counteract the effectiveness of some immune system–suppressing drugs, increase the side effects of NSAIDs, make alcohol and sedatives more powerful, hinder the absorption of select nutrients, and so on. Always let your physician know about *all* the supplements, herbs, and other substances you're taking. Consult with her before beginning to take supplements, increasing or decreasing the dosage, or discontinuing their use.

What you need to know before taking supplements

First of all, before you buy anything else, see your doctor, and bring a list of any medications, over-the-counter drugs, vitamins, minerals, herbs, or other supplements that you're currently taking. Be aware that some supplements can interact with medications, change the results of medical tests, and cause side effects. Ask your doctor if the supplement combinations and amounts that you're taking are okay for your health and your body.

Then, tell your doctor about any supplement you're planning to take and ask these questions:

- ✔ Will it interact with any medications I'm taking?
- ✔ Will it interact with any other supplements I'm taking?
- ✔ Will it have an effect on any of my medical conditions?
- ✔ Are there side effects I should watch for?
- ✔ Is there any good research that shows this supplement is safe?

✔ Is there any good research that shows this supplement is worth taking?

✔ What kind of results can I expect?

✔ How much should I take?

✔ How often should I take it?

✔ How long should I take it?

✔ How will I know when I should stop taking it?

Of course, your doctor may not know the answers to these questions. If that's the case, you might want to see a registered dietitian, or just do the research yourself. The Arthritis Foundation puts out a special Supplement Guide each year that gives the latest information on supplements and other natural remedies for arthritis. You can also contact the organizations listed in Appendix B for the latest nutrition and diet information. And you can find several excellent reference books in the library or at the bookstore on the topic of dietary supplements. Your best bet is to find something endorsed by the Arthritis Foundation, the American Dietetic Association, or the American Medical Association. Don't turn yourself into a guinea pig. Get the facts first!

What oxidants and free radicals do

Here's a short list of the damage that oxidants and/or free radicals can cause:

✔ They can attack the fatty membranes surrounding body cells. With repeated hits, the cell membrane may eventually become damaged and unable to ferry water, oxygen, and nutrients into the cells and waste products out. In short, the cell will be unable to function properly.

✔ Sometimes they harm the outer wall of the cell, and parts of the cell will leak out. In the wake of the spill, neighboring cells can be damaged.

✔ They can severely damage the DNA that makes up the genetic blueprints within your cells. When this happens, your cells may be unable to grow, function, and/or repair themselves properly.

✔ They can increase the inflammation response. (The inflammation response is the body's answer to foreign invaders, such as bacteria, and to injury. During the inflammation response, fluid rushes to the afflicted area, and the immune system is mobilized. Inflammation is a byproduct of the immune system's attempt to destroy the foreign invader or repair the damage.)

✔ They can hamper the immune system, the same internal defense system that goes awry in some forms of arthritis. (The immune system sometimes uses oxidants and free radicals to fight off certain germs. But these same "weapons" can harm the immune system: It's like a soldier being shot with his own gun.)

Fighting damaging oxidants and free radicals

Oxidants and free radicals are perfectly normal substances in the body; they're the result of normal metabolism. Unfortunately, if not properly controlled by the body, they can cause damage to cells, tissues, and organs, and have been linked to many ailments, including arthritis. Researchers can't absolutely say that they *cause* arthritis, but they're implicated in actions that lay the groundwork for trouble — or make current trouble worse.

Fortunately, many oxidant quenching and free radical–corralling substances (called *antioxidants* and *free radical quenchers*) can be found in foods and supplements. This section goes over some of the substances that may help you fight the cellular damage that can contribute to arthritis.

Vitamin C

This popular vitamin works together with vitamin E to scavenge free radicals or stabilize them so they're no longer dangerous. It also helps reactivate used vitamin E so it can charge back into the fray. Researchers have reported that vitamin C may help halt the progression of osteoarthritis. It's also been found to decrease OA pain.

Fresh fruits and vegetables, especially papaya, guava, red peppers, cantaloupe, sweet green peppers, oranges, broccoli, cauliflower, and asparagus are good sources of vitamin C. An often-suggested dose is 500 to 1,000 milligrams of vitamin C per day in supplement form.

Vitamin E

Vitamin E, like NSAIDs, slows the action of the prostaglandins that play a major role in producing pain. It also helps control the free radicals that can damage cells and tissues in and around the joint. A third way that vitamin E may help is by stabilizing the proteoglycans (the water-loving molecules in the cartilage.) Individual reports have also suggested that vitamin E may help in the treatment of Raynaud's.

Vitamin E is found in a variety of foods, including green leafy vegetables, broccoli, Brussels sprouts, seeds, nuts, green beans, and wheat germ oil. An often-suggested dose of vitamin E is 400 to 800 IU (international units) per day in supplement form.

Selenium

Selenium, an essential mineral with antioxidant properties, works together with *glutathione peroxidase* (one of the body's internal defenders) to control free radicals. Selenium also makes vitamin E more effective.

You find selenium in whole grains, fish, poultry, and meat; smaller amounts are present in fruits and vegetables. Selenium levels in food vary, depending in part on how much of the mineral was in the ground where the food was grown. An often-suggested dose is 100 to 200 micrograms per day in supplement form.

Warding off OA with boron

The vital mineral boron doesn't get much respect from the public — mostly because the public isn't familiar with it. But boron helps regulate calcium (a mineral key to bone health), keeping it from leaving the bones and the body. One way it may work is by increasing estrogen levels, helping the body hold on to more calcium and magnesium in the bones. Although boron's role in arthritis control isn't completely clear, it can help relieve inflammation and appears to be helpful in combating both osteoarthritis and rheumatoid arthritis. Studies of populations have shown that osteoarthritis was more common in areas where there were low levels of boron in the soil.

Boron is found in a variety of foods, including apples, peaches, peas, beans, lentils, peanuts, almonds, and grapes. An often-suggested dose is 3 to 9 milligrams per day in supplement form (as sodium tetrahydraborate).

Lowering homocysteine with vitamin B6 and folic acid

The combination of vitamin B6, folic acid, and vitamin B12 helps lower blood levels of *homocysteine*, an amino acid linked to a higher risk of heart attack and stroke. Homocysteine levels are often high in people with lupus. Vitamin B6 may also help to relieve the pain and stiffness of carpal tunnel syndrome and, in some cases, can make surgery unnecessary.

You'll find vitamin B6 in brewer's yeast, sunflower seeds, and brown rice; folic acid in green leafy vegetables; and B12 in meat, fish, and dairy products. An often-suggested dose of these three for reducing elevated homocysteine levels is 5 milligrams B6, 650 micrograms folic acid, and 50 micrograms B12 in supplement form.

Fighting OA and RA with vitamin D

Vitamin D helps you build strong bones by aiding in the absorption of calcium and is also vital for preventing bone loss and muscle weakness. But did you know that it may be able to ward off both OA and RA? Studies have found that getting too little vitamin D may actually triple the rate at which OA progresses! And those who get adequate amounts of vitamin D have been found to be less likely to develop OA of the hip. And if they do develop hip OA, it seems to progress at a slower rate.

A large-scale study begun in 1986 followed nearly 30,000 women (who did not have RA) over the course of 11 years. Those who took less than 200 IU of vitamin D each day had a 33 percent greater risk of developing the disease. Researchers aren't sure why vitamin D helps guard against RA — perhaps because it affects the immune system. Whatever the reason, getting ample amounts of vitamin D appears to be protective.

Your body can manufacture an adequate supply of vitamin D by getting about 20 minutes of direct sun exposure per day on an area about as big as the back of your hand. But 400 to 800 IU (international units) of vitamin D from dietary sources is often recommended. Good food sources include fortified milk, egg yolks, butter, cheese, fish oil, and fortified cereals.

Pumping up cartilage with collagen hydrolysate

Also known as hydrolyzed collagen or gelatin, pharmaceutical-grade collagen hydrolysate (PCH) may help the cartilage absorb *collagen,* the "netting" that holds the proteoglycans (*water-loving molecules*) in place. Collagen gives cartilage its elasticity and ability to absorb shock. When collagen fibers weaken and thin out, the cartilage dries out, cracks, and is more likely to show signs of wear. PCH, when taken with the hormone calcitonin, may help "plump up" the cartilage, inhibit the breakdown of bone collagen, and aid in bone repair. The effectiveness is still controversial, with much of the research coming to us from Germany.

Made from the hides and bones of pigs, cattle, sheep, or chickens, collagen hydrolysate is available in powder, tablets, and capsules and appears to be safe when taken in daily doses up to 10 grams.

PCH that comes from chickens can cause allergies in those allergic to chicken or eggs. PCH that comes from cattle has a remote chance of being contaminated due to mad cow disease. Some people taking PCH experience nausea and stomach upset.

Combating Raynaud's with niacin

Niacin is a member of the B-vitamin family. It was first noted early in the twentieth century during the battle against *pellagra,* the disease that causes blotchy skin rashes, confusion, weakness, memory loss, and other problems. Pellagra is rarely seen today, and doctors are primarily interested in niacin's ability to keep the skin, nerves, and intestines healthy, to lower cholesterol, and possibly to guard against cancer.

Niacin also has some antirheumatic properties. For example, Raynaud's patients given a niacin preparation reported fewer and shorter attacks of the disease compared to those given a placebo. OA patients experienced significant improvements in joint mobility and overall severity of the disease after three months of taking niacin. They were also able to lower their NSAID dosage by an average of 13 percent.

Nuts, liver, fortified grains and cereals, peanut butter, milk, cheese, and fish are good sources of niacin. Although a typical daily dose of niacin for health maintenance is 15 to 20 milligrams, therapeutic doses are closer to 4 grams. Niacin should be taken in the form of niacinamide to minimize side effects (for example, severe facial flushing).

Niacin can produce liver damage when taken in "therapeutic" doses. Don't take high doses of niacin unless under a doctor's supervision.

Zapping RA and psoriatic arthritis with zinc

The mineral zinc is necessary for many aspects of good health. Although no one has shown that a lack of zinc causes arthritis, researchers know that the amount of zinc in the blood is lower than it should be in at least some people suffering from rheumatoid arthritis, which suggests that zinc supplements may help some rheumatic arthritis patients.

The results of studies with zinc on arthritis have been mixed. One study of zinc sulfate showed that it improved RA, while another found that it eased symptoms of psoriasis. But others have shown that it has no significant benefit. This has led some researchers to suggest that zinc may not be helpful for everyone but can be a great aid to carefully selected arthritis patients who have low levels of the mineral. And side effects don't seem to be an issue: Hundreds of thousands of people take it every day without a problem.

You can find zinc in oysters, seafood, eggs, meat, wheat germ, and plain yogurt. An often-suggested dose is 50 milligrams per day in supplement form.

Relieving Arthritis Symptoms with Other Nutritional Substances

Omega-3 fatty acids, GLA (the "good" omega-6 fatty acid), antioxidants, free radical quenchers, vitamins, and minerals: The nutritional arsenal against arthritis is growing larger every year. And there's more. Here are a few of the nonvitamin, nonmineral, nonantioxidant substances that are gaining recognition.

Alleviating inflammation with aloe vera

Made from the leaves of the aloe plant, aloe vera juice is an ancient beauty aid, reportedly used by Cleopatra to keep her skin fresh and soft. It is also an all-purpose balm that was carried by Alexander the Great's soldiers as they conquered much of the ancient world. Today, aloe vera juice's popularity is partially due to its inflammation-relieving properties. Many people drink aloe juice as a laxative and health booster, and aloe vera creams or gels are used to treat sunburn, cuts, burns, and abrasions. Stabilized aloe vera juice contains numerous vitamins, minerals, and amino acids, which may explain its many beneficial effects.

There are reports that drinking aloe juice can help relieve symptoms of rheumatoid arthritis, as well as other inflammatory forms of arthritis. A few animal studies back up these claims, and many arthritis sufferers are eagerly awaiting human studies that will show that aloe can help knock down arthritis symptoms. Meanwhile, many people insist that moderate amounts of aloe juice relieve swelling.

You can find aloe vera in juice, cream, gel, and capsule form. An often-suggested dose is up to 200 milligrams or more per day in capsule form.

Supporting your joints with SAMe

Gaining fame as a remedy for heart disease, depression, and other ailments, SAMe (short for S-adenosyl-L-methione and pronounced *sammy*) is naturally produced by the body. SAMe helps the body manufacture a vital hormone called melatonin, which plays an important role in the sleep process. SAMe also protects DNA.

Since at least the late 1980s, SAMe has also strutted its stuff as an anti-inflammatory and painkiller that's particularly effective in osteoarthritis. In Europe, where it is sold as a drug, SAMe has been used for many years to treat OA. And no wonder. When placed head-to-head against four standard arthritis medicines (ibuprofen, indomethacin, piroxicam, and naproxen), SAMe proved to be just as effective — with fewer side effects than some of these drugs. Clinical trials involving thousands of people have shown that SAMe helps treat OA and improves the health of joints, most likely by repairing and rebuilding the cartilage. It's also been shown to counteract depression just as well as a standard antidepressant, with few side effects. An often-suggested dose is up to 400 milligrams, three times a day, for 21 days; then reduce dosage to 200 milligrams twice daily. Make sure you get plenty of B vitamins, because SAMe works closely with them. SAMe is available without a prescription in many health food and vitamin stores.

High doses of SAMe can cause headache, nausea, vomiting, diarrhea, and flatulence. SAMe can worsen bipolar disorder and Parkinson's disease, and may interact with antidepressants, especially monamine oxidase inhibitors (MAOIs).

Battling inflammation with bromelain

An enzyme found in pineapple, bromelain is often used as a digestive aid because it can help break down protein. But bromelain also has anti-inflammatory properties that may help reduce the swelling and pain of arthritis. In one study of 73 people with OA of the knee, bromelain, combined with rutin (a citrus flavonoid) and trypsin (a pancreatic enzyme), relieved pain and improved function as well as an NSAID. However, as yet there is no evidence that bromelain alone is effective.

Bromelain comes in capsule form, and an often-suggested dose is 80 to 320 milligrams per day, divided into two or three doses.

Bromelain can increase the effects of medications that thin the blood. Large doses can cause stomach upset or cramps. Avoid bromelain if you're allergic to pineapple.

Curtailing the pain with capsaicin

Chili peppers have long been used to treat numerous ills, including (surprisingly enough) indigestion! Today, researchers know that *capsaicin,* the ingredient that gives chilies their bite, can help relieve pain. Applying cream that contains capsaicin stimulates the pain impulse (it feels hot!) and then blocks it. It works by depleting the nerves' supply of substance P, a messenger that carries the pain message to the brain. Substance P also revs up the inflammation process, so decreasing your substance P stores can translate to less pain *and* less swelling.

Creams containing capsaicin are available in many drugstores without a prescription. Apply the cream to the painful area, following the instructions on the label.

Some people find capsaicin irritating, so if you decide to try it, start with a very small trial dose and work your way up.

Guarding your joints with grapeseed extract

Medical researchers haven't yet discovered all the ins and outs of grapeseed extract, a potent antioxidant that appears to help vitamin C cross into certain body cells. With a good supply of vitamin C safely tucked inside, these cells are better able to prevent and/or repair oxidative damage. Grapeseed extract may also help combat the inflammation associated with many forms of arthritis by slowing the body's release of inflammation-producing enzymes. Some evidence suggests that it can help strengthen the connective tissue.

Grapeseed extract is available as a supplement. Typically recommended is a *loading dose* (a large dose to get things going) of 75 to 300 milligrams per day for three weeks, dropping down to 40 to 80 milligrams per day for maintenance.

Don't use grapeseed extract if you're currently taking blood-thinning medication, because it increases the risk of bleeding.

Fighting disease with flaxseed oil

Many people swear by flaxseed oil, which contains many "parts" that the body can turn into the helpful omega-3 fatty acids known as EPA and DHA. Although there aren't any good studies showing that flaxseed can actually ease the symptoms RA and other inflammatory disorders like lupus, flaxseed does increase levels of EPA, while decreasing certain markers of inflammation in the blood — encouraging signs. One study found that flaxseed oil put the kibosh on autoimmune reactions just as effectively as EPA. And taking flaxseed oil brings some hefty side benefits: it helps inhibit tumor growth, balance your hormones, ward off heart disease, and reduce high blood pressure.

Flaxseed comes in oil or capsule form, and as flour or meal. Whole seeds need to be ground into meal, or your body will just pass them right through without absorbing the helpful linolenic acid. The oil spoils easily and shouldn't be heated to high temperatures (as in frying), although you can cook with it and bake with the flour or meal. An often-suggested daily dose is 1 to 3 table-spoons of the oil, the equivalent in capsule form, or up to a third cup of the flour or meal.

Giving OA pain the boot with ginger

Ginger has been used for more than 2,000 years by the Chinese to treat cough-ing, diarrhea, vomiting, and fever. Today we know that it contains ingredients that can ease nausea, alleviate motion sickness, and prevent heart attacks by thinning the blood. But it also may help ease the hurt of osteoarthritis, thanks to its pain-relieving and anti-inflammatory properties. One double-blind study found that 225 milligrams of highly purified ginger extract, taken twice daily, reduced OA knee pain.

Don't take ginger if you have gallstones or are on medications for blood pres-sure, heart problems, blood thinning, or diabetes. Ginger can cause heartburn, diarrhea, or stomach discomfort in sensitive people.

Glucosamine sulfate and chondroitin sulfate: Cures for osteoarthritis?

In early 1997, two supplements burst upon the arthritis scene: glucosamine and chondroitin sulfate. Although touted as new, veterinarians had used them for years to relieve arthritis or arthritis-like symptoms in horses and other animals.

Unlike standard drugs for osteoarthritis that are designed to relieve symp-toms, glucosamine and chondroitin (both components of human cartilage) appear to slow the progression of OA, reduce cartilage loss, and improve pain, inflammation, and joint function. Glucosamine, which in supplement form comes from shrimp, crab, or lobster shells, provides the building blocks for cartilage growth, maintenance, and repair. Chondroitin, which comes from pork byproducts or the tracheas of cattle, helps attract water to the cartilage (improving its shock-absorbing properties) and slows the action of certain enzymes that prematurely destroy cartilage.

Pulling together the results from many studies using either or both of these two supplements gives a promising picture. Here are some of the exciting results:

- ✔ Osteoarthritis patients reported significant and consistent improvement in joint function and pain — as much or more than they experienced with traditional medications (NSAIDs).

- ✔ Patients who had difficulty walking were now able to increase the rate at which they walked a measured distance by 30 percent or more.

- ✔ Symptoms such as pain sometimes disappeared altogether.

- ✔ Erosion of the cartilage was sometimes slowed or halted.

- ✔ Study participants experienced few or no side effects.

- ✔ People taking glucosamine and chondroitin sulfate were often able to reduce their NSAID dosage.

- ✔ The positive benefits did not fade with time, unlike the benefits reaped from many other medicines.

- ✔ The medicinal effect continued even after patients stopped taking the supplements.

- ✔ The two supplements were as effective as ibuprofen, an often-prescribed NSAID, but were better tolerated because they lack the side effects typically seen with drugs.

Not everyone will experience all the positive benefits of these two substances, of course, and researchers don't yet know who is most likely to benefit. Glucosamine and chondroitin are not fast acting, like pain pills, so you can expect to wait anywhere from a few days to several weeks before you feel the difference. If you don't notice any improvement within a few months, it's a good bet that the two supplements aren't for you.

Many people take these two supplements together, but no real evidence supports that they work better together than individually. A big study done by the National Institutes of Health (NIH) will address this question, with results due in 2005. There are many different brands of glucosamine and chondroitin sulfate supplements. An often-suggested dose is 500 milligrams of glucosamine three times a day and 400 milligrams of chondroitin three times a day.

There are several forms of glucosamine, including glucosamine sulfate, glucosamine hydrochloride and n-acetyl glucosamine. Although most of the studies have been conducted with the sulfate form, the hydrochloride form is believed to be just as effective. Some researchers feel that the n-acetyl form is weaker than the other two.

If you're allergic to sulfates, avoid glucosamine sulfate and chondroitin sulfate. Also, glucosamine may cause a reaction in those allergic to shellfish, and chondroitin taken with medications that thin the blood (like NSAIDs) can increase the risk of bleeding.

Looking at a Possible Link between Lupus and Food

There are no easy nutritional answers for *lupus,* one of the more puzzling and complex forms of rheumatic disease. Studies with mice suggest that a low-calorie, low-fat diet may help improve the symptoms, possibly by reducing abnormal immune system responses. And because more and more evidence suggests that lupus itself is a serious risk factor for heart disease, lowering elevated cholesterol levels, stopping smoking, and taking steps to prevent diabetes have become especially important parts of lupus treatment.

Taking certain vitamins may also be helpful. For example:

- Intravenous injections of niacin improved (but did not eliminate) skin lesions in systemic lupus patients.

- Pantothenic acid given in large doses caused improvement in patients with systemic and discoid lupus.

- Injecting vitamin B12 into three patients who had systemic lupus cleared up their skin lesions in six weeks.

- Vitamin E eased the symptoms in 9 out of 12 people with systemic lupus.

- Within one to six months, 67 people enjoyed improvement in their symptoms when given daily doses of pantothenic acid plus vitamin E.

Chapter 12

Oiling Your Joints with Exercise

*O*ur local gym has a sign that says, "Warning: Not Exercising Is Hazardous to Your Health!" This truth goes double for arthritis sufferers, because a lack of exercise can do a number on your joints, making them stiffer, less mobile, and more likely to degenerate. The old saying, "Use it or lose it!" is an appropriate one for those who live with arthritis. In this chapter, we discuss the elements of a good fitness program and give you tips on setting up a plan that can help strengthen your joints without disrupting your lifestyle.

Before you start on any kind of exercise program, consult your physician to determine whether your body can accommodate the stresses of exercise. This is especially critical when you haven't exercised in a while, you're over 40, or you have heart disease or high blood pressure.

Reaching Different Goals with Different Exercises

Every good fitness plan, no matter how simple or complex, includes three basic kinds of exercise: *cardiovascular endurance*, *strength training*, and *flexibility*. Together, these three types of exercise can build a strong, toned, and healthy body more able to withstand physical, mental, and emotional stresses.

Your initial goal should be to follow a short, easy fitness plan that includes these three kinds of exercise. Then you can slowly increase the length and intensity of the exercises as you become more physically fit.

A physical therapist or exercise physiologist experienced in working with people who have arthritis should design and supervise your fitness program. Any kind of exercise, whether cardiovascular endurance, strength training, or flexibility, can cause injury if done improperly, especially over time.

Building cardiovascular endurance

Countless studies have shown that people who do cardiovascular endurance exercises regularly have less heart disease, more energy, less body fat, lower blood pressure and cholesterol levels, faster metabolisms, higher self-esteem, and a greater sense of well-being. After you've warmed up with some moderately paced walking or calisthenics, you can safely move on to these exercises that rev up your body's motor. You have to become a heavy breather, however, because cardiovascular endurance exercises that are done properly make your breath come faster and your heart beat more quickly.

You can choose from a host of invigorating activities: walking, swimming, cycling, ballroom dancing, and so on. If you enjoy the outdoors, try a brisk walk or hike. If you prefer climate-controlled conditions, why not dance or ride a stationary bike? You can also try a water aerobics class held in a heated pool.

Take advantage of the great variety of fun and exciting cardio-endurance exercises available, and mix them up in your individual fitness plan. For example, you may swim during one session, ride a bike in the next, and take a jitterbug class in the third. Doing different kinds of exercise that work out different parts of your body is important so that you increase overall fitness and don't put too much stress on any one area.

Most people with arthritis tend to gravitate toward three kinds of cardio-endurance exercises — walking, cycling, and water exercises — because they're easy on the joints. You may want to start with these, and then begin to investigate other activities as you get stronger and more adventurous.

Walking

Unless you have severe trouble with your feet, ankles, knees, or hips, walking can be an ideal exercise. It's easy, inexpensive (all you really need is a good pair of supportive shoes and some absorbent socks), and can be done just about anywhere. It also provides the weight-bearing exercise you need to keep your bones in shape without the heavy impact on your joints delivered by running or jogging.

In order to get cardio benefits, though, you need to work your way up to *brisk* walking. Strolling is certainly pleasant and beneficial, but you have to pick up the pace if you want walking to qualify as a true cardiovascular endurance exercise. That means walking fast enough to make you somewhat winded (but not gasping for breath!).

Cycling

Whether you do it by flying through the park on an autumn day or by pumping away in the comfort of your very own bedroom, cycling can be a great way to get your heart racing without putting much strain on your joints. Start on flat ground. Then after several sessions (and if your joints permit it), you can raise the level of incline on your stationary bike or find a road that slopes upward slightly as you ride your outdoor bike. Take it easy, though. Strenuous uphill cycling is not recommended for those with osteoarthritis of the knees or hips.

As with walking, you need to pick up the pace. Coasting along is certainly pleasant but doesn't count for much if you're trying to give your heart and lungs a workout. If you're riding outdoors, look for a place free of traffic lights, pedestrians, and other impediments, because you'll have a hard time raising your heart rate and keeping it there if you're forced to stop every two minutes.

Exercising in water

Exercising in the water is just what the doctor ordered for most arthritis sufferers: It offers overall physical conditioning and great cardio-endurance with little or no pressure on the joints. With water to buoy you, you can say goodbye to gravity's woes and get your heart pumping without feeling that nagging pain in your knees or hips.

Positive side effects of exercise

If you don't already have enough reasons to exercise, here are a few more that don't directly relate to joint health but certainly boost your health in other ways. By getting regular exercise you can:

- Reduce stress
- Improve the quality of your sleep
- Increase your physical abilities
- Regain or maintain your independence
- Reduce body fat while increasing muscle mass
- Improve your balance
- Increase the activity of your immune system
- Promote relaxation
- Improve your sexual function
- Enhance your emotional health

Swimming is one of the best exercises that you can do to increase your head-to-toe fitness. When you swim, more than two-thirds of the muscles in your body go into action, giving you a good total workout in a short time. It's an efficient and enjoyable way to increase your overall strength, endurance, and flexibility — and swimming improves your posture!

For those who like the water but aren't keen on swimming, water aerobics can be a good choice. Offered by many local YMCAs in conjunction with the Arthritis Foundation, these classes are held in warm-water pools. Those with arthritis or other joint problems are led by a qualified instructor through a series of gentle range-of-motion, cardio-endurance, and flexibility exercises. Many people find that not only is their pain reduced during the time they're in the water, but also both their mobility and relief from pain are increased for hours (or even days) after a workout.

Strength training

Strength-training exercises improve the ability of your muscles to do work by increasing the force they can exert *(strength)* and the length of time that they can exert that force *(endurance)*. If you have arthritis, strength training is particularly important because strong, well-toned muscles and other supporting structures can help absorb the stress and strain placed on your joints. Weak muscles do just the opposite, forcing your joints to bear the brunt of impact, and encouraging joint misalignment or slippage. Your weight-bearing joints (those in your spine, hips, knees, and ankles) and their supporting structures (tendons, ligaments, muscles, and so on) also need to be sturdy and strong enough to take on an additional load as your body tries to protect the injured or diseased area by shifting the weight elsewhere. Performed regularly, strength-training exercises can help fight weakness, frailty, falls, and disability.

Weight and repetition are the basis of strength training. You can build your strength by gradually increasing the amount of weight that your muscles must lift, which will make your muscles bigger and bulkier. But by increasing the number of times your muscles perform a certain movement (repetitions or reps), you can increase your endurance, which is even more important. Bulkier muscles are less flexible, more likely to be injured, and less likely to improve joint range of motion than muscles that have been conditioned for endurance.

Don't be fooled into believing that you can do strength training only with a set of barbells. When a dancer slowly lifts her leg and holds it in position, she is lifting weight — the weight of her leg as gravity pulls against it. When a swimmer pulls his arms through the water, he is working against the resistance of the water. With exercises like dancing and swimming, you don't need additional weights!

You can do different strength-enhancing exercises to vary your workouts and keep your exercise plan fresh and interesting, while toning different muscle groups. Strength-enhancing exercises include the following:

- Isometric exercises
- Sit-ups
- Push-ups
- Leg lifts
- Weight training
- Swimming
- Stair climbing
- Cross-country skiing
- Dance or yoga (sustained poses)
- Running

You can do two kinds of strength-training exercises — *isotonic* and *isometric.* When performing *isotonic* exercises, your muscles move against the resistance of gravity, water, light weights, or your own body weight, and your joints bend and straighten. Weight lifting and swimming are two examples.

Isometric exercises, on the other hand, are done *without* moving your joints. Muscles are contracted and released, but the joint stays in a static position. Often, your body itself provides the resistance. For example, clasping your hands in front of you and pushing them together is an isometric exercise for your arms and pectoral muscles. These exercises are great for toning your muscles and supporting structures on days when your joints are just too painful to move.

Increasing flexibility

Flexibility exercises (stretching) increase your ability to bend, reach, twist, and stretch. They help you maintain or increase your *range of motion* — the amount of movement your joints allow in various directions. Flexibility exercises also improve the elasticity of your muscles, which makes them more resistant to injury. If you have arthritis, flexibility exercises are crucial, because pain, stiffness, and restricted range of motion tend to make you want to move your joints less, which only increases the pain, stiffness, and limited movement over time.

You may think that you already bend and stretch enough while doing housework or gardening, and that you can just skip flexibility exercises. But everyday activities don't move your joints through their full range of motion, so you need to make flexibility exercises a regular part of your daily program. Try to do them every day if possible.

Easing Joint Pain with Exercise

Countless exercises can help make you stronger, more fit, more flexible, and better able to fight arthritis. Those that you choose depend upon what you and your physical therapist feel are the best ones for your particular condition. Having said that, we include the exercises outlined in this section as good ones for stretching or strengthening the indicated areas.

For some of the exercises in this section, you need to use an exercise mat to protect your weight-bearing joints from excessive pressure when they're in contact with the floor.

Stretching your neck

Use this exercise to stretch and relieve tension in your neck muscles:

1. **Sit cross-legged on your exercise mat, hands resting comfortably on your knees or thighs.**

2. **While facing to the front, drop your head to the right side, as if trying to touch your right ear to your right shoulder.**

   Don't scrunch up your shoulders!

3. **Put your right hand over the top of your head, and your left hand on top of your left shoulder.**

4. **Exert gentle pressure with each hand, stretching your neck.**

5. **Repeat on the other side.**

Stretching your hand and wrist

This stretches and strengthens your fingers and wrists:

1. **Make a fist.**

2. **Fling your fingers out to their straightened position, fingers spread.**

3. **Return to the fist position.**

4. **Repeat five times for each hand.**

The following exercise increases finger and hand flexibility:

1. **Open your hand flat.**

2. **Touch the tip of your thumb to the tip of each of your fingers, one at a time.**

3. **Repeat ten times per hand.**

Extending the shoulder and arm

Use this exercise to strengthen your upper back and shoulder muscles:

1. **Get on your hands and knees on an exercise mat.**

   Make sure your neck is straight and parallel to the floor.

2. **Slowly reach your right arm out in front of you, keeping your arm straight, parallel to the floor and about the height of your ear.**

   Your fingers should point at the wall on the opposite side of the room. (See Figure 12-1.)

3. **Hold for five seconds, if possible, and then slowly return your arm to its starting position.**

4. **Repeat with your other arm, and then alternate, doing as many reps as you can manage.**

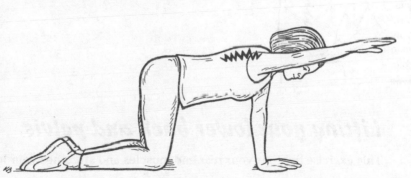

Figure 12-1: Shoulder arm extension. This exercise strengthens your upper back and improves posture.

Stretching your side

This exercise tones your side and back muscles and helps prevent sudden back spasms that can result from turning or twisting the wrong way.

1. **Stand straight with your feet about 18 inches apart.**

2. **Bend your left elbow, placing your left hand at your waist.**

3. **Straighten your right arm above your head while trying to keep your right shoulder level with the left one.**

4. **Bend slowly toward the left (toward your bent elbow), keeping your right arm above your head, as shown in Figure 12-2.**

5. **Hold this position for a count of five.**

   You should feel a pull in your right side. Be careful not to push your right hip to the side as your bend — that's cheating, and it can put stress on your knees.

6. **Slowly return to an upright position.**

7. **Repeat on the other side.**

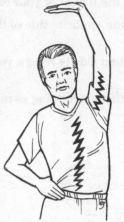

Figure 12-2: Side stretch. You should feel a nice pull in the muscles running from your upper arm all the way down to your hip.

Lifting your lower back and pelvis

This exercise tightens your rear-end muscles and stretches your lower back.

1. **Lie on your back on your exercise mat, knees bent and a couple of inches apart, with the soles of your feet flat on the mat.**

   Your arms should be straight and about 3 inches away from your sides, with your palms flat against the mat.

2. **Tighten your buttock muscles and slowly raise your pelvis, supporting your weight with your feet and your lower arms.**

   Try to keep your spine straight — don't arch up — but don't let your rear-end sag, either. You should have a nice straight line from your shoulders to your knees. (See Figure 12-3.)

3. **Hold this raised position for five seconds.**

4. **Slowly ease your back down, vertebrae by vertebrae, beginning with your upper back and ending with your tailbone.**

5. **Repeat slowly at least five times.**

Figure 12-3:
Lower back and pelvic lift. A good exercise for tightening the buttocks and releasing tension in the lower back.

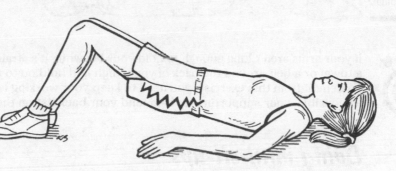

Stretching your hamstring

Use this stretch to help you loosen up your lower back and back of your thighs (hamstrings), as well as to improve your ability to bend over.

1. **Lie on your back on your exercise mat with your knees flexed and arms at your sides.**

2. **Bend your right knee and grab the back of your thigh with both hands.**

3. **Pull your knee toward your chest, keeping your foot pointed rather than flexed.** (Flexing stretches the sciatic nerve.)

4. **While holding onto your thigh, extend the lower part of your leg until your leg is completely straight, as shown in Figure 12-4.**

   If you can't straighten your leg in that position, lower your leg until you can straighten it. Hold for a count of five.

5. **Bend your knee and move your leg back to the mat.**

6. **Repeat with the other leg.**

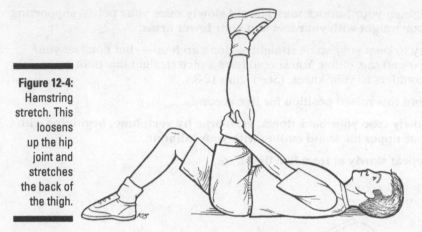

Figure 12-4:
Hamstring
stretch. This
loosens
up the hip
joint and
stretches
the back of
the thigh.

If your arms aren't long enough to hold your leg while it's straightening, slide a towel or a belt around the back of your thigh and hold on to the ends of it. To benefit from this exercise, you need to keep your working leg as straight as possible, your supporting leg bent, and your back flat on the ground.

Doing mini-sit-ups

This exercise is great for tightening the abdominal muscles, which support your lower back. The mini-sit-up causes your abdominals to contract and hold at the point of maximum resistance, without putting too much strain on your back and neck muscles.

1. **Lying flat on your back on your exercise mat, bend your knees, keeping your feet flat on the floor.**

   Your knees shouldn't be more than an inch or two apart.

2. **Fold your arms across your chest and raise your head, neck, and shoulders off the floor, as shown in Figure 12-5.**

   Your head and neck will curl forward, but they shouldn't curl so far forward that your chin is on your chest.

3. **Hold this position for a count of five.**

   Try not to let your stomach muscles pop out; instead, suck them in.

4. **Slowly release and roll back down to your starting position.**

5. **Repeat this exercise five times, if possible.**

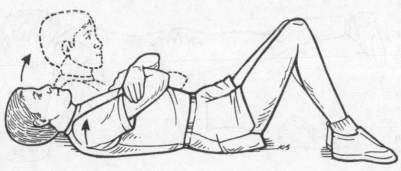

Figure 12-5:
Mini-sit-up.
This exer-
cise tightens
the abdom-
inal muscles
without
putting a lot
of stress
and strain
on the back
and neck.

TIP

If you can't get your shoulders completely off the floor at first, don't worry. Do the best you can and work toward that goal in the long run.

Extending your hip and back leg

The buttock muscles are important in maintaining good posture. When they are contracted and "tucked under," the stomach muscles automatically contract, too. This contraction helps you support your lower back, while avoiding the sway back, stomach out, knees locked position that is so detrimental to your joints. Use this exercise to tighten up your rear-end muscles:

1. **Get on your hands and knees on an exercise mat.**

   Make sure your neck is parallel to the floor.

2. **When you feel comfortable and balanced, flex the toes of your right foot.**

3. **Slide your right leg out behind you until it's straight and supported only by your toes.**

4. **Slowly lift your right leg up until it's parallel with the floor, as shown in Figure 12-6.**

5. **Hold the position for five seconds.**

6. **Lower your leg slowly, bend it, and bring it back to its original position.**

7. **Repeat exercise with your left leg.**

Figure 12-6:
Hip and
back leg
extension.
This exer-
cise helps
support your
lower back
by strength-
ening the
buttock
muscles.

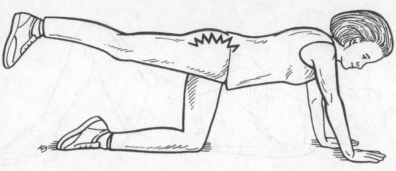

Rotating your ankle

This exercise is great for increasing the range of motion in your ankle.

1. **Lie on your back on your exercise mat, legs bent and arms at your sides.**

2. **Raise your right leg into the air, keeping it bent, and hold onto your right thigh for support.**

3. **Rotate your foot slowly in a circle to the right, as if drawing a circle in the air with your big toe.**

4. **Rotate four times to the right and four times to the left.**

5. **Repeat the exercise with your left foot.**

Using Yoga to Ease Arthritis Pain

Yoga is an ancient way of bringing your physical, mental, and spiritual "selves" into balance and harmony, thus achieving the highest form of good health. All of the many kinds of yoga involve assuming various sitting, standing, or lying-down postures called *asanas*. The postures are held for anywhere from seconds to minutes and are accompanied by deep breathing.

The benefits of yoga for arthritis sufferers are many, including relaxation, stress reduction, increased energy, improved flexibility, increased strength, and improved circulation. As an added bonus, many people find that regularly practicing yoga helps relieve depression, increase alertness, and improve overall well-being.

The snake

Use this posture, or *asana*, to stretch your chest, stomach, and upper back muscles while strengthening your arms and upper body.

1. **On your exercise mat, lie face down on your stomach with your arms bent and hands palm down resting on either side of your neck, as shown in Figure 12-7a.**

2. **Pressing your hands and lower arms into the mat, slowly raise your head and upper chest until they're completely off the floor. See Figure 12-7b.**

3. **Gradually straighten your arms as you push your head, chest, and torso as far up as you can, as shown in Figure 12-7c.**

   Be sure to keep your pelvis flat on the floor and your legs extended.

4. **Hold the position for a count of five.**

5. **Slowly bend your arms as you ease your torso down to the mat.**

6. **Gradually return to the starting position with your face on the mat.**

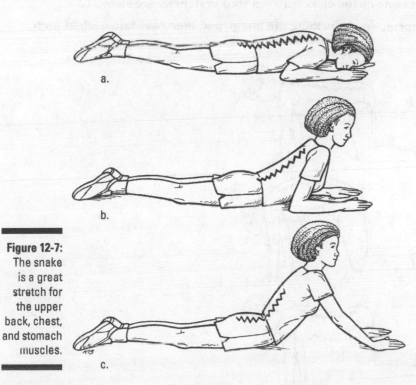

Figure 12-7: The snake is a great stretch for the upper back, chest, and stomach muscles.

a.

b.

c.

The cat

This exercise helps increase spinal flexibility.

1. **Get on your hands and knees on an exercise mat.**

   Make sure your neck is parallel to the floor. Your knees should be about 12 inches apart, with your arms straight down and your fingers pointing forward. See Figure 12-8a.

2. **Contract your stomach muscles and roll your head forward until your chin touches your chest as you round your back upward toward the ceiling.**

   Your entire torso should be contracted, forming a hollow. See Figure 12-8b.

3. **Gradually release the contraction and roll your head back to its original position.**

4. **Arch your back slightly, creating a curve going the opposite way.**

   Don't stick your rear-end out, let your stomach muscles relax, or sway your back to accomplish this position; these things can put too much pressure on the disks between your vertebrae. See Figure 12-8c.

5. **Repeat, slowly forming the hump, and then ease into a slight arch.**

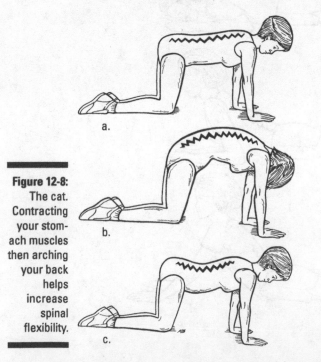

Figure 12-8:
The cat. Contracting your stomach muscles then arching your back helps increase spinal flexibility.

a.

b.

c.

The pretzel

Use this exercise to stretch your inner thigh and hip.

1. **Lie on your back on your exercise mat, legs bent and arms at your sides.**

2. **Cross your right leg over your left leg, with your right foot just clearing your left knee.**

3. **Grab your left thigh with both hands and pull it toward you while keeping your legs in the crossed position, as shown in Figure 12-9.**

4. **Hold this position for at least five seconds.**

5. **Slowly release, and then repeat with the opposite leg.**

Figure 12-9:
The pretzel.
A nice relax-
ing stretch
that loosens
the hip and
increases
the flexibility
of the inner
thigh.

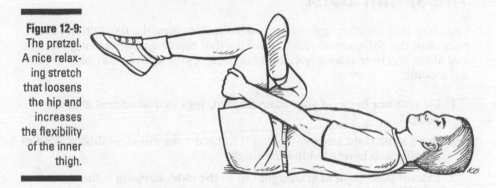

Knee-to-chest stretch

This exercise loosens up the hip joint while stretching your lower back and buttock muscles:

1. **Lie on your back on your exercise mat, legs extended and arms at your sides.**

2. **Bend your right leg, grab it with both hands just below the knee, and pull it gently toward your chest as far as it will go, as shown in Figure 12-10.**

3. **Hold your leg at its maximum position for a count of five.**

    Make sure your other leg is straight and on the floor.

4. **Slowly release and repeat with your left leg.**

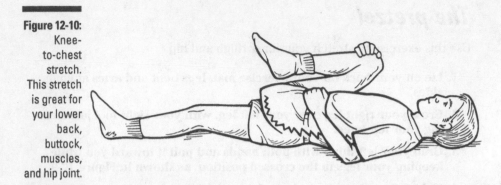

Figure 12-10:
Knee-to-chest stretch. This stretch is great for your lower back, buttock, muscles, and hip joint.

The spinal twist

Exercises that twist the spine are good for maintaining the flexibility of the spine and the oblique muscles — muscles that run diagonally along your side and allow you to reach for something in back of you without completely turning around.

1. **Lie on your back on your exercise mat, legs extended and arms at your sides.**

2. **Bend your right knee and bring it toward your chest, grabbing hold of it with both hands behind the thigh.**

3. **Extend your right arm straight out to the side, keeping it flat on the floor to make a 90-degree angle to your body.**

4. **Using your left hand, pull your right knee across your body, as if to touch it to the floor beside your left hip.**

    Your right foot should stay in contact with your left knee, and your right shoulder should stay flat on the floor. Your left leg should stay straight.

5. **Turn your head to the right, as if looking at the right wall.**

6. **Hold this pose for a count of ten, and then slowly return to your original position.**

7. **Repeat, bending your left knee this time.**

    One time on each side is sufficient.

The child's pose

This posture stretches your entire back, your buttock muscles, and your upper arms, while putting you into a dreamy state of relaxation.

1. **Sit on your mat with your legs tucked under you, heels directly under the buttocks.**

   Your knees should be about 12 inches apart.

2. **Roll your upper body head first toward the floor, until you can place your forehead on the floor in front of your knees.**

3. **Place your palms on the floor on either side of your head.**

4. **Slowly extend your arms in front of you as far as possible.**

   Your buttocks should stay in contact with your heels, and your feet should stay on the floor.

5. **Hold this position for a count of ten, then slowly return to the sitting position.**

6. **Repeat five times.**

Doing Chair Exercises to Save Your Joints

If you like the idea of exercising without putting weight on your joints, consider *chair exercises,* which are performed while sitting in a straight-back chair. The following subsections give details on some simple chair exercises that can be used for warm-ups (or, if performed more vigorously, as aerobic exercises).

Chair marching

This is a good one to do with music — try a Sousa march! Be careful not to slam your feet on the ground in your enthusiasm, though.

1. **Sit up tall in your chair with feet planted on the ground and pointing straight ahead.**

2. **March your feet in place, beginning slowly then gradually picking up the pace.**

   Be sure to lift your thighs as far off the chair seat as possible.

Chair running

Follow the directions for chair marching, but move at a much faster pace. It's fair to "run" on your toes (it's too fast a pace to put your whole foot down), and you won't be able to lift your thigh off the chair as high as you do in chair marching. But a couple of minutes of chair running are guaranteed to make you "glow" and start shedding your sweaters.

What you may *not* know about exercise and arthritis . . .

If you have arthritis, getting up and moving around may be the last thing you want to do, especially when you're in pain. But studies have shown that exercise may actually be the arthritis sufferer's best friend because it can lessen pain, improve joint function, and even protect against the development of certain kinds of arthritis. Check out the following exercise facts to find out more:

✔ Those with OA of the knee often experience less pain if they use free weights or machines with fixed weights to strengthen their knees before exercising.

✔ A team of Dutch researchers found that moderate-to-high intensity exercise (75 minutes, twice a week) performed over a two-year period helped increase functional ability in RA patients, with no additional damage to the large joints. This finding was surprising because RA patients are often told that strenuous activity can increase joint inflammation.

✔ Kids who engage in vigorous physical activity may enjoy some protection against OA later on. This is partly due to the fact that exercise stimulates the production of cartilage. An Australian study found that inactive children had 22 to 25 percent less cartilage than those who were just mildly active. But cartilage volume in the knee in children who were very active increased up to 15 percent a year in boys and 10 percent a year in girls. However, too much high-impact exercise, or sports that contribute to joint injuries, can lead to premature OA.

✔ Both high-intensity *and* low-intensity aerobic exercise seem to be equally effective in improving joint function, gait, pain, and aerobic capacity for people who have OA of the knee.

✔ T'ai chi, the ancient Chinese form of exercise that involves slow, fluid movements, helps improve physical functioning and ease the symptoms of OA. Those who participate in t'ai chi exercise programs (one-hour sessions at least twice a week) can expect to see improved walking speed, bending ability, arm function, balance, management of arthritis symptoms, control of fatigue, and ability to do household tasks. One study found that this was true even for those with severe limitations (use of a walker, use of an oxygen tank, or obesity).

Chair dancing

You can do the hora, the heel-toe polka, or the shuffle-off-to-buffalo all while sitting in a chair. Not only will it warm you up, it's fun!

In addition to the following, many more dance steps can be performed from a chair; it only takes a little imagination. Try out some of your favorites; you may be surprised how enjoyable this kind of exercise can be.

The hora

As with all dancing, the right music can make you forget that you're exercising and get you thinking that you're just kicking up your heels. Music for the hora can be found in the Jewish folk music section at your local record store.

1. **Starting with your right foot, step to the side.**

2. **Cross behind your right foot with your left.**

3. **Step to the side with your right.**

4. **Do a small kick with your left foot.**

5. **Then kick with your right foot.**

6. **Reverse it: step side with your left, back with your right, side with your left, kick right, kick left.**

Heel-toe polka

The count should go: heel, toe, step-together-step, or 1, 2, 1-2-3.

1. **Start with your right foot. Touch your right heel to the floor, and then touch your right toe to the floor.**

2. **Step to your right side with your right foot, then bring your left to meet it.**

3. **Step to the right again with your right foot.**

4. **Reverse: Left heel touches, then left toe, step side with left, bring right to meet it, step left.**

Shuffle-off-to-Buffalo

The sequence goes hop-step, cross, step, cross, step, cross, step, with a count of "and one and two and three and four."

1. **Begin with both feet all the way to the left of your chair. Lift your right foot slightly off the floor and "hop" on your left foot.**

2. **Step to the side with your right foot.**

3. **Cross your left behind the right.**

4. **Step right again, cross left behind.**

5. **Step right again, cross left behind.**

6. **Step right.**

7. **Reverse, starting with your left foot.**

Chair fencing

Although real fencing is a real strain on the knees — all that deep lunging! — chair fencing spares your knees while giving your arms a good workout.

1. **Sitting up straight, extend your right leg forward as far as you can while keeping your foot flat on the floor, toes pointing straight ahead.**

2. **Extend your right arm forward, in a thrusting position, with left arm against your side, elbow bent and fist curled against the front of your shoulder.**

3. **Reverse, extending your left leg and left arm. Continue to change positions, as if you were "fencing."**

Maximizing the Healing Effects of Exercise

Performing the proper exercises on a regular basis is a vital part of almost any arthritis treatment program. But to gain maximum benefits, you also need to be aware of proper exercise techniques, and always make sure that you're completely warmed up before exercising. A warm bath or shower can help, but you should also do some light cardio or strengthening exercises until you break a sweat. If you have painful, inflamed joints, you may find that icing them before your warm-up helps keep pain at a minimum.

As for exercising when you're in the midst of an arthritis flare, try a warm shower or bath, and then some gentle stretching to get a little circulation going. Take it easy, though. If stretching causes too much pain, stop. You can always try again later.

Warming up your muscles, through light exercise or a warm shower, is just one idea for making the most of your exercise sessions. Some other helpful tips include:

✔ Start slowly with a program that you can do fairly easily.

✔ If you feel dizzy, nauseous, faint, or tightness in your chest, stop exercising and call your doctor.

✔ Pick a cardio-endurance activity that you can do continuously for ten minutes, if possible. (If not, try five minutes or even one minute, and gradually increase your time.)

✔ Make your cardiovascular-endurance exercises vigorous enough so that you sweat, your heart beats faster, and your breath comes more rapidly. Find a pace at which you feel slightly short of breath but can maintain a conversation.

✔ Do your cardiovascular endurance exercises three days a week (every other day, with one day off per week) for at least 10 minutes, working your way up to 30 minutes.

✔ Exercise at a slower pace to cool down after doing cardio-endurance exercises. For example, you can walk slowly until your heart rate returns to normal.

✔ Do your strength-training exercises three days a week, on the days you don't do cardiovascular endurance exercises. Leave one day a week free for rest.

- Do some flexibility exercises (stretching) before your strengthening routine, and then again afterwards. This will help decrease the likelihood of injury to the muscles.

- Ask your physical therapist to supervise your stretching sessions, at least in the beginning. Incorrect stretching can cause more harm than good. Stretching sessions should last from 10 to 20 minutes, with each stretch held at least five seconds. As you become more flexible, you can gradually increase the holding time to 10, 20, or even 30 seconds. Stretch every day, if possible.

- Always stretch slowly and carefully — don't bounce. Move your body to its maximum position, hold it in place for at least 30 seconds, then ease into your stretch just a little more before releasing.

- Don't hold your breath while stretching — breathe slowly and deeply and try to relax into the stretch.

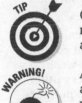

One of the most important things you can do to help make exercise a permanent part of your life is to keep a positive attitude toward yourself, your body, and your program. Remember, the more you exercise, the easier it gets.

Although we've said that exercise may help ease your current joint pain and lessen tomorrow's pain, we don't suggest that you go for a jog when your arthritic knees act up or that you do push-ups when your wrist aches. If an exercise or activity hurts or causes your joints to become inflamed, *stop immediately.* Pain is a message from your body telling you that tissue is being damaged. Respect the pain; try a different kind of exercise, or call it a day and try again tomorrow.

Designing Your Workout Program

In this section, we give you the lowdown on how to make sure your exercise program is everything it can be to improve your health, keep you safe, and maximize the benefits of exercise.

What you discover by reading this book isn't a substitute for professional advice. Doing the wrong exercises, or even the right exercises in the wrong way, can make your condition worse. Enlist professionals to help you design your exercise program so that you do the right exercises in the right way.

Your doctor can advise you as to which kinds of exercise are helpful for your condition, how much is too much, and when to stop. A physical therapist can also be extremely helpful by suggesting appropriate exercises, teaching you correct techniques and positioning, and urging you on when it's time to increase the length and/or intensity of your workout. (An *exercise physiologist* can do much of what a physical therapist does, but make sure that he or she has experience working with arthritis.) And an occupational therapist can teach you how to use your joints in the least stressful ways.

Considering the basic game plan

With the help of your health-care professionals, you can begin to devise an exercise plan. Ideally, you'll do some kind of exercise six days a week, taking one day off to rest. A good exercise session contains the following elements:

- ✔ **Warm-up:** A good warm-up lasts at least ten minutes and should make you break a sweat. If your joints can handle it, calisthenics (jumping jacks, jogging in place, and so on) make ideal warm-up exercises. If not, try doing the slow version of the activity you plan to do next — slow walking or relaxed cycling, for example — before beginning a brisk walk or bike trip.

  Don't begin your warm-up with big stretches (for example, the hamstring stretch). Stretching a cold muscle invites injury. Save your flexibility exercises until after the bulk of your exercise session has been completed. (A small amount of gentle stretching is okay during the warm-up, but be careful.)

- ✔ **Cardiovascular endurance exercises:** According to the American College of Sports Medicine, you should do at least 20 minutes worth of continuous cardiovascular endurance exercises at least three times a week. Try to get in 20 minutes of walking, cycling, or water exercises every other day. However, if you haven't exercised in a while or if you're experiencing a lot of joint pain, this may not be possible. The best idea is to start wherever you are right now. If you can do only five minutes worth of aerobic exercises, then so be it. Perhaps by next week you can increase it to six minutes. The point is to get moving and gradually improve.

  If you find that you're doing great at your present level and aren't experiencing any physical problems, you can increase the length of your cardio workout and/or the number of sessions you do per week. Just make sure you don't do so much that you exhaust yourself or cause injuries. See the earlier section, "Building cardiovascular endurance" to find out more.

- ✔ **Strength-training exercises:** On the days that you don't do cardio exercises, do about 20 minutes worth of strength training, in the form of weight training, swimming, stair climbing, or other exercises that involve pitting your muscles against some form of weight. Check out the earlier section, "Strength training" to find out more.

- ✔ **Flexibility exercises:** You should do exercises that involve stretching, bending, twisting, and reaching six or seven days a week for at least 10 minutes. To avoid muscle strains and sprains, flexibility exercises should be performed only after your body is well warmed-up. The safest strategy is to stretch at the end of an exercise session

- ✔ **Cool-down:** At the end of your exercise session, it's important to cool down for five to ten minutes to help your heart rate, breathing, and blood pressure return to normal. Begin by tapering off your activity; for example, slow your brisk walking down to an easy stroll. When your breathing has become easy again, you may want to do some gentle stretches, which will not only improve your flexibility, but reduce your risk of future injury, remove waste products from your muscle tissue, and help lower the amount of muscle soreness you'll feel later on.

Figuring out if you're working hard enough

First of all, as long as you're doing some form of exercise, you should be congratulated! A whopping 50 percent of American adults, many with no excuses for their idleness, get no exercise at all. If you're at least making an effort, especially on a daily basis, you're definitely on your way to better fitness and better health.

But to get the most out of your cardiovascular endurance exercises without running the risk of exhaustion, you need to remember two things while exercising:

✔ Your breath should be coming faster and harder, but not to the point where you're panting.

✔ Your heart should be beating faster, but not pounding in your ears!

So how do you figure out if you're doing enough, but not too much? Try using the Target Heart Rate system.

1. **First, subtract your age from 220.** (Example: 220 − 60 = 160)

2. **Then, multiply the answer by .9 and by .6** (example: 160 x .9 = 144; 160 x .6 = 99).

Your two answers indicate the upper and lower ends of your target heart rate zone. That means that for maximum cardio-endurance benefits, your heart rate should fall somewhere between these two numbers while you're exercising — in this case somewhere between 144 and 99 beats per minute.

To figure your current heart rate, all you need is a watch or clock with a second hand and your own fingers:

1. **Place your index and second fingers across the inside of your opposite wrist.** There's a little "well" on the thumb-side of the tendon that runs up the middle of your wrist. Your two fingers should easily slide over that tendon and into this "well," where it should be easy to feel your pulse.

2. **With an eye on the second-hand of your watch or clock, count the number of pulse beats you feel in 15 seconds.**

3. **Multiply by four, and you have the number of times your heart beats in a minute.**

If you do this either during or immediately after your cardio-endurance session, you should be able to figure out whether you're in "the zone" or not.

Here's an easy way to find out if you're working hard enough (or too hard) while exercising. You should be breathing too heavily to be able to sing, but not so heavily that you can't talk. If you can sing while you're exercising, you may want to step up the intensity a bit. But if you find you can't catch your breath enough to talk during exercise, you're probably overdoing it.

Taking it easy!

Whenever you start a new exercise program, add a new activity, or increase the frequency or duration of your workout, the number one rule is this: Start slowly. Many would-be exercise enthusiasts are sidelined by doing too much too soon, winding up either injured or just plain burned out! Your exercise sessions should emphasize enjoyment. They should require some effort but should never be grueling. If you're more than just a little bit sore a day or two after the workout, you've done too much.

Finding a good class

After you've done some initial training with a physical therapist or exercise physiologist, you may feel ready to join a class. You can enjoy several advantages by working out in groups — it's a lot less expensive than private instruction, classes usually have more space and a greater variety of equipment, and the friendships formed among classmates can make exercise more fun. But where can you find a class suited to the special needs of those with arthritis? The best bet is to contact your local chapter of the Arthritis Foundation and ask about its Arthritis Foundation Aquatics Program. (See www.arthritis. org, and type in **Aquatics Program** in the Search box. This takes you to a site where you can enter your zip code and find a nearby class. Or call the Arthritis Foundation at 800-283-7800.) The YMCA and the Arthritis Foundation jointly offer a warm-water exercise program at YMCAs and YWCAs nationwide. The pool is typically kept at about 83 degrees, and soft music is generally played in the background. A specially trained instructor takes the class through a variety of stretching, strengthening, and aerobic exercises, and the buoyancy of the water allows participants to increase overall fitness without putting excessive strain on their joints

The Arthritis Foundation also offers exercise videotapes for those with moderate to severe arthritis. The People with Arthritis Can Exercise (PACE) videos take viewers through both range-of-motion and strengthening exercises. Contact your local Arthritis Foundation chapter for more information.

Chapter 13

The Right Stride and Other Ways to Protect Your Joints

· ·

In This Chapter

▶ Looking into biomechanics

▶ Sitting in the least stressful, most healthful position

▶ Saving your joints with correct posture

▶ Walking correctly

▶ Sleeping in positions that protect your joints

▶ Lifting without extra strain and stress

▶ Looking at seven keys to joint health

· ·

You may not realize that how you sit, stand, and walk can help determine how healthy or hurtful your joints are today and how well they fare tomorrow.

You probably think that sitting in a chair or walking down the street is a natural behavior that you instinctively perform correctly. After all, you've been doing these things all of your life. But believe it or not, almost everybody misuses their joints by doing some of these things incorrectly. And over time, repeated abuse of your joints can cause permanent tissue damage and a lot of unnecessary pain. Luckily, by using certain joint-saving techniques, you can take undue pressure off your joints today, thereby helping to prevent tomorrow's problems. In this chapter, we tell you how you can take a load off your joints while doing everyday things that you probably don't realize can be harmful.

Believing in Biomechanics

Biomechanics is the study of how your body handles the impact of its own weight against gravity. When your body is in a "biomechanically correct" position, the force of the impact created by movement is spread out over a large area. During correct walking, for example, when your heel strikes the ground, the impact travels up your entire leg and is absorbed along the way by your foot, ankle, knee, and hip, and all their supporting tissues. But during incorrect walking, the brunt of the impact may be taken by the ankle and knee alone. By distributing the load as widely as possible and positioning the joints for maximum impact absorption, joint stress and damage can be cut.

Everybody should use correct biomechanical (joint-saving) techniques. And for those who already have joint problems, observing correct biomechanics is absolutely essential. But most people have a hard time analyzing their own posture or the ways they move, which means they also have a hard time figuring out just how they may be overstressing their joints. So you may want to be evaluated by a practitioner who specializes in biomechanics.

In addition to a physical therapist or a physician trained in sports medicine or osteopathy, you may want to consider a practitioner trained in one of the following areas to help you with overall body alignment (Appendix B tells you where to find more information about each):

✔ **The Alexander Technique:** Developed by F. Mathias Alexander, an actor who couldn't shake a lengthy case of laryngitis, the basis of this technique is that faulty posture and poor movement habits contribute to problems in both the physical and emotional realms. (Alexander found that his laryngitis was the result of tension and moving improperly.) Students are taught to stand, walk, and sit in ways that are less stressful to the body through the use of movement, touch, and awareness.

✔ **The Feldenkrais Method:** Moshe Feldenkrais, a physicist, martial arts expert, and engineer, devised this method to heal a sports-related knee injury without resorting to surgery. By changing unhealthy movement habits, breathing deeply, and improving the self-image, patients begin to ease their pain. Classes are held in which patients are taken through exercises that increase flexibility, range of motion, and body awareness.

✔ **Trager Approach:** Milton Trager, MD, believed that stress and pain originate in the mind and that bodywork can change the mental and physical habits that lead to them. Although the Trager Approach is more like massage (you lie on a table, and the practitioner manipulates your body), the gentle moving of your body (rocking, stretching, and so on) can help you relax and increase your body-mind awareness.

Although no bona fide studies prove that any of these methods work for arthritis, many physical therapists extol their benefits for rheumatoid arthritis, osteoarthritis, and fibromyalgia. In the end, you have to decide for yourself whether one of these methods is worthwhile. (Remember that it may take several sessions and a significant investment of time and money before you can come to a decision.) But if one of these methods does make you feel better, great! Just make sure you find a certified therapist (see Appendix B), listen to your body, and don't do anything that causes you pain.

Waxing Ergonomic at Your Workstation

With so many of us permanently wed to the computer, the incidence of neck, back, wrist, and hand problems has risen phenomenally, giving birth to a whole new field of study — ergonomics. *Ergonomics* involves the design of equipment that "fits" the body and allows it to function in its least stressful positions. As a result, bodily stress, strain, fatigue, and repetitive motion injuries can be reduced.

When sitting at the computer, think 90-degree angles. Your head and torso should be erect, as if a piece of string attached to the top of your head is pulling you toward the ceiling. Your chin, arms, thighs, and feet should make 90-degree angles to your body as you type. See Figure 13-1 for an example.

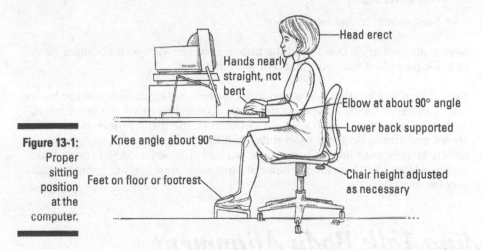

Figure 13-1:
Proper sitting position at the computer.

Head erect

Hands nearly straight, not bent

Elbow at about 90° angle

Lower back supported

Knee angle about 90°

Feet on floor or footrest

Chair height adjusted as necessary

Remember that angling your neck and head downward to read is stressful to your neck. A bookstand or a document holder that attaches to the side of your computer can help you maintain the proper position of your head and neck. When you're sitting at your desk and working at your computer, your body should be aligned as in Figure 13-1.

Take a look at your workstations (both at work and at home) and see if they meet the following requirements. If not, start making the ergonomically correct changes today!

✔ The top of your computer screen should be just below eye level.

✔ Your eyes should be 18 to 28 inches away from the screen.

✔ Your chin should be at a 90-degree angle to your neck when you look at the screen.

✔ Shoulders should be relaxed but not hunched over as you type. Forearms should be at a 90-degree angle to your body, and your wrists and hands should be flat (not bent, flexed, or curled) on the keyboard.

✔ The chair should have adjustable armrests that support both your forearms and elbows at a 90-degree angle. This eliminates neck strain and positions the wrists properly.

✔ The chair's built-in lumbar support, a rolled-up towel, or a cylinder-shaped pillow should support lower back.

✔ Knees should be bent, creating a 90-degree angle between your upper and lower legs.

✔ Feet should be flat on the floor.

Save your own neck! Don't hold the phone receiver with your shoulder as you talk. Either hold it with your hand or get a headset.

Even if your workstation is ergonomically perfect, sitting in one position for too long can wreak havoc on your body. Every 15 minutes or so, get up, stretch, and move around a little to get your circulation going and relieve muscular stress and strain. Do some head rolls, shoulder rolls, and neck stretches. Gently stretch your fingers toward the back of your wrist. Shake your arms and hands and let them dangle loose at your side. Your body is going to thank you for it!

Standing Tall: Body Alignment

You can start improving your posture right now, just by becoming aware of its general principles. Correct posture doesn't just mean a straight back; it's a group effort involving many parts of the body.

Focusing on feet

As you might imagine, standing up straight starts at the ground level. The way you position and use your feet determines how the rest of your body functions.

You should stand with your feet slightly apart and toes pointing forward or just a little turned out. *Turnout* occurs when the toes point away from the center of the body. If you think of your feet as the hands of a clock, pointing at 12 when they're straight forward, a slight turnout would put your left foot at 11 o'clock and your right foot at 1 o'clock.

Distribute your weight evenly across your heel, along the inner edge of the outside of your foot, up to the ball of your foot. (Don't walk on the outside "rim" of your foot, but don't transfer your weight in toward your arch, either.) The weight should also be borne by your big toe, second and third toes, and on the ball of the foot directly under the big toe. Figure 13-2 shows an example of the proper distribution of weight on your foot.

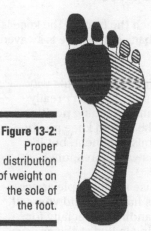

Figure 13-2:
Proper
distribution
of weight on
the sole of
the foot.

Many people carry their weight primarily on the inner edge of their feet, in a line that runs directly from the big toe down to the arch side of the heels. This causes their arches to collapse and their ankles to roll inward or *pronate*. Because the feet and ankles make up the base of the body, pronation throws the alignment out of whack all the way up. (Can you imagine the result if the Eiffel Tower had pronated ankles?) Pronation is a major cause of poor posture, and if you pronate, simply trying to stand up straighter won't solve your posture problem. You need to correct the pronation first. (You may need to see a physical therapist to help you correct the pronation.)

If you're a pronator, try rolling your weight more toward the outer edge of your feet, but not so far that your big toe is no longer bearing weight. See Figure 13-3 for the correct and incorrect position of your ankles.

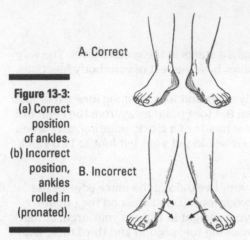

Figure 13-3:
(a) Correct
position
of ankles.
(b) Incorrect
position,
ankles
rolled in
(pronated).

A. Correct

B. Incorrect

Bending your knees — just a bit!

Another cause of misalignment is *locked knees,* in which the front of the knee is completely straight (with no give to it at all) and the back of the knee is swayed back or *hyperextended.*

Many people adopt the locked knees position, because standing this way requires less muscular effort. Your leg and rear-end muscles aren't really holding you up; your leg bones are just locked into an unbending position. It's as if your upper body is perched on two stilts. The locked knee position is tough on knee joints, because it forces them into misalignment, but it's even worse for the lower back, which automatically sways in response.

The locked knees habit is a hard one to break, because most people are completely unaware that they're doing it. If you have this habit, remind yourself to keep your knees slightly bent whenever you're standing, especially for long periods of time. This means when you're standing in line at the grocery store or the bank, and also when you're ironing, doing dishes, waiting for a streetlight to change, or standing over your child while she does homework. Standing this way takes a little more effort, but you build up your "good posture muscles" while you work on healthier joint alignment if you do it.

If you're standing in line at the movies, ease the pressure on your knees by shifting your weight subtly back and forth from foot to foot. Don't put all your weight on one foot; just transfer the bulk of the burden. If you find yourself standing for a long time (for instance, while ironing), you may try putting one foot up on a stool, which helps flatten the back and keeps you from slouching.

"Unswaying" your lower back

Your pelvic bones should face straight forward like headlights on the front of a car. If yours point slightly downward, you may have a *sway back* — a lower back with an excessive curve. Swaying your back is often the result of locked knees and loose stomach muscles. A major cause of back pain, swaying puts extra pressure on the ligaments, muscles, and joints in your spine.

If you're wondering whether you have a sway back, try this test:

1. **Stand with your back to a wall and assume your typical relaxed posture.**

2. **Slide your hand behind your lower back into the space between your back and the wall.**

3. **Your hand should almost be able to touch both your back and the wall at the same time.**

   If you have extra room between your hand and your back, you're probably swaying your back. Try contracting your buttock muscles and tucking them under in order to flatten your lower back. Contracting your stomach muscles helps, too.

Believe it or not, one of the best ways to protect your lower back is to keep your stomach muscles firm and toned. If these muscles are weak, your center of gravity is thrown off, your posture distorted, your back muscles and ligaments strained, and the discs in your lower back unduly stressed. Rather than just "letting it all hang out" when sitting or standing, contract your stomach muscles and tuck your rear-end under. Your posture improves automatically, the pressure on your lower back eases, and you give these muscles a miniworkout.

Relaxing your shoulders

Your shoulders should line up with your ears — not hunched forward but not pinned back behind you, either. Rounding the shoulders is a common bad habit that lengthens upper back muscles and exaggerates the upper back curve while causing the chest cavity to cave in. Not only is this hard on the back and neck, but it's also a very low-energy position. Your lungs can't fill to capacity when your chest is sunken.

Pull your shoulders back to a *midline position* (pulling too far back throws off your alignment), and press down the area between the neck and the shoulders, lengthening the neck. Raised shoulders are full of tension that eventually expresses itself as neck or back pain.

Holding your head high

Your head weighs anywhere from 10 to 12 pounds; no wonder your neck some-times bows under the strain of holding it up! Your neck should have a gentle forward curve to it that's similar to the shape of a banana. Many people jut their heads forward, though, distorting the natural shape of the neck and putting excessive pressure on certain vertebrae.

The "forward head" is the natural result of the round-shoulders, caved-in-chest position that so many of us assume. To correct this, first pull your shoulders back until they line up with your ears, and open up your chest. Then gently pull your chin in toward your neck — not to the point of making a double chin, but a little more than what feels natural to you. Your eyes should be straight ahead and your chin parallel to the floor as you do this.

Putting the posture points together

From stem-to-stern, here are the elements that make up the most efficient and least stressful ways to position your body:

- Head erect, with chin slightly pulled in
- Neck long
- Shoulders relaxed and slightly pulled back; they should line up with your ears
- Buttock muscles slightly tightened to counteract "sway back"
- Stomach muscles contracted
- Knees slightly bent
- Ankles directly over the feet (not pronated)
- Feet apart, weight evenly distributed across the heels, the first three toes, and the ball of the foot directly under the big toe

Now that you know how to stand correctly, you can do a lot to alleviate uneven wear and tear on your joints. But we don't just stand around all day — we move, too! And just as you can save your joints by standing correctly, you can also save your joints by moving in the right ways.

Reducing Joint Stress with the Right Stride

Our Aunt Bessie used to say, "My mother never taught me to walk correctly, and that's why I have bad ankles today." We all pooh-poohed this idea (although not to her face). How ridiculous! Walking is just putting one foot in front of another. What was Bessie's mother supposed to do, other than get her on her feet and let her go?

Today we know that dear old Aunt Bessie was right — there's a correct way to walk, as well as loads of incorrect ways. And no matter how natural it may feel to you, walking incorrectly throws off your body's alignment. The end result is pain, uneven wear and tear on your joints, and (sometimes) permanent joint damage. Think of a car that's out of alignment: Eventually some areas of the tires wear smooth, but others still have plenty of traction. If this goes on long enough, the tires become worthless, and you have to buy a whole new set. The same is true of your joints — although buying a whole new set isn't usually an option! See Figure 13-4 for the correct position of the feet when walking.

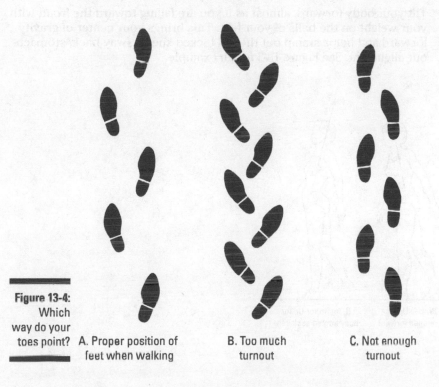

Figure 13-4: Which way do your toes point?

A. Proper position of feet when walking

B. Too much turnout

C. Not enough turnout

Correct walking is based on the principles of good posture with just a few additions:

- Turn your feet out slightly, just 15 or 20 degrees (refer to Figure 13-4). Feet that are turned out more than about 20 degrees (think ballet dancer), pointed straight ahead, or turned slightly inward (think pigeon-toed) throw off your body alignment.

- Make sure your heel is centered as it strikes the ground. (Remember: Avoid "rocking in" on your ankles.)

- Feet should be about 8 to 10 inches apart as you walk. (Don't cross one foot over the other as you step.)

- Keep your knees in an ever-so-slightly flexed position at all times (no "locking back").

- Swing your arms naturally as you walk, moving them in a straight line forward and back, not around your body. Palms should face inward toward your thighs.

- Keep your head erect, with eyes and chin just slightly lower than horizontal level.

- Tilt your body forward, almost as if you are falling toward the front, with your weight on the balls of your feet. This brings your center of gravity forward and helps stamp out the old locked-knees, sway back, stomach-out alignment. See Figure 13-5 for an example.

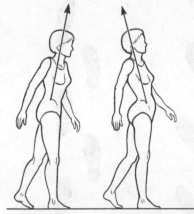

Figure 13-5: Proper angle of the body when walking.

A. Proper-Upper body angled forward

B. Improper-Upper body angled backward

Saving Your Joints When Hitting the Hay

Remember when you were a kid and one of the most fun things in the whole world was to fly through the air and belly flop on your parents' bed? That approach is the exact opposite of the way you should lie down today.

The best way to go from upright to lying flat is to follow these steps:

1. **Sit on the edge of the bed.**
2. **Support your body weight by placing your hands flat on the mattress to one side of your body.**

   You may need to bend one of your arms and lean on your elbow.
3. **Draw your legs up, knees bent, until you can lie on your side.**
4. **Adjust your arms, legs, and pillows until you are in a comfortable position.**

Although most people arise by sitting straight up in bed and then throwing their legs over the side, it's much easier on your joints if you follow these steps:

1. **Scoot over to the edge of the bed while lying on your side, facing the edge of the mattress.**
2. **Place your hands flat on the mattress and push yourself up while you simultaneously swing your legs down to the floor.**

   The weight of your legs counterbalances the weight of your upper body and helps pull you to a sitting position.

If you're lying on the floor during an exercise session and you want to sit up, don't just throw your body up like you're doing a sit-up. Roll to your side and push off with your hands. You help save your back and your neck in the long run.

Lifting Without Losing It

By now, everybody should know that you don't just bend over to pick up a weighty load. This position puts great stress and strain on your back muscles, especially those in the lower back. But if you think about how most people pick up small children, you'll realize that improper lifting goes on all the time.

Protecting your joints

According to the Arthritis Foundation, the following seven keys can help you unload a great deal of joint stress and strain, while helping to prevent further bone and tissue damage:

- Respect pain.

- Avoid improper postures or positions.

- Avoid staying in one position for a long time.

- Use the strongest and largest joints and muscles for the job.

- Avoid sustained joint activities.

- Maintain muscle strength and joint range of motion.

- Use assistive devices or splints, if necessary.

Lifting any size load (even baby-sized ones) should always be done this way:

1. **Make sure the load is as close to your body as possible before lifting it.**

   The farther away an object is, the greater the strain on your lower back.

2. **Keeping your back straight and your neck in line with your spine, bend your knees until you can get your hands under the load.**

   Use two hands for lifting instead of one.

3. **After you have a good grasp, rise by straightening your legs, keeping your back straight at all times.**

Setting down a load should be done in the same way; just reverse the process. And whenever possible, slide the load along the floor instead of lifting it.

If you feel pain while lifting, you're overdoing it. Stop immediately and find another way to get the job done.

Chapter 14

Controlling Your Stress, Aggression, and Depression

· ·

In This Chapter

▶ Understanding how your emotions may increase your pain

▶ Discovering how positive thinking helps reduce pain

▶ Using prayer to reduce pain

▶ Finding an arthritis support group

· ·

*W*e used to believe that pain was simply a matter of a hurting impulse traveling from the "ouch point" up the nerves and to the brain. For example, say the bones in your right knee were rubbing together. The nerves would send a pain message up to your brain, and you'd feel a throbbing, grinding, burning sensation in your knee.

But in 1965, two doctors decided that it wasn't quite that simple. They introduced the "Gate Theory of Pain," which suggests that "gates" exist along the nerve pathways. Like the locks on a canal, these gates can raise or lower to either let pain messages through or block them. And they *don't* automatically have to open wide to every pain message.

Several factors influence this opening and closing of the gates — including your feelings about pain and your experiences with it. Here are some of the things that get those gates swinging one way or the other:

▶ **The way you think about the pain.** Not only what, when, and where, but also your perception of its intensity, duration, and quality.

▶ **The way you feel about the pain.** Emotions that accompany your pain, such as fear, depression, anger, and despair.

▶ **Your tendency to take action in response to the pain.** For example, whether you tend to isolate yourself from others when you're hurt, immediately take pain pills, or take positive self-help measures.

▶ **Your prior experience with pain.** Memories, comparison of this pain to others, your perception of your own coping ability, and so on.

In other words, pain has more to it than the physical problem at the "ouch point." Your thoughts help determine whether the pain messages race through the gates to the brain, move at a more leisurely pace, or crawl slowly along.

Understanding Why We Hurt More Than We Have To

The bad news is that many of us hurt more than we have to, because we're quick to think the unhappy thoughts that help open the gates to pain messages. The good news is that positive thoughts and feelings can close those gates — a little or a lot — and make it harder for the pain messages to get through. Of course, pain is pain, and a brick dropped on your toe hurts. No amount of positive thinking can close the gate on that kind of pain message! But good thoughts can act as healing balms for a fair amount of the chronic pain that comes with arthritis.

Switching from one set of thoughts to another helps reduce your pain, but which thoughts are "good" and which are "bad"? The good thoughts are discussed later in this chapter. In this section, we focus on thoughts and feelings that you need to clear out of your mind to help reduce pain, namely a trio of notorious gate openers: stress, aggression (or what is called *Type A* behavior), and depression.

Ratcheting up the pain with stress

Flares of rheumatoid arthritis and certain other forms of arthritis can be (and often are) associated with stress. As a matter of fact, any kind of pain, brought about by any ailment, can be worsened by stress. Reducing and managing stress, then, can be very helpful.

In simple terms, stress is your body's response to *stressors,* which can be anything that frightens, angers, annoys, scares, or challenges you, or that forces you to change or respond to change. Cars about to ram into you are stressors, as is a nasty boss giving you a rough time. Other stressors include illness, the loss of a loved one, and a failed relationship. Even good things, like getting married or having a baby, can be stressors because they force you to respond to challenge or change.

But stressors and stress are two very different things. Nasty bosses, illness, and failed relationships are stressors, not stress. You may get tense, angry, or frustrated; you may feel helpless and hopeless when these stressors appear — now you're stressed. On the other hand, you may simply ignore the stressors, laugh them off, or find a calm way to deal with them. The facts are the same, but you're not stressed.

Stress can make the "pain gates" swing wide open. If you respond to the stressors by getting stressed, there's a very good chance that whatever already hurts is going to hurt more.

Eliminating stress doesn't magically make all your pain disappear. (And, besides, eliminating stress probably isn't even possible.) But controlling your stress can help ensure that you don't hurt any more than you absolutely have to — and most of us *do* hurt more than is necessary.

You're always going to face stressors, many of which you can't do anything about. But you *can* change your attitude toward them. Reshaping your view of events and taking a more positive approach that calms your reaction to stressors (check out the section "Discovering the Healing Power of Positive Thinking" later in this chapter) can help you reduce your stress and close the pain gates.

Increasing pain the "A" way

People often equate the hectic pace of modern life with stress: You wake up early to get the kids ready for school, hurry to work, race through errands during lunch, drive the kids around, run more errands in the evening, and then scramble to throw together something for dinner, with a cell phone glued to your ear all the while. It's no wonder so many of us are stressed out. Or is it? Several studies suggest that feeling harassed and under pressure aren't to blame. Instead, anger and hostility are the culprits.

You may have heard about the Type A personality — the often angry, hostile, hard-driving, competition-loving person who seems to relish going into battle. Unfortunately, anger, hostility, and aggression can trigger stress and open the pain gates wide.

Are you a Type A personality? Do you

- Hate to waste any time?
- Feel like you always have to be accomplishing something?
- Love to compete with others, just for the fun of winning?
- Often think about your life and accomplishments in terms of dollars earned, cases won, opponents defeated?
- Feel somewhat unsatisfied after each success and immediately begin working for the next?
- Anger easily?
- Always feel like you're behind or that you're racing against the clock?
- Leave little time for hobbies and relaxation, often taking work with you on vacation?

✔ Generally dominate conversations, finding it boring to listen to other people talk about themselves or their interests?

✔ Make snap decisions that you "know" are right?

✔ Often feel like other people are in your way?

✔ Often find yourself locking horns with others?

✔ Feel threatened when someone questions your achievements?

If you answered yes to more than a few of the questions, you may be a Type A, and this may be increasing your pain.

If you're a Type A, the odds are that you can't simply "stop acting that way." You can, however, do quite a bit toward reducing your hostility and calming both yourself and your body chemistry. Try integrating the following behaviors into your busy life:

✔ Slow down!

✔ Make it a point to find someone or something to admire every day.

✔ Take time each day to relax — really relax, not just move your work to a nicer, seemingly more relaxed environment.

✔ Make loved ones and friends a top-of-the-list priority.

✔ Go easy on others.

✔ Go easy on yourself.

✔ Have some fun!

✔ Accept things you can't change.

Heightening pain when you're feeling low

Depression, a common companion to lingering and painful arthritis conditions, can also make your pain feel worse because it affects both your body and your mind.

On the physical front, depression leads to inactivity — at times you may not even want to get out of bed — inactivity, in turn, leads to a general de-conditioning of the body, joint stiffness, decreased flexibility, and weak muscles — all of which can increase arthritis pain. Depression can also raise your sensitivity to pain because it causes insomnia, fatigue, irritability, stress, and anxiety.

On the emotional front, depression is associated with a low level of endorphins, the body's natural painkillers. Too few endorphins can mean increased pain. Your perception of pain also increases when you focus on it. Depressed people typically withdraw from life and become inactive, which increases their self-awareness and focuses their attention on their pain. In short, depression may be the result of pain, but it can cause pain, as well.

As many as 80 percent of those suffering from chronic arthritis pain become depressed about it from time to time. That's not surprising, given that doctors are unable to cure the disease. The good news is that when depression is recognized and treated, pain tends to lessen as well. A study reported in the *Journal of the American Medical Association* in 2003 found that when 1,001 older adults with arthritis received normal or enhanced depression care, more than half of them enjoyed a 50 percent drop in pain intensity, along with significant improvements in quality of life and ability to function.

Identifying the symptoms of depression

Many people don't realize that they're depressed, because the signs of depression aren't always obvious. Besides sadness and feeling low, other possible emotional symptoms of depression include

- Anxiety
- Brooding
- Difficulty concentrating
- Disturbed sleeping patterns
- Excessive or inappropriate crying
- Fatigue
- Feelings of worthlessness or hopelessness
- Irritability
- Loss of interest in formerly pleasurable activities
- Loss of sexual desire or pleasure
- Not laughing as much as usual
- Thinking and speaking slowly
- Withdrawal
- Weight gain or loss

And in some people, depression can show up as physical symptoms that can lead to expensive and unnecessary testing and treatment. These symptoms include

- Abdominal pain
- Back pain
- Headaches
- Worsening of joint pain

Any of these emotional or physical symptoms can and do strike from time to time; we all get the blues. But when several of these symptoms linger day after day for a couple weeks or more, it's considered depression. See your doctor or a mental health professional to help you get through this difficult period.

Seeking medical treatment for depression

Depression should be taken seriously. If you recognize the symptoms of depression in yourself, feel unable to help yourself, or find yourself becoming suicidal, see your doctor or a mental health professional immediately. Although many of the milder forms of depression respond well to the self-help approaches discussed in this chapter, more severe depression can require medication, face-to-face psychotherapy and careful monitoring by a mental health professional.

Lifting your mood to ease your pain

If you have arthritis or any other painful condition, you need to guard against depression and to look for ways to take control of your situation and your life. Thinking good thoughts is like a medicine for the body. It can increase your body's production of natural painkillers, help boost your immune system, and speed healing.

Depression, on the other hand, can increase the sensation of pain, weaken the immune system, and interfere with your ability to participate in treatment and rehabilitation.

Although we can't offer you an instant cure for depression, we can suggest several steps that can help lift your mood:

- **Express your feelings.** Don't pretend everything is all right to please your doctor. If you're frustrated or angry because you're stuck with arthritis and its resultant pain, say so. This doesn't mean that you should misbehave, throw temper tantrums, or break things. Look instead for the middle ground between bottling up your feelings and blowing your top.

  In other words, express yourself in an assertive, yet moderate and positive way. Tell your doctor what hurts and ask for help. If a certain pill or procedure doesn't help, say so and ask for another approach. Tell your family if your pain is preventing you from performing your normal activities and ask for help and understanding. It can also be very helpful to join a support group and express your feelings there. (See Chapter 15 for more information about support groups.)

- **Don't get caught in the "Love Me Because I Hurt Syndrome."** Some depressed people start to subconsciously enjoy what they consider the "good" parts of being depressed (for example, you get lots of sympathy, you're excused from certain chores, you're allowed to act out, you may be given extra treats, and so on). Don't get attached to these secondary gains from depression. Remember, depression can breed more depression, so you need to break the cycle as soon as possible.

- ✔ **Exercise regularly, even when you don't feel like it.** Take brisk walks, ride a bicycle, or otherwise rev up your body and your body chemistry to increase the production of *endorphins,* which are the natural feel-good hormones.

- ✔ **Try to avoid seeing yourself as a victim.** Some forms of arthritis are still mysterious to us, but they're physical diseases, not the results of curses or black magic. New breakthroughs are constantly happening; new therapies and drugs are constantly being developed. At the very least, you can manage your disease. And you can always hope that someone will discover a cure in the near future.

- ✔ **Walk, talk, and act positively!** Even if you don't feel good, approach life with a positive attitude. If possible, don't shuffle. Instead, walk tall and with vigor. Don't mumble; speak clearly and enthusiastically. Don't look down at your feet; look up. Don't avoid other people's gazes; look them straight in the eye. Even if you're only pretending, always walk, talk, and act positively. You may be surprised to find that soon you're not acting anymore — you're really feeling better.

Discovering the Healing Power of Positive Thinking

Stress, Type A behavior, and depression can change your perception of pain, pushing the pain gates open and making you hurt more than you have to. That's one of the reasons why doctors have trouble dealing with pain: They can tell how much cartilage has been worn away and can guess how much it *should* hurt, but they can't gauge whether your attitude is making the pain better or worse.

Just thinking positively may help you close the pain gates, a little or a lot. For example, researchers found that people who had positive expectations before going into hip replacement surgery were more satisfied with their results than those who doubted they'd benefit. And those who imagined that they would enjoy complete relief of pain actually *did* experience significantly less pain and better physical function than those who weren't so optimistic. So maybe you really can make good things happen just by expecting them.

Thinking positively doesn't mean you have to love everyone you meet and everything that happens to you. You can be a positive thinker and still get upset now and then, and you can avoid people or situations you don't like. In fact, letting off a little steam once in a while or staying away from annoying people can be a good idea.

The next few sections present a few of the many techniques you can use to make yourself better equipped, emotionally, to deal with physical pain, and to keep from making that pain worse than it has to be. Which approach is best for you? The one that works. Give them all a try; the ones that help you control your stress and your pain most effectively are the ones you should use.

Relaxing the pain away through biofeedback

Although the body usually runs things as it sees fit, you *can* override some of its instructions. Biofeedback operates on the premise that "seeing" what's happening inside your body may help you control it. During biofeedback sessions, you're hooked up to sensitive electrical equipment that monitors your blood pressure, heart rate, muscle tension, body temperature, and so on. The machine(s) may beep or flash a light every time your heart beats. A continuous display may show fluctuations in your body temperature or blood pressure, and lights may change colors in response to changes in your skin temperature.

These numbers, displays, lights, and beeps give you something tangible to work with as you try to control what's happening inside your body. After figuring out these relaxation and visualization techniques, you may be able to alter these bodily functions for the better — and see the results on the monitors. For example, with practice, many people can lower their heart rates and otherwise calm themselves, even in the midst of stress.

Biofeedback is a wonderful teaching tool that gives immediate reinforcement as you practice relaxation techniques. Eventually, you can apply these techniques in your daily life without the equipment.

You can find a biofeedback practitioner in the yellow pages or by contacting the Association for Applied Psychophysiology and Biofeedback (see Appendix B.) The best plan, however, is to get a referral to a biofeedback technician from your physician. Or your HMO or insurance plan may have a list of biofeedback technicians covered under your plan.

Quieting your mind with meditation and programmed relaxation

Practiced in many different forms, meditation helps you quiet both your body and your mind. Some forms of meditation are exotic, using chants, incense, and foreign terms, but others are plain and simple. However, all forms have one thing in common: a strong, deliberate focus on something outside of the self. Meditation reduces stress by giving you a break from your thoughts, problems, and the stressors in your life.

In basic meditation, you focus strongly on a *mantra,* a special word that is believed to have mystical powers. Repeating your mantra over and over again in your mind is a way of keeping your mind still. As thoughts and images drift into your mind, you simply ignore them and concentrate on your mantra. Soon, they just drift right out again.

Programmed relaxation, also known as the relaxation response, is another form of meditation. But instead of focusing on a mantra, you tune in to your muscles, feeling them tighten and relax in a programmed manner. Programmed relaxation can help relieve the stress that accompanies chronic pain, reduce your overall pain load, and help you sleep better.

You can find out more about meditation and programmed relaxation from many sources, including psychologists, other mental health experts, and meditation centers. Some HMOs and hospitals offer courses in meditation, and some large companies offer them for their employees. You can also find a meditation or programmed relaxation practitioner through the yellow pages or by contacting the organizations listed in Appendix B.

Moving to a stress-free place through guided imagery and hypnosis

Although no hard scientific data proves that guided imagery can dramatically change body chemistry and conditions, many people have benefited from finding out how to put themselves in a better place by imagining happy scenarios. For example, you may imagine yourself relaxing on a beautiful tropical beach when you're actually caught in bumper-to-bumper, rush-hour traffic. You manage to remain calm, at ease, and even happy while those around you are ready to scream with frustration.

The same effect can be accomplished with hypnotherapy. Hypnosis doesn't cure arthritis, but it can help you handle emotional upsets caused by pain, which can help ease the sensation of pain. Hypnosis can help you relax in the face of pain and stress, reduce your stress and anxiety, and make you feel as if you're no longer a prisoner to your pain.

You can find hypnotherapists listed in the yellow pages, or you can contact the organizations listed in Appendix B. The best approach, however, is to get a referral from your doctor or psychologist. (Many psychologists practice guided imagery and hypnotherapy.)

Controlling your breathing

Think about your breathing when you're stressed: You probably take short, shallow breaths. But when you breathe in the opposite manner, with long, deep breaths, your body naturally moves toward a relaxed state. Making it a point to breathe slowly and deeply when you feel stressed can help short-circuit the stress cycle. And by focusing on your breath rather than your fear, frustration, anger, or pain, you can also help derail negative feelings.

Using cognitive behavioral therapy

Cognitive behavioral therapy (CBT) is a form of psychotherapy that helps you discover how certain thinking patterns can exacerbate your problems, and it teaches you how to change your habitual reactions to these problems.

A study of 53 RA patients (reported on in the journal *Rheumatology* in 2003) found that CBT not only helped the patients deal with their anxiety and depression, but also decreased their disability and significantly improved their joint function. CBT fostered more positive attitudes in the patients toward the illness and challenged erroneous beliefs that tended to drag them down (in other words, "I'm going to end up in a wheelchair, so why should I make things worse by exercising?") The patients found out how to couple optimism with realism and to manage their conditions more effectively.

Many (but not all) psychologists use cognitive behavioral therapy in their practices. To find one in your area, access the following Web site: www.nationalregister.org. Click on **Online Searchable Database.**

Laughing your way to relaxation

Undoubtedly, the most enjoyable stress reliever is laughter. A good, hard laugh is believed to lower the levels of cortisol, one of the stress hormones. It also helps you relax all over. Laughing takes your thoughts away from whatever is going wrong in your life, so you can't stew in your own negativity. In fact, many health experts believe that a good sense of humor is like a vitamin for body and soul. And laughter heightens the activity of the body's natural defenses. So the more time you spend laughing, the better your health!

The laughs may not just come to you, so be ready to find the funny if you have to. Spend time with the friends who make you laugh and, most importantly, look for the funny side of whatever life throws you. If you can laugh at your problems, they can't control you. There's almost always something funny in a situation — if you look hard enough.

Forgetting all about it

Even something as simple as distracting yourself from your problems can be helpful. Instead of focusing on your pain, which only increases your stress, try going for a walk with a friend, doing an arts and crafts project, volunteering, going to a singalong, taking a fun class, watching an interesting movie or television show, reading an engrossing book, or listening to some great music. Distraction doesn't cure arthritis, but it does help prevent the stress caused by focusing on pain.

Easing Depression and Anxiety with Prayer and Spirituality

Several studies have shown that people who belong to religious groups and regularly attend services are less depressed and anxious than those who don't. Studies with hospitalized patients support the notion that religion is an antidepressant. We can't be certain why this is so, but it may be because being religious makes you feel that

- Someone very important (a higher power) is looking out for you.
- You belong to something large and wonderful.
- You have a role to play in life.
- You're loved.
- You belong to a community of people who can help support you.

You can also find plenty of opportunities to help others through your church, temple, or mosque; there's nothing like reaching out to others to help you forget about your own pain and feel better about yourself.

Hand-in-hand with religion goes prayer, which itself is often an antidote to stress. The simple act of praying can relieve stress, and the thoughts expressed in many prayers can also have a calming effect. A favorite of many is the Serenity Prayer:

> God grant me the serenity to accept the things I cannot change, the courage to change the things I can, and the wisdom to know the difference.

Of course, you needn't be religious to be spiritual. Spirituality is the quest for a connection with a higher power, however you define that. You can also think of spirituality as a search for meaning in life and as an attempt to understand the world and your place in it. You can express your spirituality through religion, or you can find your own path. Some people approach spirituality through meditation or yoga. Others commune with nature, write poetry, or do charitable deeds. The road to spirituality that you take is yours to choose; you may even define a new one all your own. However you approach spirituality, you may find it a helpful balm for your pain.

Dealing with "helpful" loved ones

As if you didn't have enough in your life to make your blood pressure rise, well-meaning friends and relatives are likely to make you crazy by "helping" you deal with your arthritis. Mary Dunkin (writing in *Arthritis Today*) describes the types of helpful loved ones who may be driving you crazy with their advice. Beware of the following types:

✔ **The caretaker:** This person hates to see you suffering and tries desperately to get you to try one treatment after another. That's because *she* needs to see you well again; what *you* want takes second place in her mind. You gotta love her, but she can drive you crazy.

✔ **The blamer:** This one insists that things would be much better if you would just stop doing things a certain way or thinking certain "silly" thoughts. This may be her way of getting out of helping you. After all, if you'd just shape up, everything would be fine (according to her).

✔ **The evangelist:** This exceedingly "helpful" person absolutely, irrevocably, and unshakably knows exactly what will cure you — and insists you try it. Maybe she was cured by the same thing, is making money off the therapy she's pushing, knows someone who was cured this way, or just believes in it wholeheartedly. And she never lets up about it. This is the helpful loved one that's most likely to make you run and hide when you see her.

✔ **The minimizer:** This person has a very simple cure, even though you have a very complex problem. But no sweat — she knows exactly how to set things right in one fell swoop. Of course, it doesn't wipe out your arthritis, but she continues to insist that it will, if you'll just give it a fair try. (She also thinks that the answer to the nation's drug problem is "just say no.")

What do you say to the caretaker, blamer, evangelist, or minimizer and everyone else who offers unwanted advice? Just say *no!* Gently but firmly tell them you appreciate their concern, but you're following your doctor's advice. If they're really annoying, you can say, "Thanks for your concern, but I've got my own thoughts about my illness. But you're a sweetheart to care so much." That ought to do it!

Chapter 15
Day-to-Day Living with Arthritis

....

In This Chapter

▶ Finding out how to help yourself

▶ Using assistive devices to simplify your life

▶ Reaching out to a support group

▶ Working when you have arthritis

....

rthritis or not, you have a life to live! Like everybody else, you probably have a lot on your plate — a job, family responsibilities, household and gardening chores, a social life, a romantic life, pets, hobbies, and maybe more. But some days, the twin demons pain and fatigue may make you wonder if you can even make it into the next room. On these days, you need to find the most efficient, least stressful ways of accomplishing your goals. But don't wait until you're having a rough day before beginning to think about how to simplify your life. Start today by making a list of the things that you typically need to accomplish each day. Then read this chapter to find ways to take on those tasks with greater ease and efficiency. Jot down ideas as you read and start to make a plan.

Studies have shown that people who take an active part in managing their arthritis and finding new ways to cope with physical disabilities do better and feel less pain and fatigue. Don't let yourself be sidelined as life's parade marches by! In this chapter, we show you how to wrest control of your life away from arthritis by applying these three watchwords to your daily activities: *organizing, planning,* and *prioritizing.* You may be surprised at how much you can accomplish and how good you can feel about yourself, even on a bad day.

Taking Care of You

When you've got arthritis, everyday stresses and activities can become twice as hard to handle. But you can help yourself by visiting an occupational thera-pist to learn the easiest, most efficient ways to get through the day, figuring out how to make the best use of your precious energy, and getting a good night's sleep. Another important part of taking care of yourself is taking care of your sex life, which can still be a happy, healthy, and fulfilling part of life.

Working with an occupational therapist

The occupational therapist (OT), a vital part of your treatment team, helps you get through your everyday activities despite your arthritis. A licensed health care professional, the OT interviews and examines you to determine how your arthritis affects the things you do on a daily basis, such as getting into and out of bed, dressing, grooming, eating, drinking, cooking, getting around, shopping, doing housework, and working.

After the OT gets a sense of where and when you may be having trouble, he comes up with ideas and recommendations. An OT can design splints or supports that conform to affected body parts, recommend and locate a wealth of assistive devices, and come up with plans to help you get through the day with greater ease and efficiency. The OT can also show you joint-protection techniques that reduce joint strain and help prevent further damage.

Many people are tempted to skip occupational therapy, thinking it not really necessary. But those who do so cheat themselves of a great opportunity to attack the practical problems posed by arthritis. Even though medical attention and physical therapy are vital parts of the treatment program, they don't help you figure out how you're going to change a light bulb in the ceiling when you can't raise your arm, or how to get yourself a decent meal when you can barely shuffle around the kitchen. Occupational therapy exists to help you discover easier, more efficient ways of getting through the day. But possibly the most important thing that occupational therapy can show you is how to conserve your energy.

Coping with arthritis when you're pregnant

Becoming pregnant when you've got arthritis can affect your body in several ways. You may find that your joints are less stable and "looser." The additional weight may increase symptoms of osteoarthritis to the knee. Your back tends to sway in response to the additional weight of the baby, so back pain, muscle spasms, or numbness and tingling in your legs can occur. An increase in water weight can increase stiffness in the hips, knees, and ankles (the weight-bearing joints) and can worsen carpal tunnel syndrome.

On the bright side, some forms of arthritis seem to improve during pregnancy. Rheumatoid arthritis, for example, often improves before the beginning of the fifth month, with a decrease in joint swelling. Sometimes lupus and scleroderma improve as well. However, you may experience a flare soon after the birth of the baby.

See both an obstetrician and a rheumatologist during the course of your pregnancy. You should also continue to take your arthritis medicines (if advised to do so by your doctors); exercise to keep your weight under control, your joints flexible, and your muscles strong; follow a nutritious eating plan; observe the rules of joint protection; and use stress management techniques to control mood swings and encourage relaxation.

Conserving your energy

Even if you're the most organized person in the world and you follow absolutely every principle of arthritis management, you only have so much energy. After that runs out, you're like a car that's out of gas — you have to pull over and stop. Don't waste your precious energy; conserve it so you have the "gas" to get through the day's most important tasks.

The Arthritis Foundation suggests the following ideas for conserving your energy:

✔ **Balance activity with rest.** Don't try to do everything at once; work in some breaks between activities. When tackling chores, don't do two difficult ones in a row. Alternate heavy chores with light ones. In the long run, you accomplish more tasks and experience less fatigue by pacing yourself.

✔ **Plan ahead.** Find shortcuts, combine activities that can be done simultaneously, figure out what you can skip, and organize the execution of tasks for maximum efficiency.

✔ **Do the most important things first.** If something absolutely *has* to be done, do it first to make sure it doesn't fall by the wayside as your energy wanes.

Getting a good night's sleep

The best fatigue fighter in the world is a good night's sleep. If you sleep well, you find yourself better able to handle pain, less stressed and less depressed, and more energetic. Unfortunately, many people develop trouble sleeping as they grow older, especially if they're suffering from pain. To give your body the best possible chance of a good night's sleep, follow these sleeping guidelines:

✔ **Go to bed and get up at the same time every day (even on weekends).** Getting up at 7:00 a.m. Monday through Friday and then at 10:00 a.m. on Saturday and Sunday throws off your body's internal clock.

✔ **Keep your sleeping area as dark and as quiet as possible.** Block the light with heavy drapes or blackout shades. Get a white noise machine or turn on a fan to cover up noises that may disturb your sleep.

✔ **Make sure your mattress and pillow are comfortable.** A mattress that is either too hard or too soft and a pillow that doesn't support your head and neck comfortably can interfere with your sleep more than you may realize. If you think you need to make a change, understand that you have loads of options. Ask your OT for recommendations.

✔ **Use your bed for sleep and sex only.** Some people use their beds as the Grand Central Station of their lives — they eat, watch TV and videos, pay bills, read, play with the kids, do office work, and perform beauty routines while firmly ensconced between the sheets. Then they wonder why they can't fall asleep there, too. Your bed should be associated with just two activities — sex and sleeping. It should be the place you go to relax, not to get on with the business of living.

✔ **Get some exercise every day, but not in the latter part of the evening.** Exercising after dinner tends to rev up your body, making it harder for you to fall asleep. Finish your heavy exercise by about 6:00 p.m. (Light exercise, like a stroll or some yoga before bedtime, is fine.)

✔ **Relax for about an hour before bedtime.** Doing yoga, meditating, reading, taking a warm bath, or listening to soft music or a relaxation tape are all good, relaxing activities to help you wind down before going to sleep. Don't try to do 101 chores before falling into bed. You may be exhausted, but your mind is going to be racing and unable to relax.

✔ **Stay away from caffeine in the evening (this includes coffee, tea, soft drinks, and cocoa).** Caffeine is a stimulant and can keep you awake, even if you ingested it hours earlier. A good rule of thumb is to avoid caffeine after 6:00 p.m.

Holding on to your sex life

Having arthritis doesn't mean you can't have a romantic relationship. Nonetheless, you may find that sex takes a back seat when you're trying to manage pain, medication, emotional issues, and physical limitations. You may have become more dependent on your partner, which can change the nature of your relationship. Perhaps physical limitations and/or deformities caused by arthritis have altered your self-image. Medications also may put a damper on sexual desire or performance.

You may also be worried that physical lovemaking is going to be painful: This fear alone can cause a lack of lubrication and/or orgasm in women and problems getting and maintaining an erection in men. Both partners may be acutely aware of the "pain factor," and even when everything seems to be going along okay, as soon as one partner winces, the other immediately becomes concerned rather than desirous. Lubrication stops, erections disappear, and the thought of sexual relations goes out the window.

Fortunately, satisfying and pleasurable sex can still be yours. The most important thing is to focus on the intimacy and closeness that sexual relations can bring, rather than on some preordained standard of performance. Gentle stroking, kissing, caressing, and massage are wonderful ways of expressing sexuality and nurturing one another at the same time. In most cases, intercourse is also possible, although it may require careful positioning and gentle technique.

To make sex easier and more pleasurable, try the following suggestions:

- ✔ Take a warm bath beforehand to relax your joints and muscles and ease pain. This can also help increase circulation to your fingers and toes, which is particularly important for those with Raynaud's. (Light exercise and stretching may help, too.)

- ✔ Take your pain medication so that it kicks in before your session.

- ✔ Some medications can bring on chemical imbalances that cause yeast infections. If you get one of these infections, ask your doctor to prescribe treatment.

- ✔ Talk to your partner about what feels good and what doesn't. Explore various methods of achieving mutual satisfaction. Good communication is an important part of any sexual relationship, and it's vital when difficulties exist.

If you have sexual problems that you and your partner can't seem to resolve by yourselves, seek help from a counselor, doctor, or nurse experienced in dealing with the problems of living with arthritis.

Finding an Easier Way to Get Through the Day

For many people, one of the most frustrating things about arthritis is that it can get in the way of their daily activities, making it hard or even impossible to do certain things that used to come easily to them. When arthritis pain strikes, it can be a big effort to get something off a high shelf or to bend over to make the bed, and just getting dressed can be very tiring. That's why it's important to learn how to simplify everyday tasks so you can conserve your energy.

Simplifying your household

You can also take steps to make other areas of your home easier to manipulate and deal with on a daily basis. Do the following:

- ✔ If you have trouble closing the door behind you, install two cup hooks — one in the door, near the doorknob, and one in the door frame, just outside the hinge area. (Position the cup hooks so they're level with each other.) Run a string or elastic cord between the cup hooks. You now have a cord that's easy to grab and pulls the door shut behind you.

- ✔ Wrap rubber bands around a doorknob that is difficult to turn. This gives you a better grip.

✔ Try using a beaded seat cover on your car seats. The beads roll and make it easier for you to get in and out of your car and then to adjust yourself after you settle in.

✔ Instead of the traditional lace-up style of tennis shoes, try the kind with Velcro closures.

You can also make your kitchen more functional and personalized for you. Personalizing your kitchen makes your daily tasks easier and helps you cope. A few ideas include:

✔ Screw a cup-hook underneath one of your cupboards and use it to pry open pull-tab cans. (In order to get the pull-tab started before the hook can grab it, slide a dinner knife or spoon under the tab and push it up slightly.)

✔ Put Lazy Susans (turntables) on your refrigerator shelves, in your cupboards, and in any other storage areas. This eliminates reaching, straining, and shuffling things around as you try to get an item that's in back.

✔ If dialing a phone is difficult, get a phone with an extra-large keypad or use a pencil to push the buttons. Most phones offer an automatic dial feature so you can call frequently dialed numbers with the touch of a button.

✔ Single-arm faucets (the kind often found in kitchens that let you control the temperature and the amount of water with just one lever) are easiest to use and don't require two hands. Consider getting your kitchen and bathroom faucets converted to this style. If you want to keep your double-arm faucets, try getting wing-type handles that can be operated with your hand, wrist, or forearm.

✔ Use the pointed tip of a can opener to open boxes of hot cereal mix with a "press here" type of opening or to get the metal spouts started on boxes of nonfat milk powder.

✔ If you can find them, get kitchen utensils (carrot peelers, can openers, stirring spoons, and so on) with extra large, rubber-covered handles for easier gripping.

Making household cleaning easier

Back in the 1960s, a popular household cleaner claimed it was so fast and versatile that it could whip through your house like a "white tornado," cleaning everything in sight in no time at all. Although the tips that follow won't exactly make a "white tornado" out of you, they may reduce the time and effort you spend on household chores. Remember to spread your chores out; don't try to get the whole house clean in one day!

If bending over while doing chores is difficult for you, use these tips to make cleaning easier:

- If it's easier for you to sit while sweeping, cut down the length of your broom handle or use a child's broom. The broom does a better job of collecting dust and dirt if the bristles are sprayed with water or furniture polish first.

- For a dirty bathtub, mix together ¼ cup of automatic dishwashing detergent and 2 cups of hot water. Plug the tub, add the mixture, and swirl it around with a long-handled mop. Let it stand for 20 minutes, and then rinse thoroughly with cold water from the shower.

- Stop bending over to plug and unplug your vacuum cleaner! Add a 30-foot extension cord instead.

If you have arthritis in your hands, you want to eliminate chores that involve scrubbing with "elbow grease" or using intricate movements. Here are a few things you can do:

- Cleaning the fireplace is a dirty, unpleasant job, but you can make it easier if you line the fireplace with aluminum foil before you put in the grate and add the wood. After the ashes have cooled, spritz them with water (to keep ashes from flying), remove the grate, carefully pull the foil toward you, and put the whole mess in the trash!

- Instead of scrubbing a pot that has burned-on food, sprinkle ½ cup baking soda in the pot, add a cup or two of water, and simmer for 20 minutes. Allow to stand for two hours. The burned stuff should wipe right off.

- If clutching a dusting rag hurts your hands, try putting old socks on both hands, spraying with a small amount of furniture polish, and then wiping off tabletops and counters with ease.

- Foam pipe insulation is great for covering the handles of tools to make them easier to grasp. You can find it in the hardware store in several sizes and slip it on the handles of your knives, carrot peelers, screwdrivers, mops, or anything else that has a tendency to slip out of your hands.

Using assistive devices

One of the best ways to conserve your energy and keep from putting undue stress and strain on your joints is to use assistive devices — equipment that can make performing a task easier, safer, and more comfortable.

Assistive devices run the gamut from long-handled shoehorns to hydraulic seat lifts that boost you out of a chair, and from bathtub benches to computerized wheelchairs. Some of these devices may require professional installation; others are ready to use upon purchase. You can find many assistive devices at medical supply houses and in mail-order catalogues, or your occupational therapist can steer you to reputable sources. The hardest part is probably deciding which ones are right for you, and your OT also can help you with that task. Here's a partial list of what's currently available:

✔ **Bathing and grooming:** Bath and shower grab bars, toilet safety frames, bathtub benches, foam tubing for handles (for example, toothbrush, hair brush, and so on), raised toilet seats, toothpaste tube squeezers, long-handled bath sponges, and makeup and razor holders are just a few items that can make bathing and grooming easier to accomplish.

✔ **Dressing:** Button hooks, zipper pulls, sock aids, long-handled shoe horns, shoe removers, cuff extenders, stretch shoe laces, and watch winders can help simplify dressing.

✔ **Food preparation and eating:** Large grip utensils (knives, carrot peelers, silverware, and so on), jar openers, can openers, pull-tab can openers, plastic bag openers, nonslip grips for plates and cups, easy-hold cups, and glass holders (with two handles) can aid in meal preparation and eating.

✔ **General household:** Doorknob turners, key turners, car door openers, faucet turners, voice-activated telephones or speaker phones, telephone headsets, voice-activated computer programs (for correspondence), reachers (long-handled devices that grab items), grips for phone receivers, and long-handled sponges and dusters for cleaning can make the handling of household tasks much easier.

✔ **Cleaning the house:** Use tools with long handles whenever possible. A long-handled mop can be used to clean the bathtub or shower, a long-handled feather duster can get those cobwebs out of the corner, and floor wax can be laid down evenly with a long-handled paint roller.

✔ **Getting around:** Canes, crutches, stair walkers, walkers, portable stools, scooters, and wheelchairs can help you become more mobile.

For a list of mail-order catalogues featuring assistive devices, see Appendix B.

Getting help from other people

If you live alone and don't have the luxury of assistance from family and friends, you can handle personal care, household, gardening, and transportation chores in several ways — without trying to do everything yourself. Home health care workers can come to your home and help you dress, bathe, do housework, prepare meals, get to the doctor's office, or do just about anything else you can imagine. Housekeepers and gardeners can take care of cleaning, laundry, and yard work. But if that kind of help is too pricey, look to the less expensive sources of assistance:

✔ Teenagers (either your own or your neighbor's) are often willing to do yard work or other chores for a small fee.

✔ A stay-at-home parent in your neighborhood may be willing to make some extra money by preparing meals or taking you to the doctor.

✔ Your church or synagogue may have volunteers who are willing to help you out for free.

✔ Your doctor, social worker, or other health care workers may be able to refer you to various nonprofit organizations that can offer either inexpensive or free services. Just ask!

Joining an Arthritis Support Group

Support groups are as individual as the people who join them. Some are quite structured, emphasizing education, but others stress emotional support and the sharing of experiences. Some may be designed for those with a particular kind of arthritis, such as osteoarthritis or rheumatoid arthritis, but others are all-inclusive.

Support groups generally have a leader, who may be either a medical professional (for example, a doctor, nurse, psychologist, or social worker) or simply a member of the group. Groups run by their members are often called self-help or peer groups.

If you think you'd like to try a support or self-help group, keep in mind that it may take some detective work and a sizable investment of time before you find the one you really like. Visit several groups and go to each one at least twice. The one-time meeting you observe may be an off night for an otherwise dynamic and helpful group. (Or a good night for an otherwise disorganized and not-very-helpful group.)

One of the great things about support groups is they remind you that you're not alone! You needn't try to master all the arthritis terms and treatments by yourself, because thousands of experts are waiting to help you. Who are these experts? Other people who have arthritis, like the ones in your group.

Finding help and hope through the group

Joining an arthritis or pain support group can be both educational and comforting. Within these groups, you can find the following:

- A chance to talk about your feelings
- A good reason to get out of the house and interact with people
- Encouragement
- Information
- People who can tell you what to expect from a certain test or treatment, because they've already been through it
- People who understand exactly what you're feeling
- Role models — people who are much more "advanced" in their arthritis than you are, but who are living happy, productive, and wonderful lives
- Sympathy

Locating a support or self-help group

To find a support or self-help group (or a pool of groups from which to choose), ask the members of your health care team for referrals. You can also call the Arthritis Foundation at 800-283-7800, or contact any of the other arthritis organizations in Appendix B. If all else fails, you may try looking in the yellow pages under *Psychologists' Information & Referral Services*. Someone listed there may know of an arthritis support group in your area.

And for those of you who don't want to leave the comfort of your desk, you can even find support groups on the Internet; see www.SupportPath.com. If you want information on how to start your own self-help or support group, contact the National Mental Health Consumer Self-Help Clearinghouse, 1211 Chestnut Street, #1207, Philadelphia, PA 19107; phone (800) 553-4539; Web site www.mhselfhelp.org.

Dealing with Arthritis in the Workplace

When you have arthritis, you have some days when you just don't feel like going to work. But you may not have the luxury of staying home every time you have a flare, especially if they happen often. That's why it's important to simplify your tasks at work, just like you did at home, to make them as easy on your joints and as energy-efficient as possible.

If your pain seriously interferes with your ability to do your job and you've done all you can to control it, you may want to consider leaving work behind and applying for disability insurance benefits.

Easing the pain when you work

Many of us spend our workdays sitting down in an office. It sounds easy, but working on a computer, handling correspondence, and doing other paperwork can be difficult if your hands hurt or you can't sit comfortably in a chair. Look into these ideas for streamlining paperwork and making desk duties easier:

- Large scissors with well-padded handles can make cutting easier.
- A rubber grip that fits around the barrel of a pen or pencil makes it easier to hold and less likely to slip.
- Rubber fingers (they look like a thimble made of rubber) can help you turn pages or thumb through a sheaf of papers without fumbling. Or you can twist a rubber band around the end of your finger for the same effect.
- Seam rippers are a nice substitute if you have trouble handling scissors.
- Tape dispensers with some weight and rubberized bottoms make it easier to pull off a piece of tape using just one hand, because they won't move.

If you have Internet access and your employer doesn't object to your handling some office tasks with online business transactions, you can cut down on the time you spend standing in long lines (putting strain on your joints) by doing the following:

- Bank by computer or through the mail. Find out if your bank offers these services. (Most do.)
- Buy your stamps online (www.stampsonline.com) or through the mail. (Call your local post office for details.)
- Buy books, vitamins, gifts — even houses and cars online. The days of pounding the pavement to do your shopping are gone!

Applying for disability benefits

According to the Social Security Administration, if you can no longer do the kind of work you've been accustomed to doing, *and* you can't engage in any other kind of "substantial gainful activity" (anything that pays you more than $740 a month) because of your age, education, and work experience, you may be eligible for disability insurance benefits.

To apply, get a claim form from your doctor, hospital, or your local employment development department office. Your doctor needs to state the exact nature of your medical condition and affirm that, in his opinion, you're unable to work at your present job. But getting disability benefits doesn't mean you can't still work. If you don't relish the idea of sitting at home, look into a special program run by the Social Security Administration that can help you find a job suited to your abilities while you continue to collect your disability benefits. Your local Social Security office can provide you with more details.

Part IV

Is Alternative Medicine for You?

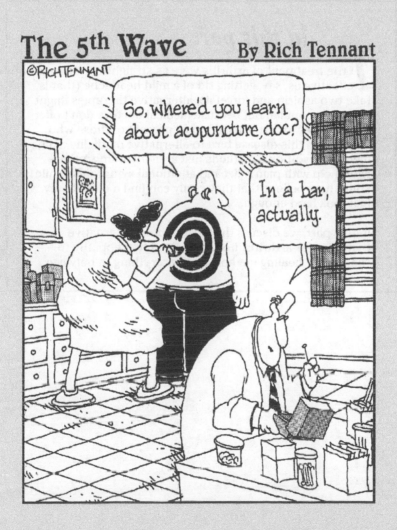

The 5th Wave   By Rich Tennant

So, where'd you learn about acupuncture, doc?

In a bar, actually.

In this part . . .

If the treatment of arthritis were as straightforward and effective as, say, getting rid of a mild headache (that is, take two aspirin and forget it), alternative therapies might not be so popular. But because medical doctors don't offer a real "cure" for arthritis, up to 60 percent of those who suffer from this disease turn to alternative medicine. Some feel that traditional methods just aren't working, others want help with pain relief and additional symptoms, while still others believe that they really can find a cure if they just look hard enough.

In this part, we discuss the most popular alternative therapies for arthritis, from herbs and homeopathy to "hands on" healing methods, and everything in between.

Chapter 16

Exploring Alternative Medicine

Alternative medicine is going mainstream — well, sort of, and only a tiny step at a time. But there has been a major change in the way those who are firmly entrenched within the world of traditional Western medicine view therapies generated by anyone outside their realm. In the early decades of the 20th century, Western medical doctors positively vilified other therapies and crusaded to make practicing other approaches illegal. In fact, well into the 1960s, talking to a chiropractor was considered unethical for a medical doctor!

Fortunately, the attitude that everything Western medical doctors do is great and that other therapies are, by definition, evil, is falling by the wayside. As a society, we've figured out that our medical doctors don't have the cures for all our ills and that other approaches can offer a lot. But the alternative approaches aren't perfect. In fact, many alternate theories and practices aren't backed by enough scientific proof to be declared valid, and some things that alternative healers do have proven to be dangerous. Regardless of the debates surrounding these therapies, however, alternative medicine has become very popular. Countless testimonials to the effectiveness of almost all types of alternative therapies exist, and a fair number of studies indicate that some of these approaches work as well as standard medicines — or even better.

Understanding the Many Faces of Alternative Medicine

Alternative, complementary, holistic, unorthodox, integrative, and preventive medicine: Many similar terms are used to describe the various approaches in medicine. But what do they mean?

CAM you dig it?

Nearly half of all Americans have used at least one kind of complementary alternative medicine (CAM) at one time or another, and more than 80 million are expected to use CAM this year — sometimes to complement and sometimes to replace standard treatment. All told, Americans pay more visits to complementary and alternative healers than to primary medical doctors. According to the *Los Angeles Times,* relaxation and herbs are the most popular CAM therapies.

Who sees CAM healers? Baby boomers make up the largest chunk of patients, especially those who have graduated from college and earn more than $50,000 a year. But the popularity of CAM is steadily growing, and according to a 2002 government survey, more than a third of American adults are now using alternative practices such as yoga, meditation, herbs, natural products, prayer, and special diets.

Defining modern Western medicine (the drugs-and-surgery approach used by medical doctors) as *conventional medicine* is the first step in deciphering the many names of alternative medicine. Anything that's not conventional is considered *unorthodox medicine. Alternative medicine* is an approach used in place of conventional medicine, but *complementary medicine* works with conventional therapies. The concepts of *holistic* and *integrative medicine* are related to each other. Instead of focusing only on the symptoms or the damaged part of the body, the idea behind holistic and integrative medicine is to examine and treat the entire person, including the body, mind, emotions, and spirit. With *preventive medicine,* the goal is to close the door on disease and keep it from striking in the first place. Education, lifestyle changes, and buffing up the body, mind, emotions, and/or spirit are parts of this preemptive campaign.

The most recent term used to describe alternative approaches to conventional medicine is *complementary and alternative medicine,* or CAM for short. According to the National Center for Complementary and Alternative Medicine, which is a part of the National Institutes of Health, CAM incorporates a variety of healing approaches that are, generally speaking, not taught in many medical schools, not used in many hospitals, and not covered by insurance companies. The mere fact that the National Institutes of Health has a division dedicated to complementary and alternative medicine means that acupuncture, massage, nutritional healing, herbology, chiropractic, and other therapies have finally gained a measure of popularity and recognition. Establishing the Center for Complementary and Alternative Medicine legitimized various therapies, and some money (not a lot, but some) is being spent to research these alternative and complementary therapies.

Another indication of the acceptance of complementary and alternative medicine is the fact that two-thirds of United States medical schools offer at least one course in complementary and alternative medicine. Most of these courses are electives (not required classes), but it's a start.

Easing Arthritis Through Alternative Approaches

Look into the medicine cabinet of just about anybody who has arthritis and you're bound to find at least a few bottles of herbs, vitamins, or other supplements that promise to relieve arthritis symptoms. Because there is no real cure for arthritis, alternative approaches to treating this disease are wildly popular and run the gamut from bee venom to prayer. And in most cases, they work — at least to some extent.

In Chapters 17, 18, and 19, we discuss some of the most popular alternative approaches to treating arthritis-related pain, inflammation, and joint dysfunction. We also touch on a few in Chapter 14 — positive thinking, prayer, and spirituality.

Check out the following overview of the alternative techniques most often used for easing arthritis pain:

- **Acupuncture/acupressure:** Releasing energy blockages and pain by inserting fine needles or exerting pressure with the fingers, hands, or special tools on specific areas of the body

- **Aromatherapy:** Using fragrant aromas of substances called "essential oils" to calm the mind and the body

- **Bee venom therapy:** Alleviating arthritis pain with venom from bee stings

- **Chiropractic:** Realigning the spine to relieve pressure on the nerves that may be increasing arthritis pain

- **DHEA:** A hormone that may help ease fatigue, pain, and inflammation in women with lupus

- **DMSO:** A colorless liquid that passes easily through membranes and is used as a topical analgesic to block pain signals

- **Herbs:** The roots, stems, or leaves of plants that can act as anti-inflammatories, antirheumatics, sedatives, muscle relaxants, or pain relievers

- **Homeopathy:** The "like cures like" method of showing the body what's gone wrong so that it can correct itself

- **Hydrotherapy:** The use of hot or cold water, ice, and steam to stimulate or soothe the body and ease pain

- **Massage:** Rubbing, stroking, or kneading the muscles to ease muscular tension and pain

- **MSM:** An odorless crystalline powder, taken in capsule or tablet form or applied to the skin in a lotion or cream to ease arthritis pain (see Chapter 19)

✔ **Polarity therapy:** Balancing the body's energy systems through touching that ranges from light to firm

✔ **Reflexology:** Applying pressure to specific points on the soles of the feet to relieve pain in a corresponding part of the body

✔ **Reiki and touch therapy:** Two ways of channeling healing energy from the hands of the practitioner to the body of the patient, without actually touching

Finding a Reputable CAM Practitioner

You should select a CAM practitioner with the same care that you give to finding the right medical doctor. You can find the names of practitioners of various alternative forms of health care in several ways:

✔ Look for listings in the phone book.

✔ Ask for recommendations from friends or alternative healers who you're already seeing.

✔ Check the list of approved practitioners that your HMO or health insurance company may offer. (Some HMOs and health insurance companies now pay for chiropractic or acupuncture services, and perhaps for other forms of alternative care.)

✔ Get names from the various societies to which practitioners belong. (See Appendix B for the names of some of these organizations.)

✔ Ask your doctor or check with your local hospital. A small number of medical doctors practice one form of alternative medicine or another, and those who don't may make recommendations.

After you put together a list of possibilities, treat them just as you would a list of physicians you're considering. Ask the practitioners you're interested in the following questions:

✔ Where did you study?

✔ Do you have a license or certification?

✔ What is your treatment philosophy?

✔ What does treatment consist of?

✔ What benefits can I expect from treatment?

✔ What are the side effects and how do you recommend handling them?

✔ How will I know whether the treatment is working?

If you feel that your questions aren't answered forthrightly, or that you're being given the runaround, run out the door.

Checking credentials and certifications

Complementary and alternative medicine has a lot to offer, and it can fill in some of the gaps in conventional medical care. Unfortunately, CAM suffers from a lack of standardization. Herbs, for example, may vary greatly in purity and potency. Likewise, although some CAM healers are incredibly knowledgeable and skillful, others are not.

Before selecting a complementary or alternative healer, make sure you do the following:

✔ **See a physician (a medical doctor) to get an accurate diagnosis.** Some forms of arthritis are easy to recognize; others aren't. You need to know exactly what you're dealing with before undergoing any kind of treatment, conventional or CAM.

✔ **Educate yourself.** Gather and study all the information you can about any given CAM therapy before subjecting yourself to it. Read books and articles, get information from the Internet, talk to people, and contact the professional organizations associated with the particular CAM that interests you.

Take all information with a grain of salt until you consider its source carefully. Is the person or group that offers this information knowledgeable? Does she have a solid educational background and/or practical experience? Is she an unbiased source or a salesperson?

✔ **Ask for credentials.** Ask the CAM therapist where he studied, whether he's licensed by the state, certified by a board, and so on. Don't be shy or afraid to ask questions. Any healer — conventional or CAM — who won't happily review his or her background with you isn't a good prospect. And don't be afraid to ask for the name and phone number of the school or society that issued the credentials so you can investigate that organization.

✔ **Ask for references.** Ask the CAM therapist for the names and phone numbers of people he has already worked with. Contact these people; ask them what they were suffering from, what the CAM practitioner did for them, how well the therapy worked, what the side effects were (if any), and so on.

✔ **Ask about the price.** Insurance doesn't cover most CAM therapies.

Identifying false claims

Everyone wants a miracle pill that can cure his ills. And everyone would like it even better if that pill were tiny and easy to swallow, worked instantly, didn't cost more than a pack of bubble gum, and had to be taken only once.

Unfortunately, such a cure doesn't yet exist for arthritis. This fact hasn't stopped some people from claiming that they have miracle cures for all your aches and pains, however. Most alternative practitioners are honest and sincere, but hucksters always happily tell you tales to take your money. So safeguard your health and pocketbook by watching for the following warning signs.

✔ **The "secret formula" trap:** Be wary if the cure offers no list of ingredients or is based on a secret formula. Claiming that something is secret can be an easy way for hucksters to avoid admitting that their "cure" doesn't contain anything remarkable. Reputable healers, on the other hand, are happy to tell you exactly what they're proposing that you take. And knowing what you're taking is important, for even if the stuff in the secret formula is helpful, it may interact dangerously with a medicine or supplement you're already taking. Or perhaps you're allergic to the secret stuff, or it's just not right for you.

✔ **One-study wonders:** Proceed with caution if the health practitioner bases all the claims for the treatment on only one study. It's true that only one study may be necessary to establish that a treatment works, but it's better if the therapy has been studied many times, with different patients and under different conditions. A therapy may work in one study with, say, elderly and bedridden osteoarthritis patients, but not work so well when tested again with younger or more active subjects. The more studies, the better. Reputable healers know this, which is why they want to cite as many studies as possible for their therapies.

✔ **Catch-all cures:** Avoid cures that purport to work for all types of arthritis — and other diseases as well. Nothing is a cure-all. As you recall from the discussion of arthritis early in this book, the many different forms have widely different causes and symptoms. How could one remedy work for all of them?

✔ **The case-history game:** Be wary of any therapy if its proof of effectiveness is made up entirely of case histories. Although the case histories may be absolutely genuine, they aren't as valid as large-scale, long-term, carefully controlled scientific studies. After all, the patients in the case histories may not have had the same form of arthritis as you do, may have had complicating conditions, and may not have been given uniform doses of the therapy. The placebo effect may also account for the good results in the case histories. (That is, some of the patients may have gotten better primarily because they *believed* in the therapy.)

A lack of studies doesn't mean that a therapy is bad, and good study results by themselves don't guarantee that a treatment or therapy can work for you. Having a combination of both studies and case histories to review is best.

✔ **Miracle cure myths:** Steer clear of practitioners who promise that their approach is the long-awaited *miracle cure,* the magic potion that erases all your problems. Some standard and alternative cures are amazingly effective, but no one has yet developed a miracle cure that eases all our ills.

✔ **Shady demands:** Avoid practitioners who tell you to throw away your crutches, stop taking your medicine, or ignore your physician's advice. Likewise, be wary of those who demand large amounts of money in advance or who don't want you to tell your physician what they're doing for you. In general, trust your instincts and don't do anything that you don't feel good about.

Working with Your Doctor

At least 40 percent of patients use alternative therapies, but perhaps three-quarters of them don't tell their physicians what they're doing. Many patients don't inform their physicians because they're afraid that their doctors may pooh-pooh their ideas, tell them that they're foolish, try to talk them out of it, or even refuse to continue working with them if they insist on using CAM.

You, too, may be tempted to keep what you're doing a secret from your physician, but don't. Telling your physician everything you're doing, from taking herbs to using bee venom therapy, is important, because you may inadvertently do something that clashes with one of your medical treatments. For example, combining St. John's wort with antidepressants can cause severe central nervous system depression and can even be deadly.

Talking to physicians about alternatives can be difficult. They have the weight of medical authority on their side. They've gone to medical school and can speak a language that you may not understand. But don't be intimidated. Doctors work for you; they're here to serve you. You have the right to ask questions and receive complete answers. To practice medicine effectively, a doctor must also practice good communication. A physician who closes his ears tosses away an important tool for understanding what his patients need. For more information about finding a doctor with great qualifications — and great ears — turn to Chapter 6.

Try these tips for discussing CAM with your physician:

✔ **Begin with the assumption that your physician is supportive.** If you open your conversation with a challenge or disparaging remark, you probably won't get very far. Make it clear up front that you're not challenging or rejecting your doctor's ideas, but that you're simply looking for more information and help.

✔ **Ask your physician what she knows about the CAM that interests you.** Ask her whether the CAM is appropriate for your ailment, whether you need to watch out for anything while participating in the alternative therapy, and so on.

- ✔ **If your physician doesn't know about the CAM that interests you, offer her information.** Go online and get studies about the CAM, copy pages from articles and books, ask the CAM's professional organizations to supply you with information, and then help your doctor find out more about the CAM that you're considering.

- ✔ **If you don't have time to discuss CAM during this visit, ask for another appointment.** Offer to pay for the extra appointment, if necessary.

- ✔ **If your physician gives you trouble, ask why.** Does he know that this CAM is dangerous? Has he had a bad experience with it? Has he seen patients in which the CAM had negative or dangerous results? Is his objection based on knowledge or simply a feeling that anything unconventional is bad?

- ✔ **If your physician refuses to discuss CAM with you or refuses to work with you if you're using a CAM, get a new doctor.** Closed-mindedness is a terrible trait in any healer and may limit your road to recovery.

Be as open-minded as you want your physician to be. Take into consideration any bad reports about the CAM that interests you, as well as the good reports. No healing art, conventional or unconventional, is perfect. Each has its strengths and weaknesses, and it's best to know what your CAM can do for you — and what it can't.

Figuring Out Whether Alternative Medicine Is for You

Deciding whether to experiment with alternative therapies is a very individual matter and depends on many things: How dissatisfied you are with traditional Western therapies, how adventurous you are, how willing you are to try unproven or controversial methods, what your inner voice tells you, and how your body responds.

If you opt for alternative treatments, always remember that many of them aren't supported by reams of scientific studies, so you're taking a chance. Always research any therapy you'd like to try, find yourself the most qualified and highly recommended practitioner, consult with your physician before and during treatment, and make sure that your physician monitors your progress. But perhaps the most important thing you can do is listen to your body: Are you feeling better? Does this approach seem to be working? Sometimes even the most scientifically sound method won't help you, whereas something strange and virtually inexplicable does. Your body possesses its own brand of wisdom — when it speaks to you, make sure you listen.

Chapter 17

Discovering Herbs and Homeopathy

In This Chapter

▶ Knowing the difference between herbs and drugs

▶ Treating arthritis with herbs

▶ Delving into homeopathy and how it works

▶ Combating arthritis with homeopathic remedies

Many people are frustrated by the inability of standard Western medicines to cure their arthritis or relieve their symptoms completely, so they look for relief from some of the older, more "natural" remedies. Two of the most popular remedies are herbal medicine and homeopathy.

Herbal medicine uses plants and plant parts to stimulate the body to return to a state of internal balance. Herbs used to treat arthritis generally fall into the classes of anti-inflammatories, antirheumatics (which are immunosuppressive and inflammation-fighting), sedatives/muscle relaxants, and pain relievers.

Homeopathy, on the other hand, is a system of medicine based on the idea that medications should be given to stimulate the body to cure itself, rather than to counteract the symptoms of an illness. So a tiny bit of the "disease" is introduced to the body, which prompts the body to get to work on healing itself. Homeopathic remedies for arthritis usually target the swelling and tenderness caused by inflammation.

Digging Into Medicinal Herbs

Ever since man began roaming the earth, healers have been using *herbs* — any plant whose leaves, seeds or flowers can be used for medicinal, flavoring, or aromatic purposes — to cure or at least alleviate what ails us. Some herbs are eaten in their natural form. Others are ground into powder, crushed, or squeezed to make oil or extract; brewed with boiling water to make tea; or mixed with beeswax, petroleum jelly, or cream to make ointments or balms.

What's the difference between a healing herb and a drug? Drugs are often stripped, highly refined versions of herbs. About one quarter of all our modern medicines come from herbs. To turn an herb into a drug, pharmacological researchers work with the herb, refining it and homing in on the main ingredient that produces the herb's effect. This ingredient is separated from the rest of the plant, modified in some way, perhaps concentrated, and standardized so that each pill or capsule delivers an exact amount. Then it's sold as a drug.

The good part about this approach is that it allows us to extract the special part of the herb, like a great soloist in an orchestra, that cures a particular ill. The bad part is that herb refinement lets us have only that soloist, casting aside the rest of the orchestra.

Doctors say drugs are better than herbs because the active ingredient is isolated, drugs are modified and pure, they're served up strong, and they work much faster than herbs.

Herbalists (those who practice the medicinal and therapeutic use of plants) say that herbs are better than drugs because the so-called active ingredient is only one of many substances that work in concert to relieve or cure ailments. Modifying and purifying the active ingredients makes them overly strong, dangerous, and more likely to cause side effects. Herbalists point out that some of the alleged impurities in herbs can actually make them gentler and safer. And although speed is sometimes necessary, many times it's not essential to effective treatment. Furthermore, drugs that work fast can also be overly harsh.

Herbs: Everything old is new again

No one knows exactly when people began using herbs or who realized that eating certain leaves could help stop an ache in the head and that drinking the liquid made from boiling roots in water could bring on sleep. But once the connection was made, people undoubtedly gathered whatever they could find and started experimenting. Some results worked well, and others sent them back to the drawing board. Herbs were a vital part of ancient medicine. The Egyptians used garlic and other herbs as medicines as early as 1800 B.C. Hippocrates, the Greek known as the father of medicine, developed a way to classify herbs based on qualities, such as heat versus coldness, and dampness versus dryness. Herbs were the backbone of medicine until the development of modern pharmaceutical-based medicine in the 19th and 20th centuries, and herbs continue to be a mainstay of Native American, Ayurvedic, and Oriental medicines.

Although herbs, like homeopathic remedies and other therapies, were swept aside by the tidal wave of pharmaceutical drugs pouring out of laboratories during the 20th century, they were certainly never forgotten. Indeed, herbs still serve as the source of one-fifth of all modern drugs. Even today, pharmaceutical companies are scouring the world (especially the tropical rainforests), looking for previously unknown plants that may have medicinal properties. They also routinely ask herbalists and traditional healers about herbs in their quest for new sources of drugs.

Although many pharmaceuticals are more potent and potentially more dangerous than most herbs, all herbs should be considered "drugs" as well because they are a concentrated source of active ingredients. The fact that something is natural does not guarantee that it's safe. (Just think of arsenic.)

Getting the Lowdown on Herbs for Arthritis

Which herbs have medicinal value? How much should be used? Which are good for osteoarthritis and which for rheumatoid arthritis and gout? Should they be taken in powder form, rubbed on as ointment, or sipped in the form of tea? The answers you get to these and many other herbal questions may depend on whom you ask, and whether he is a doctor of Oriental medicine, an herbologist, a naturopath, a chiropractor, or the clerk at the vitamin store. Unfortunately, no national board of herbology exists to set standards and doses, so the advice you receive about herbs to treat arthritis undoubtedly varies from one healer to another. A variety of herbs may be prescribed, some specifically for your type of arthritis, others for joint problems in general, and still others for pain, depression, or strengthening the immune system.

Keep in mind that some of these herbs have been subjected to scientific studies of their effects on arthritis. The following herbs have been proven to ease the symptoms of arthritis:

- Aloe
- Angelica
- Boswellia
- Capsaicin
- Cat's claw
- Chinese Thunder God Vine
- Devil's claw
- Ginger
- Kava kava
- Stinging nettle
- Valerian

Inside the herbalist's toolbox . . .

Herbal medicine is used to treat just about anything that can go wrong with the human body — from hemp for treating glaucoma, to fringe tree bark for fighting liver disease, to Essiac tea for combating cancer. A tremendous number of herbs are at home in the herbalist's little black bag, including:

- *Agrimony* for allergies
- *Cayenne pepper* to strengthen the immune system
- *Celery* for arthritis
- *Feverfew* for migraine headaches
- *Fringe tree bark* for liver disease
- *Garlic* for elevated cholesterol and blood pressure
- *Ginger* for nausea

- *Ginkgo biloba* for problems with memory and circulation
- *Goto kola* for varicose veins
- *Hemp* for glaucoma
- *Hyssop* for asthma
- *Kava kava* for anxiety and insomnia
- *Linden* for tension
- *Sambucol,* an elderberry extract, for the flu
- *Skullcap* for asthma
- *St. John's wort* for insomnia and depression
- *Turmeric* for inflammation
- *Valerian* for asthma
- *Vervian* for headaches

The following herbs may or may not have benefits for arthritis sufferers but have not yet been tested:

- Alfalfa
- Black cohosh
- Bladderwrack
- Burdock
- Celery seed
- Centaury
- Fennel
- Meadowsweet
- Mustard
- Sarsaparilla
- Wild yam

Even though many people consider herbs to be safe, it's best not to self-medicate. You could do more harm than good to yourself, especially under the following circumstances:

- You may have an allergic reaction.

- The herb may interact with another medicine that you're taking, which could increase the intended effect of either, create the opposite effect, produce a toxic effect, or otherwise affect the body in harmful ways.

- You may have a medical condition that makes it dangerous for you to take a particular herb.

- The herbal concentration is too strong, too weak, or the herb is mixed with other ingredients that your body cannot handle. (The U.S. government does not regulate the content and quality of herbs, supplements, vitamins, and other non-drug alternatives, so you really *don't* know what you're getting.)

Avoid potential risk by checking with your health advisor before taking any herbs. Make sure your physician knows that you are taking herbs or planning to take them. Even if he is not an advocate of alternative healing methods, your physician should be aware of everything you're taking.

Anti-inflammatories

Inflammation, when a part of the body becomes reddened, hot, swollen, and painful, is a major problem in several forms of arthritis and related conditions. Doctors have powerful anti-inflammatory drugs, like the corticosteroids, but many people prefer the gentle relief offered by herbs such as those listed below. Anti-inflammatory herbs don't suppress inflammation on their own as much as they help the body reduce the inflammation naturally.

Alfalfa

Rich in minerals, alfalfa is a folk remedy for arthritis favored in the Middle East for its ability to reduce swelling and inflammation. Alfalfa is scientifically known as *Medicago sativa*.

Angelica

Angelica, or *Angelica archangelica,* has been used to treat the inflammation associated with rheumatism. This herb is also believed to purify the blood and protect against contagious diseases.

Black cohosh

Scientifically known as *Cimicifuga racemosa,* black cohosh is a Native American remedy taken to reduce the inflammation and pain of rheumatoid arthritis.

Bladderwrack

Rising to prominence in the early 1800s, Bladderwrack was originally used as a source of iodine. Today the herb, known by the scientific name *Fucus vesiculosus,* is used in compresses to help reduce arthritis inflammation.

Boswellia

Known scientifically as *Boswellia serata,* boswellia comes from India, where its gummy resin has been used for thousands of years as an anti-inflammatory. Substances in boswellia, called *boswellic acids,* are believed to reduce inflammation and help relieve the pain of osteoarthritis and rheumatoid arthritis. It has also been used to treat psoriasis, ulcerative colitis, and allergies, and may also help lower high cholesterol and high triglyceride levels. Boswellia is used as an extract, cream, or ointment.

Cat's claw

The extract of the bark of a vine native to the Peruvian rainforest, cat's claw was used for generations by the Ashanica Indians of South America to treat colds, tumors, and cold sores. Known scientifically as *Uncaria tomentosa,* the herb is considered useful in combating arthritis symptoms in several ways; it may be recommended by herbalists to reduce inflammation, boost the immune system, and ward off free radical damage to the cells. Cat's claw is taken in the form of tea or capsules. The herb may also help counteract gastrointestinal damage caused by NSAIDs, discussed in Chapter 8.

Centaury

Also known by its scientific name, *Erythrina centaurium,* centaury was used by the ancient Egyptians to reduce high blood pressure, and later by German herbalists for anxiety and melancholy. Today, it's often recommended for cases of gout and rheumatism because of its ability to help relieve inflammation.

Devil's claw

Devil's claw, or *Harpagophytum procumbens,* is the root of an herb grown in Africa. An infusion made of devil's claw, which is believed to reduce joint inflammation and pain, is a folk remedy for arthritis, rheumatism, and gout. This herb is most commonly used in capsule, tea, and tincture form. Devil's claw contains harpagoside, which has pain-relieving and inflammation-reducing qualities that have been compared to cortisone and phenylbutazone.

Sarsaparilla

With the official name of *Smilax officinalis,* sarsaparilla originated in the New World and was brought to Europe in the 1600s. There, the herb was used to treat inflammation due to rheumatoid arthritis. Herbalists still use it today to relieve the pain and swelling of arthritis and to enhance overall well-being.

Wild yam

Known scientifically as *Dioscorea villosa,* wild yam is perhaps most famous as a traditional "female remedy," used for menstrual ailments and to prevent miscarriage. It also has anti-inflammatory properties, which is why herbalists recommend it for rheumatoid and other forms of inflammatory arthritis.

Antirheumatics

Several herbs seem to be especially helpful in reducing the symptoms of rheumatoid arthritis (joint inflammation in a majority of joints, swelling in two matched joints, fever, fatigue, and so on) and related conditions. Here are a few of the better-known antirheumatics.

Bogbean

Once used to prevent scurvy, this pretty wildflower is renowned for its ability to relieve the pain of rheumatism. Known to scientists as *Menyanthes trifoliate,* bogbean has mild sedative properties.

Be careful, however, because large doses of bogbean may cause vomiting. It should not be used if you have inflammatory bowel disease.

Celery seed

Scientifically known as *Apium graveolens,* celery seed was used by Oriental healers to reduce elevated blood pressure. And the celery stalk was prized by Americans during the 1800s because it was so expensive. Today, celery seed and celery juice are used to rid the body of excess water and aid in digestion. The seed is also believed to ease both rheumatoid arthritis and gout.

Chinese Thunder God Vine

Used medicinally in China for over 400 years, an extract of the root of the toxic Thunder God Vine *(Tripterygium wilfordii)* eases pain and inflammation safely and effectively in patients with treatment-resistant rheumatoid arthritis. The extract helps to "turn off" an overactive immune system and tone down the activity of certain inflammatory genes. Researchers believe that Chinese Thunder God Vine also has potential as a treatment for lupus, although more study is needed.

Meadowsweet

Meadowsweet *(Filipendula ulmaria)* contains a substance with aspirin-like properties. The herb has been used for hundreds of years to relieve arthritis pain and help combat rheumatic conditions.

Sedatives and muscle relaxants

Sleep can be a major issue for those with some forms of arthritis. How well can you sleep if you hurt, if movement is difficult, or if you're worried and stressed? The herbs in this category can help you relax and sleep better.

Kava kava

A popular treatment for insomnia and nervousness, kava kava *(Piper methysticum)* promotes relaxation of the muscles and nervous system without diminishing mental alertness. By helping you relax and perhaps sleep better, this herb can help you deal more effectively with the stress of arthritis.

Valerian

Known as *Valeriana officinalis,* valerian comes from the rootstock or roots of a perennial herb. It is typically used in the form of capsules and extracts. Valerian is recommended for arthritis patients because it helps ease pain and tension, and it also encourages sleep. In Germany, valerian is used as a mild sedative, and one study showed that it worked as well as a standard sedative drug with the added advantage of being non-addictive.

Tea, please

Not all herbs are taken as pills or capsules. Some are taken in the form of teas or, more accurately, *infusions.* (Technically speaking, the only true "tea" is one made from tea leaves, or the leaves of the *Camellia sinensis* bush.) To make an infusion, the herb is submerged in water that is just slightly cooler than boiling, and then left to steep as its health-promoting ingredients seep into the water. After a few minutes, the herb is skimmed out, and the liquid is ready for drinking.

Try infusions of any one of these or a combination of a couple, as they suit your mood:

- ✔ **For a pick-me-up:** basil, borage, ginseng, Hawthorne berry, bilberry, cinnamon, yarrow

- ✔ **For depression, stress, or tension:** borage, catnip, jasmine, hops

- ✔ **For a digestive aid:** ginger, juniper berry, Iceland moss, alfalfa, angelica

- ✔ **To strengthen the immune system:** elderflower, green tea, goldenseal

- ✔ **To promote sleep:** chamomile, orange flower, valerian

Don't take more than the recommended dosage — very high doses can cause a weakened heartbeat and even paralysis. Check with your physician to see how much you should take.

Pain relievers

Pain is perhaps the most significant symptom of many forms of arthritis. Dull or sharp, constant or intermittent, achey or gripping, pain can make your life miserable. Here are some of the better-known herbs that can help relieve pain.

Aloe

Used internally or externally, aloe is a popular herbal cure for the pain of wounds, burns, and arthritis. Known to the scientific community as *Aloe vera* or *Aloe barbadenis,* it can also be used in the form of a fresh leaf, a gel, capsule, lotion, or liquid. In addition to relieving arthritis pain, aloe has been used to treat gastrointestinal problems and ulcers, as first aid for wounds and burns, and as a mild laxative.

Taken internally, aloe may hamper or increase the action of certain medications and cause uterine contractions or miscarriage in those who are pregnant.

Burdock

Burdock *(Arctium lappa)* is an ancient remedy that has been used to treat snakebites, dog bites, and a variety of other conditions thought to leave impurities in the blood. Today's herbalists have found that burdock has a diuretic effect and may ease arthritis pain as well as skin irritation due to psoriasis, eczema, and canker sores.

Capsaicin

Capsaicin, which comes from chili peppers, is the ingredient that makes the spice cayenne so darn hot. Capsaicin is believed to prompt the release of endorphins, the body's natural, built-in pain relievers, and to interfere with substance P, which helps transmit nerve signals through the nervous system. Known scientifically as *Capsicum frutescens,* capsaicin is used to treat pain. It's typically applied as a cream or taken as a tea or capsule.

Fennel

Well-known among chefs, fennel has also been used to relieve stiff, painful joints. Herbalists and folk medicine healers often suggest that their patients apply fennel oil directly to their distressed joints and rub it in. This herb's scientific name is *Foeniculum vulgare.*

Ginger

The aromatic root of a tropical herb, ginger has been used by the Chinese to treat indigestion, stomach cramps, and stomach upset for over 2,000 years. Scientifically known as *Zingiber officinale,* ginger may be recommended by modern herbalists for arthritis patients. Studies have shown that taking ginger supplements or eating fresh ginger can help ease the pain, morning stiffness, and inflammation associated with some forms of arthritis, while increasing flexibility and range-of-motion.

Ginger is typically taken as a powder, capsule, extract, tea, or tincture. It can also be freshly grated and added to food or eaten as a side dish. Ginger compresses may be applied to painful joints.

Mustard (black)

A preparation of mustard, or *Brassica nigra,* has long been a favorite remedy for painful joints. Sometimes it's taken internally (often with honey), and sometimes it's applied directly to the joint. (Mustard oil plus rubbing alcohol can be applied to the skin to increase circulation to the affected area.) Black mustard is generally considered stronger and more effective than white mustard.

Knowing tincture from extract

A lot of terms are casually tossed about by herbalists and herbal enthusiasts: *extract, infusion,* and so on. Here are a few definitions to help you find your way through the sometimes-confusing world of "herbal speak."

✔ **Botanical medicine:** The use of plants or plant parts to treat or lessen the symptoms of illness, ease aches and pains, and/or restore health.

✔ **Extract:** A key ingredient of an herb or plant is isolated and drawn out using steam or water; then the ingredient is condensed into liquid or powder form, known as an *extract.*

✔ **Herb:** A plant or part of a plant valued for its medicinal, aromatic, or savory qualities.

✔ **Infusion:** Boiling water is poured over an herb or plant part and then allowed to steep to release the plant's useful qualities into the liquid.

✔ **Nutraceutical:** Any food or component of food that has a therapeutic or medicinal effect.

✔ **Raw herbs:** Fresh or dried parts of plants, plucked right from the ground, bush, vine, or tree.

✔ **Standardized extract:** An herbal extract manufactured to deliver an exact concentration of the desired ingredient.

✔ **Tincture:** Herbal preparations made by steeping herbs in alcohol.

Stinging nettle

A prickly plant with stinging hairs that "inject" an irritant into the skin, stinging nettle has traditionally been used to treat allergies, insect bites, and wounds. Today it may be recommended to relieve joint pain and swelling; laboratory studies suggest that stinging nettle can counteract at least some part of the inflammatory response. A German study found stinging nettle plus a small amount of an NSAID to be as effective as the full dose of the NSAID in relieving symptoms of osteoarthritis. In addition, stinging nettle contains boron, a mineral important for bone health. Known scientifically as *Urtica dioica*, stinging nettle is typically taken as a capsule or extract. A poultice of cooked leaves may be applied to the painful area.

In addition to the preceding herbs, your herbalist may suggest black willow, caraway seed, cinnamon, clove, couchgrass, dandelion, juniper berries, oats, nutmeg, poke root, prickly ash, skullcap, spearmint, star anise, wintergreen, wormwood, yarrow, and more. Suffice it to say, herbalists can draw from a lengthy list of herbs when recommending treatment for arthritis pain, inflammation, anxiety, depression, insomnia, skin rashes, muscle pains, and other symptoms!

Stimulating the Body to Heal Itself with Homeopathy

Before drugs and surgery came to dominate Western medicine, healers called *homeopaths* flourished in the United States and Europe. Their guiding philosophy was *homeopathy,* which means "similar suffering."

The idea behind homeopathy, which was created by Dr. Samuel Hahnemann in the 18th century, is to stimulate the body's natural healing mechanisms by, in a sense, "showing" it a piece of what's wrong. This may sound odd; after all, we're accustomed to modern Western medicine killing disease with strong medicines. But Dr. Hahnemann believed that "like cures like." If large amounts of a substance could cause the symptoms of a disease in a healthy person, he reasoned, then very small amounts of the same substance should be able to help the body eliminate the same ailment. These small doses would act something like vaccines and gently stimulate the body to heal itself.

For example, suppose that a large amount of Substance X caused constipation in healthy people. According to Dr. Hahnemann's homeopathic theory, a very tiny dose of the same Substance X would unlock the bowels in people who were already constipated. This idea was codified as homeopathy's *Law of Similars.*

Determining remedies according to your symptoms

While medical doctors try to suppress symptoms, doctors of homeopathy look upon them as helpful signs that the body is trying to heal itself. To the homeopath, symptoms are more than simply indicators that a certain disease is present. Instead, they are the body's way of describing what has gone wrong on a physical, mental, and emotional level. Probing beyond the symptoms (where Western medicine stops), homeopaths look for the essence of their patients. Thus, they ask what the patients like to eat and drink, when and how well they sleep, whether they're day or night people, what they wish for and what they fear, what kind of weather they prefer, how they respond to stress, and so on.

If you complain of pain, a good homeopath looks beyond its location, intensity, and number of occurrences. He or she asks additional questions, such as:

- ✔ When does it hurt?

- ✔ What are you doing when it starts to hurt?

- ✔ How are you feeling, emotionally, before the pain strikes?

- ✔ What does the pain feel like? Is it sharp? Throbbing? An ache? Does it radiate? Is it constant? Does it come and go?

- ✔ What makes the pain feel better? A warm bath? Eating certain foods? Going to work?

- ✔ What makes it feel worse? Movement? Cold temperatures? Stress? Work? Family gatherings? Holidays?

These kinds of questions are designed to get to the essence of the problem: the physical and emotional state that allowed the disease to take hold and grow.

After the homeopath identifies the essential problem, it can be treated — but not with a medicine designed to destroy anything. Instead, the homeopath looks for the single best remedy (homeopathic "medicine"). What remedy is most effective depends mostly on the patient. If a patient has joint pain, for example, not just any remedy for pain will do. It has to be the remedy that best matches the patient's *constitutional makeup*. Every one of the 2,000 or so homeopathic remedies closely matches a particular temperament — a person's fears and hopes, likes and dislikes, and sleep and behavior patterns.

In *classical homeopathy,* only the absolute minimum dose of a remedy is given, and only one remedy is prescribed at a time. If the right remedy is given, the patient's symptoms begin to clear up in a few days. If not, a different remedy is selected. No new remedies are used after the body has begun to heal itself. Practitioners of *complex homeopathy*, however, prescribe more than one remedy at a time.

Discovering recipes for remedies

Homeopathic remedies are derived from a variety of sources: leaves, berries, fruits, bark, roots, minerals, and sometimes animals. But no matter where they come from, they're all processed in a very special way.

In keeping with the idea that small amounts are best, the remedies are diluted over and over again in solutions made of water and alcohol, lactose, or other diluents. And each time they're diluted, they are shaken and struck in a special way. The more diluted, shaken, and struck, so the theory goes, the stronger the remedy becomes. Indeed, a finished remedy may only contain one part per million of the active ingredient. Critics charge that very little or even none of the active ingredient remains after these successive dilutions, so the remedy couldn't possibly work. Supporters believe that either 1) what's left over is enough to do the trick; or 2) that the fluid retains a "molecular memory" of the medicinal substance and acts accordingly.

Remedies are rated according to their potency. When one drop of the medicinal substance is shaken and struck into 99 drops of diluent, the remedy has a potency rating of 1c. (This mixture is sometimes written as 1CH.) If one drop is taken out of this mixture and added to 99 drops of new diluent, the new remedy has a potency rating of 2c. If one drop of the 2c remedy is then diluted with 99 drops of a new diluent, the potency rating rises to 3c, and so on.

How potent the remedy should be depends on the state of the disease. Here are the general guidelines used in the United States and many other countries:

- ✔ **Low potency:** Up to 6c, used when only physical symptoms or severe changes in the disease state exist.

- ✔ **Medium potency:** From 12c to 30c, used when physical and mental/emotional symptoms exist.

- ✔ **High potency:** Up to 200c or greater, used when the problem is long-standing or acute, or the symptoms are mental/emotional.

Another, very similar rating system is based on 10 drops of diluent rather than 99. Instead of shaking and striking one drop of substance into 99 drops of diluent, you use only 9 drops of diluent. In this method, based on 10 drops, potencies are rated 1x (or D), 2x, 3x, and so on.

Homing in on homeopathic remedies for arthritis

Most homeopathic remedies come from minerals or plants, and only a few are derived from animals. Homeopathic remedies are not highly concentrated; in fact, they're diluted again and again until only minuscule amounts of the original substance are left.

This method is counter-intuitive to practitioners of Western medicine, who believe that medicines should have more of the active ingredient, not less. But remember, homeopaths argue that smaller portions are better, because larger portions can cause the arthritic problem. The tiny portions, they insist, help the body heal itself.

Self-medicating is never a good idea and can lead to unintended consequences, interactions with other substances, and possible damage to your health. No matter how much you may have heard about the safety of homeopathic remedies, working with a medical doctor or doctor of homeopathy is essential when you're using them. If you are using any homeopathic remedies, be sure your physician knows exactly what and how much you're taking. Even if he or she doesn't believe in homeopathy, your physician should be aware of what you're taking.

The purpose of the homeopath is to find the best match between remedy and patient. The remedy that the homeopath selects depends as much on the patient's constitutional makeup as it does on the symptoms, which is why you can't just pull any old arthritis remedy off the shelf. The following are some of the homeopathic remedies used for arthritis:

- *Aconitum napellus:* May be indicated for gout. The pain grows worse at night or when temperatures rise, and gets better when the patient rests or gets fresh air. The patient is anxious and imagines terrible things are happening.

- *Actea spic:* May be indicated when the joints are swollen and pained, and the focus of the arthritis is in the hands and feet or the smaller joints.

- *Ammonium carbonicum:* May be indicated when poor circulation to the hands exists, as in Raynaud's phenomenon (see Chapter 5).

- *Apis mellifica:* May be indicated when the joints are stiff and swollen, when pressure makes the pain worse, and when the skin over the swollen joints feels stretched and tight.

- *Arnica montana:* May be indicated when the patient has rheumatoid arthritis linked to cold and dampness, and soreness and bruising are problems. The patient is nervous and extremely sensitive, prefers to be alone, and denies that anything is wrong.

- *Belladonna:* May be indicated for sudden, sharp pain, and red, swollen joints. Getting wet or chilled makes the pain worse, and the patient usually avoids any kind of stimulation.

- *Benzoic acid:* May be indicated when rheumatoid arthritis settles in the smaller joints, and nodular swellings exist.

- *Bryonia alba:* May be indicated for gout with greatly swollen joints. Heat, movement, or touch makes the pain worse; cold, rest, and pressure help.

- *Calcarea carbonica-ostrearum:* May be indicated for rheumatoid arthritis in the shoulders and upper back. Wetness and dampness worsen the pain, and fear and perhaps confusion engulfs the patient.

- *Causticum:* May be indicated when arthritic joints are stiff and tight. Lying on the afflicted joints increases the soreness, and the patient is restless at night.

- *Chamomilla:* May be indicated for severe pain when anger and restlessness are present.

- *Cimicifuga racemosa:* May be indicated when pain is centered more in the muscles than the bones. Restlessness, talkativeness, and an unstable mood often accompany the pain.

- *Ledum palustre:* May be indicated when pain is primarily in the smaller joints and travels up the body, with little or no swelling. Pain is worse when patient is in a warm bed.

- *Ruta graveolens:* May be indicated when the patient suffers from bursitis (see Chapter 5).

- *Sabina:* May be indicated when the patient is suffering from gout, and the gouty joints have nodules. The pain worsens with heat and movement, feels better with cool air, and is usually accompanied by depression.

- *Sambucus:* May be indicated when the patient is suffering from poor circulation to the hands, as in Raynaud's phenomenon. The hands are blue and cold, and the patient sweats excessively while awake, but not while sleeping.

Finding homeopathic help

No one has proven why or how homeopathy may work, and while some studies suggest that it's significantly more effective than a placebo, others have found it unimpressive. Although all the evidence is not yet in, many people are convinced that homeopathy is right for them. Homeopathy is practiced by a variety of healers in the United States: naturopaths, chiropractors, herbalists, dentists, acupuncturists, and even certain medical doctors and doctors of osteopathy (DOs). The level of training and skill, however, varies from healer to healer, so be forewarned!

The National Center for Homeopathy (see Appendix B for contact information) offers a directory of homeopaths in the United States. You can also find homeopaths by asking for referrals from certain physicians and other health professionals, reading the ads or listings in alternative health newspapers and magazines, or contacting homeopathic pharmacies.

Chapter 18

Hands-On Healing Methods

. . . .

In This Chapter

▶ Exploring the different types of Eastern and Western touch therapies

▶ Understanding the theory behind the therapy

▶ Knowing what to expect during a therapy session

▶ Getting to know the possible benefits of each therapy

▶ Finding a competent practitioner

. . . .

For thousands of years, healers have known that the "laying on of hands" can have a powerful therapeutic effect on the body. And why wouldn't it? Human beings are made to be touched. Babies fail to thrive if they're not touched enough. Huddling together against the cold was undoubtedly a survival technique for scores of our ancestors, and lovemaking is perhaps one of life's most fulfilling, restorative activities. Therefore, looking to hands-on methods for healing your body when it's ill or in pain makes sense. This type of therapy doesn't necessarily cure the disease, but it can help relieve pain, increase vital circulation, ease mental stress, relax tensed muscles, increase overall relaxation, and aid the body in its struggle to rebuild itself.

The various methods of hands-on therapy, from the ancient acupressure to the relatively new trigger point therapy, are explored in this chapter. Keep in mind, however, that if you decide to engage in any of these therapies, you should use them in addition to — not in place of — standard medical treatment, and you should first discuss your preferred therapy method with your physician.

Unblocking the Energy Flow: Eastern Hands-On Healing Methods

These therapies, which are rooted in either Chinese or Japanese medicine, are designed to remove blockages and restore balance in the body's energy flow. After balance is restored, the body can begin to heal itself.

Pinpointing the pain with acupuncture

An important part of traditional Chinese medicine, *acupuncture* has been used for thousands of years to prevent and treat disease by balancing the body's energy flow.

In traditional Chinese medicine, disease is thought to be the result of an imbalance or blockage of energy or *chi* (pronounced "chee") in one or more parts of the body. (Air and food supply us with energy, while the stresses and strains of living diminish this energy.) Acupuncturists believe that manipulating specific points on the body can unblock the energy flow and restore the body's balance.

According to traditional Chinese medicine theory, energy flows through the body along invisible channels called *meridians.* Twelve major meridians run through your body to deliver energy and sustenance to your tissues, but these channels can become obstructed. When they do, the obstructions act like tiny dams, blocking or slowing the flow of energy and serving as a major cause of pain and disease. Luckily, the meridians touch the surface of your skin at some 300 different points called *acupuncture points,* and by manipulating and stimulating these points, the acupuncturist can remove the obstructions and reestablish the healthy flow of chi throughout your body.

When you first visit an acupuncturist, she will probably interview you extensively about your symptoms, level of pain, medical history, diet, bowel habits, quality of sleep, and so on. She may also examine your eyes, tongue, skin, or fingernails; take your pulse; and listen to your voice, breathing, and bowel sounds.

During your visit, you either lie or sit on a padded table for the treatment, but you won't have to remove all your clothing, just loosen it and uncover the areas to be treated. Your acupuncturist then stimulates and manipulates certain acupressure points, but just a few — not all 300 of them! The following list explains the various methods your acupuncturist may use to do this:

✔ **Inserting fine needles:** Your acupuncturist may insert anywhere from 2 to 15 hair-thin needles into certain points and leave them standing for a period of time (usually 20 to 40 minutes). He won't necessarily insert the needles directly into the area that's bothering you, but rather along the meridian that affects that area. So don't be surprised if your feet are manipulated to ease your back or neck pain! The needles are so fine, you may not feel them, but if you do, you usually feel just a moderate sting that disappears quickly. Your acupuncturist may insert needles shallowly (just under your skin) or as deep as an inch or more.

- **Adding a low-level current (electro-acupuncture):** Many acupuncturists have found that the addition of a low-level electrical current can make the treatment more powerful. Wires are attached to the acupuncture needles after the needles are inserted, and these wires are hooked up to a box that delivers an electrical current. Your acupuncturist adjusts this current by turning a dial. You should feel a light buzzing at your acupuncture points. If the buzz is annoying or uncomfortable, tell your acupuncturist, and he can turn down the "juice" until it no longer bothers you.

- **Using heat and herbs (moxibustion):** To stimulate your acupuncture points, your acupuncturist may burn a small amount of an herb called *mugwort* (or *moxa* in Chinese) over your acupuncture points, being careful not to burn your skin.

- **Cupping:** Small glass cups are heated and placed over your acupuncture points where they create a vacuum-like effect. As they cool, the cups invigorate these areas.

Discovering what acupuncture can do for you

More than 15 million Americans have used acupuncture to treat ailments ranging from asthma to ulcers, but its primary use is for pain relief. Many people with osteoarthritis, rheumatoid arthritis, gout, fibromyalgia, and Raynaud's phenomenon swear by acupuncture, and some studies have shown that it can relieve pain caused by osteoarthritis and/or fibromyalgia. Although no scientific explanation for its effectiveness exists, acupuncture does produce real responses in the body, including stimulation of the immune and circulatory systems and the release of endorphins, the body's natural painkillers.

You may require several acupuncture sessions (perhaps as many as six) before you begin to notice a difference, but once the beneficial effects set in, they often last for weeks, months, or even longer. Unfortunately, acupuncture doesn't work for everyone.

Finding a good acupuncturist

To find a good acupuncturist, begin looking for one who is licensed by the state, if your state happens to be one that licenses acupuncturists. (Some states don't.) It's also a good idea to look for a practitioner certified by the National Certification Commission for Acupuncture and Oriental Medicine (NCCAOM), acupuncture's equivalent to the American Medical Association. Some 13,000 practitioners have been certified by the NCCAOM, so you can probably find at least one in your area. Or, if you like the idea of receiving acupuncture from someone with a medical degree, contact the American Academy of Medical Acupuncture. It can provide you with a list of MDs or DOs (doctors of osteopathy) who have completed 200 hours of medical acupuncture training, had two years of medical acupuncture clinical experience, and performed at least 500 medical acupuncture treatments. (See Appendix B for more information.)

Finally, ask the members of your health care team for referrals, because more members of the traditional Western medical community are becoming aware of the benefits of acupuncture. (Who knows? Maybe some of them see acupuncturists themselves!) It doesn't hurt to ask, and your medical team members may be able to give you some good leads.

Pressing your buttons with acupressure (shiatsu)

Acupressure (which the Japanese call *shiatsu*) is a lot like acupuncture, but instead of needles, the therapist presses on your acupuncture points using the fingers, hands, or special tools to unblock your energy flow and restore balance. Because acupressure involves hands-on manipulation, it's often considered another form of massage instead of a version of acupuncture. Because it's actually a combination of these two methods, both acupuncturists and massage therapists often use acupressure.

Instead of lying on a padded table as you do during an acupuncture session, during acupressure you lie on a mat on the floor for better resistance against the pressure exerted during treatment. Using the thumbs, fingers, whole hand, elbows, or feet, the practitioner applies pressure and manipulates your body along meridians to improve your flow of *chi* (energy). He may also use tools, such as wooden rollers, balls, or pointers. As the practitioner works to unblock your *chi,* he also works to transmit some of his own energy into your body. Your acupressure session may include stretching or other kinds of massage, and some practitioners also give diet and lifestyle tips.

Discovering what acupressure can do for you

Acupressure is designed to produce the same pain relieving and energizing results as acupuncture — without the needles, of course! Like massage, acupressure has a calming and soothing effect, and that alone may help ease some of your symptoms almost immediately. Although good studies demonstrating its effectiveness don't currently exist, acupressure does work for some people, without side effects (when it's properly done). At the very least, your acupressure session should be a pleasant experience.

Finding a good acupressurist

Contact the National Certification Commission for Acupuncture and Oriental Medicine (NCCAOM) to find a certified acupressurist. (See Appendix B for more contact information.)

Many massage therapists also use acupressure techniques. To find one that does, check out the American Massage Therapy Association (AMTA) Web site. (See Appendix B.) At the top of the AMTA homepage, click **Find a Massage Therapist**. Click on **Search Engine**, and then enter your city, state, and (under modality) click on **acupressure**. If nothing comes up, try eliminating the city.

You may also find referrals through your health care team, rehab center, pain management center, or chiropractor.

Restoring healing energy with Reiki

The word *reiki* (pronounced "ray-kee") is a combination of two Japanese words — *rei*, meaning a higher intelligence or spiritual consciousness, and *ki* (or chi in Chinese), meaning the life force or energy that animates all plants and animals. Therefore, *Reiki* is a healing energy guided by a higher intelligence or a spiritual power.

A Reiki practitioner administers the treatment by laying his hands on specific parts of your body and applying little or no pressure. (You remain fully clothed.) Some practitioners don't actually touch, but rather place their hands directly above the patient's body. The practitioner then channels healing energy into you, which helps to relieve energy blockages and balance the life force within your body. This technique is sometimes used along with some form of massage. The basic principle of Reiki is that universal life energy, which creates and maintains all forms of life, can be channeled into a patient by the practitioner as a force for healing.

Discovering what Reiki can do for you

Enthusiasts say that Reiki can help ease the pain and other symptoms of virtually every kind of illness and injury while increasing the effectiveness of all kinds of therapy. Although the practitioner may not actually touch the patient, those who have experienced Reiki say that they feel a glowing radiance flowing throughout their bodies after a 60- to 90-minute session. Stress reduction, relaxation, and an increased sense of well-being are typical benefits of a session.

Finding a good Reiki practitioner

Check out The International Association of Reiki Professionals Web site. (See Appendix B for more information.) Click on **Locate a Reiki Practitioner or Teacher**, and then click on your state to get a list of Reiki practitioners in your area.

Realigning and Releasing Tension: Western Hands-On Healing Methods

While Eastern therapies are based on releasing energy blockages and restoring the chi, Western therapies contain a potpourri of approaches, ranging from manipulating the alignment of the spine to applying pressure to specific points on the sole of the foot. Each is based on a different theory, and each takes a completely unique approach to pain relief.

Realigning the spine with chiropractic

First introduced to the Western world in the late 1800s by Daniel David Palmer, chiropractic is based on the belief that the body has the power to heal itself, and that power is concentrated in the central nervous system, extending from the brain down through the end of the spine. According to Palmer, disease is the result of the spinal vertebrae causing undue pressure on nearby nerves. This pressure interferes with the healthy functioning of the tissues or organs served by those nerves, causing disease or damage. According to the chiropractic theory, manipulating the spine to relieve nerve pressure can eliminate illness and restore health.

Misalignments in the spine that put pressure on the nerves are called *subluxations* and can be caused by injury, poor posture, stress, lack of exercise, or genetic problems, just to name a few. You won't necessarily be able to feel that you have a subluxation (they're often very minor imbalances), and you probably won't realize that a misalignment in your back could be causing the pain in your kidney. That's why you visit the chiropractor. She can tell by touch or other simple tests where your spine is out of alignment and then adjust it accordingly.

When you visit a chiropractor, she asks you about the location, duration, and intensity of your pain and how long you've had it. If it seems appropriate, she may take an X-ray of the area.

After your X-ray, you go to the adjustment room where you lie face down on a padded table. The chiropractor feels along your spine looking for vertebrae that are out of line, tension in the muscles, swelling, or any other abnormalities. Then, she may use a variety of methods to apply controlled, directed forces to your spine, including straight massage, acupressure, trigger point therapy, and myofascial release. All these methods fall into the category of *spinal manipulative therapy* (SMT) and aim to release stress, improve alignment, relieve pain, and improve function. Many chiropractors also use a tool called an activator that resembles a tiny, rubber-tipped pogo stick. The activator delivers a precise, measurable force that, when applied to specific points on your body, helps adjust misalignments. And, of course, the chiropractor may "crack" your back or neck to relieve pressure within a given area of your spine.

The term subluxation has different meanings in Western medicine and in chiropractic. In Western medicine, *subluxation* refers to the incomplete or partial dislocation of a joint, in which the bony surfaces no longer face each other. No such condition can be corrected by chiropractic treatment. In chiropractic, a *subluxation* refers to subtle, minor imbalances in a joint, usually those involving the spinal vertebrae, which interfere with the spinal cord and/or spinal nerves, causing pain.

Discovering what chiropractic can do for you

Chiropractic can be a very effective treatment for acute lower-back pain, as well as a faster, better way to treat certain types of neck and back pain than standard Western medicine, massage, or acupuncture. Chiropractic may be a useful way to treat headaches, muscle spasms, knee pain, and shoulder pain. It is also used occasionally to relieve pain in the hip, knee, or shoulder, although it doesn't usually work as well in those areas as it does in the neck and spine.

Manipulating already-damaged joints can make them worse. Consult your physician before trying chiropractic, and make sure you let your chiropractor know that you have arthritis.

Finding a good chiropractor

Begin your search for a chiropractor through referrals from friends, especially if you know someone who has been treated by several chiropractors over the years and can compare their strengths and weaknesses. Otherwise, check the American Chiropractic Association's Web site (see Appendix B for more information), click on **Find a Doctor** and enter your city, state, and zip code for a referral list. Then start making trial visits. Many types of insurance now cover chiropractic if you go to one of their designated practitioners, so you may want to get a list from your insurance company. After you narrow your choices, look for a chiropractor who:

- ✔ Has had experience in treating patients with your type of arthritis.
- ✔ Spends at least 20 minutes with you each session, performing hands-on work.
- ✔ Doesn't pressure you to buy vitamins or supplements.
- ✔ Doesn't rely on gadgets, such as back massaging beds, infrared lamps, waterbeds, or vibrators.
- ✔ Takes few, if any, X-rays.
- ✔ Performs myofascial release or some other soft-tissue massage before adjusting your spine.

You may need several treatments before you see a noticeable improvement. However, if you aren't getting results after five or six treatments, chiropractic (or your current chiropractor) may not be for you.

Rubbing away muscle tension with massage

Massage is the manipulation of body tissues by rubbing, stroking, kneading, or tapping using the hands or other instruments such as rollers, balls, or pointers. For most kinds of massage, you lie on a padded table, wearing little or no clothing, covered by a soft flannel sheet. Your body remains covered by the sheet throughout the massage, except for the area that's actually receiving the treatment.

If you're uncomfortable with the idea of disrobing in front of the therapist, remember that you only need to take off enough clothing to reveal the areas that you want massaged. Keeping your underwear on is definitely okay! It's also possible to be massaged while sitting in a chair, completely clothed. (Sometimes this is done in the workplace.)

The therapist asks you what kind of massage you'd like (invigorating, relaxing, and so on), if and where you're experiencing any pain, and how firm or soft a touch you'd prefer. If you like, the therapist may darken the room and play soft music during the massage. Oil or lotion (usually pre-warmed) is used so that the therapist's hands glide over your skin without causing friction.

Speak up! It's not necessary to get a whole body massage unless that's what you want. If you just want work done on your neck, feet, and hands, for example, say so. And don't be afraid to give your therapist feedback during the massage: Tell him or her what's painful, what's soothing, what you'd like more or less of, what kind of pressure feels best, and so on. The therapist adjusts the technique and pressure accordingly. The whole point of massage is for you to relax and feel comfortable, so be clear about what you need.

Many kinds of massage are available, but here is a list of some of the most popular:

✔ **Swedish massage:** Also known as *effleurage*, Swedish massage involves the gentle kneading and stroking of muscles, connective tissue, and skin, using oils or lotions. Sometimes clapping or tapping movements are also used. Therapists can make this method of massage as gentle or as vigorous as you like. If you have fibromyalgia, rheumatoid arthritis, or another particularly painful form of arthritis, a gentle Swedish massage may be just what you need to help you relax.

✔ **Shiatsu:** Also known as acupressure. (See the section titled "Pressing your buttons with acupressure (shiatsu)," earlier in this chapter.)

✔ **Deep tissue massage:** This method of massage involves the exertion of intense pressure to relieve chronic tension deep within the muscles. Using fingers, thumbs, and sometimes elbows, aching, knotted, or chronically tense muscles are slowly stroked across the grain to release tension and induce relaxation. Deep tissue massage can be painful and may cause soreness during and after the session. But if favoring your painful joints causes chronic tension to develop in other parts of your body, deep tissue massage may be a way to release the tension.

Make sure you consult your doctor before trying deep tissue massage.

✔ **Rolfing:** Rolfing was developed in the 1950s by Ida P. Rolf, a biochemist who discovered therapeutic bodywork when an osteopath successfully treated her for a respiratory problem. Dr. Rolf's treatment is based on the idea that both physical and psychological health are affected by the alignment of the body. If the body is out of line, poor physical, mental, and emotional health results.

To correct body misalignment, the Rolfing practitioner stretches and manipulates the thin membrane called the *fascia* that covers each bone, muscle, organ, nerve, and blood vessel. The fascia can become tight in response to stress, injury, or chronic misuse. To release this tightness, the practitioner uses his or her fingers, knuckles, or elbows to apply intense pressure. Administered in one-hour sessions once a week for ten weeks, Rolfing is uncomfortable at best; at worst, it's quite painful. But proponents of this method claim that it can produce marked improvement in muscle function and reduced strain on the joints. Combined with special breathing techniques, Rolfing may also help release the buried emotions that create chronic physical tension.

✔ **Myofascial release:** Myofascial release is a milder form of Rolfing in which the practitioner applies gentle but steady pressure to the fascia to stretch it and release tension.

Rolfing and/or myofascial release may be too painful for many arthritis patients. Make sure to get your doctor's permission before trying out either of these kinds of massage.

✔ **Sports massage:** This form of massage is intended to ease soreness; assist in healing sports injuries such as sprains, strains, tendonitis, or muscle soreness; and prevent future injury. Like Swedish massage, sports massage involves kneading and stroking the muscles and connective tissue, with an emphasis on the areas of your body most affected by the sport (for example, the shoulder and arm of a baseball pitcher or the knees and legs of a football player). If you have an injury or an inflamed joint, make sure that your massage therapist is a qualified expert in this type of massage.

✔ **Trigger point therapy:** Using the fingers to apply prolonged, deep tissue pressure to specific points on knotted, painful muscles, trigger point therapy relieves tension and helps muscles relax. This therapy causes the pain sensors in the pinpointed area to "overload," so they either send fewer pain messages or stop sending them altogether. In some cases, trigger point therapy can be a helpful treatment for fibromyalgia.

Trigger point therapy is a treatment that feels so good — when it stops! Let's say, for example, that you have chronic tension in your neck that you just can't seem to release. To perform trigger point therapy, your massage therapist or chiropractor asks you to lie face down on a padded table and then proceeds to apply intense thumb pressure to a specific point where your neck and shoulders meet. (Yes, it hurts!) Your therapist maintains this pressure for a good 30 to 45 seconds (or as long as you can stand it), but after the pressure is released, your chronic neck tension should be gone (or at least, greatly reduced).

As with deep tissue massage, Rolfing, and myofascial release, you should check with your doctor before engaging in trigger point therapy.

Injured and/or inflamed joints should not be massaged directly, as injured tissue may be further damaged, and the increased circulation brought about by massage may make swelling worse.

Discovering what massage can do for you

Like most kinds of hands-on therapy, massage can significantly affect your well-being — at least temporarily. A slower heart rate, increased endorphin levels, decreased pain levels, and improved relaxation are just a few of the positive results. Like a nice warm bath, a good massage can increase your circulation and then go two steps further. It helps your body clear away by-products of metabolism that can irritate nerve endings, and massage eases pain by increasing your level of endorphins — the body's natural morphine.

Some types of massage may not be appropriate for your type of arthritis. Consult your doctor for guidelines before getting massage therapy, especially if you have rheumatoid arthritis, osteoarthritis, or ankylosing spondylitis. Also, avoid massage if you've got a fever or infection, if you're having an arthritis flare, or if you're coming down with an acute illness.

Be sure to drink plenty of water prior to and following a massage. Massage can help release built-up toxins in the muscles, and you can help your body flush them out by keeping well-hydrated during this period.

Finding a good massage therapist

Locating a skilled massage therapist who is experienced in treating clients with arthritis should be one of your top priorities. Fortunately, your physical therapist or doctor may be able to steer you to someone suitable.

For a therapist who specializes in a particular type of massage, consult the Web site of the American Massage Therapy Association (see Appendix B for more information). At the top of the AMTA homepage, click **Find a Massage Therapist**, click on **Search Engine**, and then enter your city, state, and (under modality) the kind of massage you prefer. If nothing comes up, try eliminating the city and run another search.

You can also get referrals from the National Certification Board for Therapeutic Massage and Bodywork Web site (see Appendix B) or from your health care team, rehab center, pain management center, or chiropractor.

But just as important as technical qualifications is the chemistry between you and your therapist. The sex of the therapist, in fact, is an issue for many people. If you feel a little strange about being massaged by a man, for example, you should automatically narrow your search to include women only. Remember, if you don't feel completely comfortable with the therapist you choose, you won't be able to enjoy all the benefits of massage. So shop around; you may want to try several therapists before deciding on one person. Keep in mind that many massage therapists come to your home with their massage tables and all the accoutrements in tow. All you have to do is pick up the phone!

Promoting energy balance with polarity therapy

Like traditional Eastern systems of healing, *polarity therapy* is based on the belief that the body contains energy systems that must remain balanced because unbalanced or blocked energy leads to pain and disease. The aim of polarity therapy is to find these blockages and release them by using the hands to touch specific points on the body, which should help restore balance. After balance is achieved, the body should return to a healthy state.

During your first visit, the practitioner interviews you, observes your body and the way you move, and manually feels certain areas of your body to determine the location and degree of your energy blockages. The therapy itself involves touches that can vary from light to firm, but you don't have to disrobe, and the touching involves your verbal feedback. A typical session lasts from an hour to an hour and a half.

Discovering what polarity therapy can do for you

Your polarity therapy practitioner works to help you increase your awareness of *subtle energetic sensations*. For example, you may feel mild waves of energy coursing through your body, tingling, warmth, or general relaxation. Your practitioner may also offer advice on diet and lifestyle. The aim of polarity therapy is to relieve your pain and help your body heal itself, but currently no studies confirm that polarity therapy actually achieves these goals.

Finding a good polarity therapy practitioner

To find a practitioner of polarity therapy, call up the Web site for the American Polarity Therapy Association (see Appendix B). Click on **Find a Practitioner**, and then click on your state to get a list of referrals.

Relieving pain and encouraging healing with reflexology

Reflexology involves applying pressure to specific points on the soles of the feet, the palms of the hands, or the ears that are thought to correspond with various organs and other parts of the body. Reflexology theory maintains that the body is divided into ten zones, each running lengthwise from head to foot and down one arm through one of the ten fingers. Applying pressure on one part of the zone is believed to help relieve pain and encourage healing in another part of that zone.

The reflexologist manipulates a specific area — most commonly on the bottom of the foot, but sometimes on the palm of the hand or the ear — that corresponds to the diseased or painful area. He uses a map of the foot, hand, or ear that indicates the points that can stimulate healing in the heart, stomach, lung, pancreas, kidney, colon, eyes, ears, throat, and even the tonsils. For example, your reflexologist may press an area just outside the middle of the ball of your foot to stimulate your lungs. Reflexologists use special thumb, finger, and hand techniques, without the addition of oils or lotions, to stimulate your body parts. For most people, reflexology is a relaxing and pleasant experience.

Discovering what reflexology can do for you

No studies exist that prove that reflexology is an effective treatment for arthritis. But, like most kinds of massage, reflexology may be helpful in reducing the stiffness seen in osteoarthritis and rheumatoid arthritis. It may also help increase circulation, which is helpful if you have Raynaud's phenomenon.

Finding a good reflexologist

Take a look at Web site for the Reflexology Association of America (see Appendix B). Click on **Find a Reflexologist**, and then enter your state for a list of referrals.

Transmitting healing energy through touch therapy

In *touch therapy,* also known as therapeutic touch, energy is transmitted from the practitioner's hands to the patient's body in order to speed the healing process and ease pain. Like certain Eastern philosophies, therapeutic touch is based on the belief that the body possesses an energy field and that the energy within this field must be ordered and balanced to maintain health. When the energy in this field becomes unbalanced, disease results.

Although the practitioner won't actually touch your body, he can discern where problems exist in your energy field by meditating while holding his hands over your body to feel the vibrations. The practitioner then channels energy into your body to help ease the pain and speed healing. One session usually takes about 30 minutes.

Discovering what touch therapy can do for you

Some studies have found that therapeutic touch is effective, including one study performed on 25 patients with osteoarthritis. The participants in this study were divided into three groups: One received standard Western medical care, another received therapeutic touch, and a third received a simulated version of touch therapy. Those participants who actually received touch therapy experienced a significant decrease in pain along with an increase in mobility, while the other participants did not. However, other studies have shown that touch therapy has little or no effect. In spite of this finding, therapeutic touch is taught at more than 80 different universities, is used by many nurses, and is the subject of a great deal of scientific research. If you're in pain, you may want to give it a try.

Finding a good touch therapy practitioner

To find a good touch therapy practitioner, find the Web site for the Nurse Healers — Professional Associates International, which is the official Therapeutic Touch organization. (See Appendix B for more information.) Click on **Online Listings**, and then on your state for referrals.

Chapter 19

Other Alternative Approaches

*Y*ou're probably familiar with herbs and homeopathy (and if you aren't, check out Chapter 17), but many people are currently using additional alternative methods to ease the symptoms of arthritis. In this chapter, we introduce you to some of the latest and greatest therapies, how they're performed, what some say these methods can do for you, and where you can begin your search for a competent, qualified therapist.

Even if you're lucky enough to find both a therapy that works and an excellent practitioner, you still need to continue to work with your physician and the other members of your health care team. Studies have shown that people with arthritis who completely ignore traditional medicine in favor of alternative methods find that their health deteriorates at an alarming rate. An alternative therapy should be used as a *complement* to traditional medicine, not as a substitute for it.

Breathing In the Healing: Aromatherapy

Aromatherapy uses a wide variety of fragrant substances called *essential oils* to treat physical and emotional ills. These oils are taken from the fruit, flowers, bark, or roots of plants, producing deliciously enticing smells that include the aromas of basil, bergamot, black pepper, camphor, cedar wood, chamomile, fennel, frankincense, hyssop, jasmine, juniper, lavender, patchouli, and rose. The unique aroma of each essential oil, when inhaled, is believed to trigger beneficial physiologic and emotional responses. Lavender, for example, is believed to be soothing and relaxing, which is why it's recommended for people who are stressed or anxious. Ginger, on the other hand, is thought to be energizing and warming and is sometimes used as a mild aphrodisiac.

Understanding how it works

Massage is perhaps the most effective delivery system for aromatherapy, using *carrier oils* that contain a small amount of one or more essential oils. Carrier oils are plain, unscented oils that do not irritate the skin (such as soy oil or corn oil) that make up the majority of the solution and are applied to the skin, with only a drop or two of essential oil added for aromatic purposes. (With the exception of lavender oil, essential oils are never applied directly to the skin in their undiluted state because they are too strong and irritating.)

As pleasurable as an aromatherapy massage may be, it's certainly not the only way to enjoy the benefits of essential oils. Aromatic oils can also be dropped into a pot of boiling water and allowed to escape into the air in the form of steam, or the steam itself can be inhaled after the solution has cooled somewhat.

When inhaling steam, be sure to remove the pot from the stove and allow it to cool until the steam can be inhaled comfortably. Inhaling the steam from a boiling pot can cause burns!

Discovering what aromatherapy can do for you

Aromatherapy is an ancient healing art, dating back over 4,000 years to the ancient Egyptians who used fragrant oils to cure the ills of both mind and body. Plant oils were used throughout the Middle Ages to treat wounds and help heal disease. And modern proponents of aromatherapy insist that it can help treat acne, arthritis, bronchitis, poor circulation, skin problems, and many other conditions. Because it acts on the central nervous system, aromatherapy may also help to ease anxiety and depression, reduce stress, induce relaxation or sedation, ease pain, give you a lift, or even act as a mild stimulant.

The essential oils most often prescribed for arthritis pain include benzoin, birch, black pepper, chamomile, eucalyptus, ginger, and juniper. One study found that arthritis patients who used aromatherapy were able to reduce their intake of painkillers while maintaining their current level of comfort.

Finding out where to get aromatherapy

Many people perform aromatherapy on their own, but it's a good idea to see a professional first to find out how to do it safely and effectively. You can find a certified aromatherapist by contacting one of the aromatherapy organizations listed in Appendix B.

Fighting Pain with Bee Venom Therapy

Believe it or not, this therapy uses the venom from bee stings to help alleviate your pain. Although the preferred method involves the sting of a live bee, the venom can also be administered via injection. But there are a few drawbacks to the injections — the FDA hasn't approved bee venom therapy as an antidote to pain, so you may have trouble finding a physician to treat you, and injections are believed to be less effective than the sting of a live bee.

Understanding how it works

The bee venom is administered either directly on or near the site of your pain, or on specific acupuncture points or trigger points. While the injections are pretty straightforward, applying the live sting of a bee is an interesting procedure. The bee, held in long tweezers, is placed on the designated spot and allowed to do its thing. (The area to be stung may be iced beforehand to dull the pain.) But this process may need to be repeated several times before you see any arthritis pain-relieving results. And, as you can imagine, it hurts.

Discovering what bee venom therapy can do for you

Surprisingly, bee venom has powerful pain-relieving and anti-inflammatory effects. There are no human studies currently available to document its prowess, but it has been shown to help prevent induced arthritis in rats. Bee venom therapy is quite popular in Asia and Eastern Europe, and many people swear by its ability to ease the symptoms of their arthritis.

This treatment can be fatal if you develop an allergic reaction to the bee venom. Before beginning bee venom therapy, ask your doctor to test you for an allergy to bee stings. If you are allergic, do not use this treatment! And even if you aren't, it's imperative that you always have someone else present when you are stung, as well as an anaphylaxis emergency treatment kit (available by prescription only) in case you suddenly develop an allergic reaction.

Finding out where to get bee venom therapy

It's best to start with a physician who will give you bee venom injections, because the injections are less painful than the bee stings, and in case anything goes wrong, you'll already be in the presence of medical personnel. But bee venom isn't FDA-approved for this kind of therapy, so you may need to rely on word-of-mouth referrals or recommendations from a pain clinic to find a willing physician.

For live bee sting therapy, contact a beekeeper or other proponent of bee venom therapy. The American Apitherapy Society (see Appendix B) can provide you with information on this unusual therapy, how to administer it safely, and a list of members you can talk to who are familiar with the procedure.

Replacing the Hormone DHEA

This therapy is based on the belief that some kinds of arthritis may be related to a lack of a hormone called DHEA (dehydroepiandrosterone). Although DHEA is a male hormone (an androgen), it's manufactured in both male and female bodies. The body then uses DHEA to make several other hormones, including estrogen and testosterone. Levels of DHEA have been found to be low in some people with lupus, juvenile arthritis, and rheumatoid arthritis.

So far, results have been positive when DHEA was given to women with mild to moderate forms of lupus. In one study of 191 women with lupus, 200 milligrams of DHEA per day helped ease fatigue, pain, and inflammation, allowing the women to cut back on their medication. Unfortunately, no scientific studies have yet shown the same positive results for rheumatoid or juvenile arthritis.

Understanding how it works

Researchers don't know exactly how DHEA works against lupus. What they do know is that the immune system "goes wild" in lupus, and that androgens tend to suppress immune function. And, in both test tube and animal studies, DHEA reduces the production of cytokines, which promote inflammation. Thus, DHEA may help combat some symptoms of lupus by keeping the immune system's "bad behavior" in check.

Discovering what DHEA can do for you

Besides helping to relieve symptoms of lupus, high levels of DHEA in the blood have been linked to a lower risk of heart disease, stroke, cancer, diabetes, Alzheimer's disease, and Parkinson's disease. Blood levels of DHEA decline rapidly after the age of 30, so keeping them high may help ward off degenerative diseases and age-related problems.

DHEA is a drug and may cause side effects, like increased testosterone levels and acne, so a physician should always monitor its use. In some people, DHEA may actually *increase* the risk of cancer and heart disease. Also, because DHEA is converted to androgens (male sex hormones), it may promote the growth of prostate cancer and breast cancer cells. Don't take DHEA if you're currently taking azathioprine (Imuran) or methotrexate, as the combination can cause liver damage.

Finding out where to get DHEA

Ask your doctor about DHEA. If she agrees that it may be worth a try, get a prescription. (DHEA is a drug, and a physician should always monitor its use.) Some people need a dose of about 200 milligrams per day to see positive results, but try starting on a lower dose and see what happens.

DHEA is available in health food stores and other commercial enterprises, but steer clear of these varieties. Some of them contain significantly less DHEA than they claim. (The FDA does not test supplements to ensure that they actually provide what they say they do.) If you do decide to buy over-the-counter DHEA, however, check out the content and quality of the supplements on www.consumerlabs.com.

You may see wild yam products in health food stores and catalogues that claim to be natural, unprocessed sources of DHEA. Although these products may be natural, your body can't absorb DHEA until it has been chemically altered, so don't waste your money.

Another form of androgen supplementation is a transdermal patch. The patch is placed on your skin, and your body absorbs the hormone at a steady rate. You replace the patch every three days. Testosterone is the main hormone delivered in this manner, but others may soon be available.

Although doctors have much more to learn about the benefits and risks of this supplementation, there seems to be a possible benefit for certain people with the rheumatic diseases, specifically those whose androgen levels are decreased. Benefits include fewer flares, increased bone mineral density, less depression, and improved joint function. The main areas of concern are increased risks of cardiovascular disease and cancer. The first step is to have the levels of the androgen hormones measured in your blood

Easing Inflammation with DMSO

DMSO (dimethyl sulfoxide), a colorless liquid that easily permeates membranes when applied to the skin, is actually a by-product of wood pulp processing. In its strongest form, it's used as an industrial solvent in paint thinner and antifreeze. But in its milder, medical-grade form, it's an FDA-approved preservative for transplant organs and a treatment for a bladder disease called interstitial cystitis.

But DMSO can also help ease arthritis symptoms by reducing inflammation, stabilizing membranes, and slowing or stopping leakage from injured cells. Its most important arthritis-fighting characteristic, though, may be its ability to fight free-radical damage to the joints. Studies in Japan concluded that DMSO relieved joint pain and increased both range of motion and grip strength. Other studies have shown that DMSO can ease muscle and joint pain, relax the constricted blood vessels seen in Raynaud's phenomenon, heal the skin ulcers seen in scleroderma, and soften scleroderma's hardened collagen deposits.

Understanding how to use DMSO

DMSO can be applied externally, swallowed, or injected into veins or muscles. It can be rubbed onto the skin to ease inflammation of the joints and soft tissues. It can help other drugs cross cell membranes and can even soften collagen. But whether taken internally or externally, DMSO has a couple of unpleasant side effects, including skin rash, headaches, sedation, nausea, and vomiting. Also, those who take DMSO often find that it leaves a bad taste in their mouths and makes them smell like a combination of oysters and garlic — a smell so intense that many regret using it.

Discovering what DMSO can do for you

DMSO was considered a revolutionary new treatment for arthritis when it was introduced back in the early 1960s. But in the mid-1960s, animal studies involving very high doses of DMSO showed it also caused damage to the lens of the eye (although no studies have shown eye problems in humans). Although many studies since have shown that DMSO appears to have few side effects, even at very high doses, it fell out of favor. Today many American physicians don't use it except to treat a bladder ailment. DMSO is still being used regularly to treat osteoarthritis and rheumatoid arthritis in Russia and some other countries, however.

Finding out how to get DMSO

You and your physician need to have an in-depth discussion about the pros and cons of DMSO usage before you decide whether you want to try it. If you do decide to try DMSO, ask your doctor to write you a prescription and to monitor your progress while you use it. Although DMSO can be purchased over the counter, chances are it's not in the purified form used in the prescription variety, which can make it overly strong and possibly detrimental to your health.

Fighting the Pain and Disability of RA with MSM

When DMSO is broken down within the body, about 15 percent of it becomes MSM (methylsulfonylmethane), an organic, sulfur-containing compound. MSM has many of the same benefits of DMSO but fewer detriments. For example, it doesn't produce the oyster/garlic smell on the breath, it doesn't appear to damage the body in any way, and it doesn't require a prescription. Yet it does seem to help fight inflammation, and it may help alleviate some of the symptoms of RA. Animal studies have shown that osteoarthritic joints have a lower sulfur content than normal joints and that mice with arthritis given MSM had less joint deterioration. One study found that 2,250 milligrams of MSM per day reduced pain in people with OA after six weeks.

Understanding how MSM is used to treat arthritis

MSM is available in capsule or lotion form. The recommended standard dose for capsules is 500 milligrams twice a day. You might start by taking 250 milligrams or less twice a day, and watch for side effects. If all goes well, gradually increase the amount until you reach the standard dose. In some people, individual doses as low as 50 milligrams are effective, and up to 1,500 milligrams may be well tolerated, although for severe conditions, even higher doses may be needed to achieve relief. Consult your physician before taking MSM, however, and don't stop taking your other arthritis medication(s) unless she advises you to do so.

MSM and DMSO may produce blood-thinning effects, and if used in conjunction with blood thinners such as heparin, aspirin, or certain herbs, can cause excessive bleeding or prolonged clotting time. Consult your physician about adverse interactions before taking either MSM or DMSO.

Discovering what MSM can do for you

When James Coburn won the Academy Award for Best Supporting Actor in 1999, he gave the marketing campaign for MSM a real shot in the arm by claiming that MSM had made it possible for him to fight the pain and disability of rheumatoid arthritis and continue working. Since then, MSM has been touted as a pain-relieving and inflammation-fighting treatment for osteoarthritis, rheumatoid arthritis, gout, and fibromyalgia. Its advertisers also claim that it can neutralize an acid stomach, fight allergies, and ease constipation, among other things. The problem is, no real scientific proof exists for any of these claims. And much more research is needed before it can be deemed safe.

Finding out how to get MSM

MSM is widely available in vitamin stores, health food stores, and on the Internet. Before you buy, you may want to check out the content and quality of various brands of MSM at www.consumerlabs.com.

Whirling the Pain Away with Hydrotherapy

Hydrotherapy is an ancient treatment using water (both hot and cold), steam, and ice to stimulate and soothe the body, thus rearranging its energies and encouraging healing.

Understanding how hydrotherapy is used to treat arthritis

Water is either applied to the entire body or to specific areas in the form of liquid, steam, or ice. It may be delivered via showers, baths, *sitz baths* (baths in which you're immersed only up to waist level), warm and cool compresses, wet sheet wraps, hot blankets, saunas, and other techniques. Hydrotherapy can also be performed internally by drinking water and/or taking colonics (enemas that flush out the colon).

Discovering what it can do for you

Hydrotherapy is an age-old therapy for arthritis. The Romans were famous for their public baths, where people "took the waters" to ease the pain of arthritic joints. A modern hydrotherapist may recommend a variety of treatments, including colonics to rid the body of toxins, drinking plenty of distilled water to flush toxins away, taking short cold baths or showers to increase circulation, using warm baths, saunas, or steam rooms to increase circulation and sweat out toxins, and applying cold compresses to ease joint pain.

Although bathing in mineral waters (and sometimes drinking them) has long been touted as a health aid, evidence suggests that bathing in plain old warm water works just as well!

Finding a good hydrotherapist

To find a specialist in hydrotherapy, contact one of the alternative medicine organizations listed in Appendix B. Be sure to look for someone experienced in treating arthritis, as some forms of hydrotherapy may be detrimental to your condition (for example, cold water therapy for Raynaud's may further constrict blood vessels that are already overly-constricted).

Peering into the Possibilities of Prolotherapy

Prolotherapy, which involves injecting an inflamed joint or the area surrounding a joint with dextrose (sugar) water, is a nonsurgical way to treat several musculoskeletal conditions. "Prolo" is short for "proliferation," and this therapy is believed to promote the proliferation (growth) of new ligament tissue surrounding joints where weakened and damaged tissue is causing joint instability and chronic pain.

Understanding how it works

Prolotherapy fights inflammation by creating even more inflammation — much like fighting fire with fire. Ligaments, the structures that connect the bones within a joint and hold those bones in place, can become injured and have a hard time healing. The blood supply to the ligaments is limited, so the healing process can be slow and incomplete, leaving the ligaments loose, damaged, and weak. Unfortunately, the ligaments do have plenty of nerve endings, ensuring that you'll feel plenty of pain. Injecting sugar water into the area surrounding the ligament where it attaches to the bone increases inflammation, bringing extra blood, nutrients, and oxygen to the weakened tissue, which may help the healing process.

Discovering what prolotherapy can do for you

Although there are only a few small studies on prolotherapy, it appears to improve joint function and ease pain in a lot of different conditions, including osteoarthritis; ligamentous laxity (loose or improperly healed ligaments), and chronic back and neck pain.

Finding out where to get prolotherapy

If you're interested in prolotherapy, ask your doctor if this treatment is appropriate for your condition and, if so, if she is willing and able to provide it. If you need to find a doctor who specializes in prolotherapy, go to www.getprolo.com to find a listing of prolotherapy physicians.

Part V
The Part of Tens

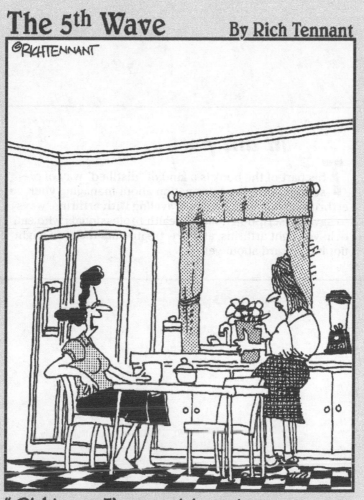

The 5th Wave
By Rich Tennant

"Right now I'm exercising pain management through medication, meditation, and limiting visits from my pain-in-the-butt neighbor."

In this part . . .

This part of the book is a kind of "distilled" way of presenting some key information about managing your arthritis. We include tips for traveling with arthritis, ways to save prescription dollars, health professionals who can help you fight arthritis, and new treatments that you might not have heard about yet.

Chapter 20

Ten Tips for Traveling with Arthritis

F ew things are more exciting and invigorating than packing your bags and hitting the road, bound for some exotic destination or just getting out of Dodge for a while to clear your head! But traveling with arthritis can be a whole different animal, what with the additional strain on your joints, sky-rocketing stress levels, change in routine, long hours sitting in cramped seats, jet lag, and having to haul loads of luggage and other travel paraphernalia. But don't worry — you *can* still travel when you've got arthritis, and you can even have a good time! You just need to plan a little more carefully than you may have in the past. Consider this chapter the Ten Commandments of Traveling with Arthritis.

Talking to Your Doctor

Tell your doctor about your travel plans: where you're going, for how long, what you plan to do, the kind of climate you're traveling to, and the kinds of foods you plan to eat. Then ask if she has any cautions for you. Should you limit yourself to certain kinds of activities? How much time should you spend resting every day? Should you be responsible for carrying your own luggage or ask others to carry it? Should you arrange for a wheelchair at the airport? Is pain the best gauge of when to stop an activity? Or should you stop before the pain sets in?

It could also be helpful to find out whether a good doctor or health facility is near your destination. Ask your doctor about the possibility of carrying along a prescription for any medicines you may need in case you run out, and get a letter from him describing your condition (just in case).

You may also want to check with your insurance company to find out if you're covered during travel and after you've arrived at your destination. If so, how does your insurance work? If, for example, you have an arthritis flare in Belgium, how do you pay for a visit to the doctor, and how do you get reimbursed? If your insurance doesn't cover you, find out about purchasing additional coverage for the short-term.

Reviewing Your Medications and Supplements

Make a list of every medication, vitamin, mineral, herb, supplement, potion, cream, rub, or liniment that you use. Then bring all of them! Try to follow your normal routine as closely as possible; don't just start tossing out what seems to be superfluous right before you go on a trip. That "superfluous" item may be just the thing that can help you avoid or clear up a flare. Bring along familiar over-the-counter aids for pain, so you don't have to start experimenting with strange brands when you're in unfamiliar territory. If you're flying, pack your medications in a carry-on bag so you have them with you even if your luggage gets lost.

After you have everything assembled, count the days you're going to be gone and make sure you take enough of everything to last the entire trip. Then pack a little extra. They may not have what you need where you're going!

Before you travel to another country, try to find out which drugs it considers illegal. For example, Japan frowns on stimulants, while Greece and Turkey are strict about opiates like codeine. Be sure to carry all of your medications (prescription, over-the-counter, and even vitamins) in their original containers. If you're taking along syringes or narcotic drugs, get a letter from your doctor explaining why you need them. The last thing you want is to undergo endless delays and interrogations because you're carrying the "wrong" medication!

Preplanning to Reduce Stress

Think through your trip and try to anticipate and solve any problems before you leave, so you can travel without worry. For example, if you have trouble walking, request a wheelchair or motorized cart in advance. Keep your carry-on bag light and easy to manage, and make sure all of your luggage has wheels and is well-balanced. (Imagine the aggravation caused by a rolling suitcase that keeps toppling over!)

Make a daily plan that includes periods of activity, periods of rest, and plenty of time to sleep. Schedule some time to exercise and some time to soak in a hot bath, if you find these activities helpful. Build in an extra day to give yourself time to recover from jet lag. In other words, don't just rush headlong into the unknown (your trip) without a plan. If you do, your body may not be getting all that it needs. And that can translate to arthritis flares and pain.

Finally, plan an "emergency exit" procedure in case you need to cut your trip short. For example, purchase trip insurance, if it's available. Or get open-ended plane tickets. Trust us, you won't enjoy being far away and unable to go home when you're not feeling well.

Eating Wisely and Well

Eating a healthful, balanced diet is always important, but especially when your body is stressed by an ongoing condition (arthritis) compounded by the strain of traveling. Arthritis sufferers need to be especially careful about what they eat, because some foods can actually make their conditions worse. Luckily, other foods can help relieve some of their symptoms.

In general, no matter where your destination, you should try to do the following:

- ✔ Eat a wide variety of foods, focusing on whole grains, fresh fruits, and fresh vegetables, with smaller amounts of meat, fish, poultry (4 to 6 ounces per day maximum), and dairy products.

- ✔ Limit your intake of cholesterol, fat, sugar, and salt (sodium).

- ✔ Take it easy on the alcohol.

- ✔ Use olive oil, canola oil, flaxseed oil, and others high in the "good" fatty acid (linoleic acid), which can help lessen inflammation.

- ✔ Watch your intake of foods that contain the "bad" fatty acid (arachidonic acid) such as meat, poultry, egg yolks, and full-fat dairy products.

- ✔ Eat fish that contain omega-3 fatty acids (mackerel, herring, salmon, and so on) a couple of times weekly.

Exercising, Even Though You're on Vacation!

We just can't stress this enough! Regular physical activity strengthens joint support structures, helping them take some of the pressure off the joint itself, while nourishing and moisturizing the cartilage. Aerobic activity can tone you all over, strengthen your heart, increase bone density, and help you keep your weight under control (very important, especially for those with arthritis of the knee). Flexibility (stretching) exercises increase and maintain your range of motion, loosen up your muscles, and make your tendons and ligaments more resilient. At the same time, these exercises help release tension and promote relaxation — translating into less pain and stiffness, greater ease of movement, and an improved mental attitude. In addition, exercise can increase your physical abilities, help prevent joint deformities, boost your immune system, improve your balance, and help you maintain your independence.

Plenty of exercise before you leave will help carry you through a short trip. If traveling by car, get out and stretch every 90 minutes or so. If traveling by plane, try to get out of your seat and walk up and down the aisle every so often to ease joint stiffness and prevent *deep vein thrombosis* (a potentially life-threatening condition in which a blood clot forms in one of the deep veins of the body, usually in the leg). If you can find room, try a few stretches and some range-of-motion exercises. Set aside some time each day to stretch and do relaxation exercises in your hotel room (or wherever you're staying). And if your trip doesn't include plenty of walking, start each day with a brisk 20- to 30-minute walk. It's a great way to greet the day, and the scenery will be brand-new to you!

Using Joint-Protection Techniques

When traveling, the way you use (or abuse) your joints becomes crucial. Remember (and apply) these joint-protection techniques recommended by the Arthritis Foundation:

- ✔ Respect pain.
- ✔ Avoid joint-stressing postures or positions.
- ✔ Avoid staying in one position for a long time.
- ✔ Use the strongest and largest joints and muscles for the job.
- ✔ Avoid sustained joint activities.
- ✔ Maintain muscle strength and joint range of motion.
- ✔ Use assistive devices or splints, if necessary. (See the next section.)

Using Assistive Devices

Splints, supports, canes, pillows, carts, and anything else that takes a load off your joints can be invaluable when you're traveling. Take advantage of the many "little helpers" designed to make your life easier and more comfortable:

- ✔ Use a horseshoe-shaped pillow to support your head and relieve neck pain while riding in the car or flying.

- ✔ Support your back by wedging a lumbar pillow between the back of your waist and the seat.

- ✔ A small pillow atop the armrest in a plane or a car can make it easier and more comfortable for you to prop up the upper body.

- ✔ Wear your knee supports, or wrap your affected joints in elastic tape for greater stability.

- ✔ If you're planning on visiting museums but your knees hurt when you stand for long periods of time, bring along a small campstool so you can pull up a chair whenever you want.

- ✔ Use canes, walkers, motorized carts, and wheelchairs as needed.

Renting an Arthritis-Friendly Car

The right car can minimize physical exertion, ease joint stress and strain, and make a driving trip a whole lot more comfortable. Call your rental car company at least six weeks before your trip to request a car that has these arthritis-friendly features:

- ✔ Automatic seat belts
- ✔ Cruise control
- ✔ Easy-access gearshift and ignition
- ✔ Four doors
- ✔ Hand controls
- ✔ Lightweight doors
- ✔ Plenty of legroom
- ✔ Power brakes
- ✔ Power locks
- ✔ Power seats
- ✔ Power windows
- ✔ Tilt steering wheel

Flying with Finesse

Flying is sometimes uncomfortable even for those who don't have arthritis, but it can be torture for those with chronically stiff, achy joints. To make your flight as tolerable as possible, try the following:

- ✔ If your budget allows it, flying first-class is a lot more comfortable — from the seats and the amount of space you have, to the service. But flying first class is mighty costly.

- ✔ If you're flying coach (like most of us), make your reservations early and request a seat in the first row or in an exit row, to ensure more legroom.

- ✔ Spend the extra five bucks and get a skycap to handle your luggage.

- ✔ Request a wheelchair or motorized cart in advance if walking is a problem for you.

- ✔ Ask that you be allowed to preboard so you can take your time to get settled. The airlines will be happy to accommodate you.

- ✔ Arrange for a nonstop flight when possible to avoid the hassle of getting on and off two planes.

- ✔ Get up and move as much as possible during the flight to ease joint stiffness.

- ✔ Drink plenty of water during the flight, because the atmosphere inside the plane is extremely dehydrating.

- ✔ Travel during the less busy times (midweek or midday, evening, and late at night) to avoid the crush of a crowd.

Taking a Test Run

If you're concerned about taking a long trip, try a smaller one first. Think of it as a test run. You find out what works for you and what you need to work on to make a bigger trip more successful. Make a detailed list of what you brought and what you were lacking. When you get home, revise your list so you know exactly what to take next time. Each time you travel, make a note of what was missing and revise your list when you get home. Then refer to the list the next time you pack. You can become a seasoned traveler in no time. Happy wandering!

Chapter 21

Ten Ways to Save on Prescriptions

In This Chapter

▶ Gaining access to free or less expensive medications through your doctor

▶ Finding out about public and private drug assistance programs

▶ Cutting drug costs by buying generic, buying in bulk, or splitting pills

▶ Finding reputable mail-order pharmacies

The high cost of prescription drugs can be a real problem if you've got a chronic condition like arthritis that requires a steady supply of medication. Luckily, you can do several things to lower the cost of your meds, beginning with sorting through what you're already taking to see what you really need, buying generic forms of the drugs you need, buying in bulk, and splitting pills. Then take a look at the many programs available that may let you buy your medications at a considerable discount, or even get them for free. Other good ideas include shopping around for the best price, getting a pharmacy discount card, and buying from certain reputable mail-order or online pharmacies. You may be surprised just how much you can do to slash the cost of your prescription drugs.

Review Your Medications

Over time, the assortment of medications you're taking can start to resemble an overstuffed closet. You may have some meds you no longer need, some that no longer fit your condition, some that are duplicates, and some that clash with others. For the sake of both your health and your pocketbook, write up a complete list of every drug you're currently taking and ask your doctor to go over it. Find out which, if any, can be eliminated and which can be replaced with over-the-counter varieties. (Over-the-counter versions sometimes cost less than your prescription drug copayment.)

If you pay for your medications out of your own pocket or your copayment is a hefty one, be sure to tell your doctor. He may be able to prescribe a less expensive version of the same drug. And because many insurance companies have a preapproved list of medications that they cover, you should get a copy of the list and show it to your doctor. If she prescribes a drug that's not on the list, you're going to have to pay more than your usual copayment — or you may even have to pay the entire cost of the medication! When your doctor knows which drugs are on the "green-light" list, chances are good that he will be able to prescribe one that's appropriate for your needs and won't break the bank.

Ask Your Doctor for Free Samples

Almost all doctors have closets full of drug samples that are routinely handed out by pharmaceutical companies. Instead of investing a lot of money in a medication that may not work for you or may have side effects that you just can't tolerate, ask your doctor for some free samples. Free samples not only save you money, but they also save you a trip to the pharmacy.

Check Out Medicare's Drug Discount Program

A comprehensive Medicare prescription drug benefit program designed to help reduce drug costs for seniors begins on January 1, 2006. In the meantime, if you're a Medicare beneficiary, you can take advantage of a temporary Drug Discount Card Program that can save you up to 25 percent on individual prescription drugs and 10 to 15 percent on total drug spending. Medicare contracts with private companies to offer drug discount cards that are good until the new prescription drug benefits start in 2006. (This program doesn't apply to those already receiving Medicaid or Tricare prescription benefits.)

You can enroll in this program as early as May 2004. See the Medicare Web site at www.medicare.gov for more information, or call 800-633-4227 or 877-486-2048 (for the hearing impaired).

You may also consider joining a Medicare HMO if one is available in your area, because it provides drug benefits that require a small copayment.

Be careful! If you purchase the Medicare Drug Discount card, there are *strict limits* on the use of other discount cards you may have. Do your homework to find what works best for your situation.

Find Out Whether You Qualify for a Drug Assistance Program

If you can't afford to buy the medications you need, some public and private resources are available. See the RxAssist (Accessing Pharmaceutical Patient Assistance Programs) Web site at www.rxassist.org. Click on **State Programs** to find contact information for the Statewide Drug Assistance Program in your state (if one exists).

Many major drug companies have established programs to give discounts or free medication to those who can't afford to pay. The Pharmaceutical Research and Manufacturers of America has set up a special Web site designed to help people get the medication they need, no matter what their financial circumstances. See www.RxHope.com, and click on **Patient Assistance Information**. You can search for patient assistance programs via drug name, companies, or the state you live in.

Get a Pharmacy Discount Card

AdvanceRX offers a free discount card for the uninsured and underinsured that covers all drugs dispensed at a pharmacy and can save you up to 20 percent. (Go to www.advancerx.com and click on **RXSavings Plus**; or call 800-238-2623.)

AARP offers a Prescription Discount Program to its members (MemberRX Choice) for a yearly fee of $19.95 that can save you from 20 to 47 percent on prescription costs. MemberRX Choice cards are accepted at pharmacies across the nation, or you can order medication online. For a list of participating pharmacies and information, see its Web site at www.aarppharmacy.com/aarpnet/mc/mcDefault.aspx.

Certain pharmaceutical manufacturers offer drug discount cards to Medicare recipients with limited incomes who have no other prescription coverage. To view a chart comparing the requirements and benefits of different drug discount programs, see www.RxAsst.org and click on **Drug Discount Cards**.

Buy the Generic Version

A generic drug is the identical twin of a brand name drug. It has the same potency, chemical makeup, dosage, quality, intended use, and performance. But it can cost between 30 and 50 percent less! So instead of buying brand name medications, ask your doctor about getting the generic equivalent. Pharmacists are legally allowed to substitute generic drugs for many brand name products, but they must first ask if this is all right with you.

Buying generic is also a great way to save money on over-the-counter medications. For example, Advil or Motrin, the brand name versions of ibuprofen, are much more expensive than the generic equivalent (often the store name brand) even though both contain exactly the same active ingredients.

Buy in Bulk

If you will be taking a medication for more than a month (for example, you have a chronic disease or condition like asthma or allergies), you may consider ordering a bulk supply of your drugs to save money. Most pharmacies charge less per individual pill if you buy a 90-day supply instead of a 30-day supply, and mail-order pharmacies are famous for selling medications in bulk supply.

Of course, there's a small catch: Most insurance companies only let you get a 30-day supply per copayment. However, getting a 90-day supply and paying the cost of the drugs yourself (that is, not using your insurance) may actually be cheaper than paying the cost of three copayments. But before you make a bulk order, speak with your doctor to make sure that he is not going to be adjusting the dose of your medicines.

Double the Strength and Split the Pills

Getting medication at a higher dose and splitting the pills is a good way to save money. In fact, in some cases it can result in a 50 percent savings! It's not appropriate for all medications though. Time-release medications and pills in capsule form should not be split. Although you can buy a pill splitter and cut each pill in half yourself, it's safer to get the pills split by your pharmacist.

Compare Prices at Different Pharmacies

If you're paying more than a set copayment for your medications, it may be worth your while to shop around for the best price. That's right — pharmacies don't necessarily charge the same prices for the same drug! Some offer discounted prices, because they don't provide extra services like consultations or home delivery. Others may have special deals on certain drugs.

To find out what a pharmacy charges, simply call and ask. Be sure to have the exact name, amount, and dosage of your medication. If you find a cheaper price at the pharmacy's competition, the pharmacy may try to match it.

Consider Online or Mail-Order Pharmacies

Unbeatable convenience and considerable discounts have made ordering medications online or through the mail an attractive prospect to many people. In fact, the Pharmaceutical Care Management Association has estimated mail-order pharmacies have cornered up to 12 percent of the total prescription market. But how do you know which pharmacies are legitimate and trustworthy and which aren't?

To answer this question, in 1999 the National Association of Boards of Pharmacy (NABP) developed the Verified Internet Pharmacy Practice Sites (VIPPS) program. To become VIPPS certified, a pharmacy must meet the licensing and inspection requirements of its state and all states in which it dispenses medications; it must adhere to certain standards of quality, authentication, and security of prescription orders; and it must offer patients the opportunity to consult with a pharmacist.

To find a VIPPS pharmacy site, go to www.nabp.net/vipps/intro.asp and click on **List of Pharmacies**.

For better or for worse, many people are looking to Canada as a source of less expensive drugs. Although driving across the border to buy prescription drugs directly is legal, importing them by other means is illegal in most cases and could be dangerous. You may get the wrong product, an incorrect dose, a contaminated product, or nothing at all. In some cases, people believe they are ordering drugs on the Internet from Canadian pharmacies, but the medicines are actually coming from India (or another foreign country with standards and practices that are different from ours) with a fake return address.

If you should decide to order from a Canadian pharmacy Web site, pick one of the duly registered and regulated Canadian Internet Pharmacies recommended by the North American Pharmacy Accreditation Commission. (Go to www.napac.org and click on **Search the NAPAC Database**.)

Chapter 22

Ten Professionals Who Can Help You Fight Arthritis

You probably know that taking charge of your arthritis isn't just a matter of seeing your doctor once in a while and popping a few pills. Because arthritis is a multi-faceted disease, your war against it must be fought on many fronts, involving the physical, the mental, the emotional, and the practical day-to-day business of living. To be effective, you probably need to assemble a team of health care professionals (think of them as "generals") to help you attack arthritis in several ways.

The most important member of the team (after you) is the *rheumatologist,* a doctor who specializes in arthritis and other diseases of the joints, muscles, and soft tissues. But other members of the team, including the pharmacist, physical and occupational therapists, social worker, massage therapist, and others also play vital roles. Assembling a team is up to you, so research all you can about what they do and find the best you can to help you win your battles against arthritis pain and joint destruction.

Rheumatologist

A *rheumatologist* is a doctor who specializes in diseases of the internal system (an *internist*), who has additional training and experience in the diagnosis and treatment of arthritis and diseases of the joints, muscles, and soft tissues. The rheumatologist treats arthritis and related diseases, such as fibromyalgia, lupus, scleroderma, and Sjögren's syndrome. The goal is to alleviate pain, ease inflammation and other symptoms and, as much as possible, ward off further damage to your joints.

Treatment by a rheumatologist can be particularly crucial for those with rheumatoid arthritis. Taking DMARDs (disease modifying antirheumatic drugs; see Chapter 8 for details) is considered a first-line treatment for newly diagnosed RA patients. Studies have shown that those treated with DMARDs have less joint damage and better joint function, and they tend to live longer than those who aren't treated with these medications. But RA patients seen by a family practitioner or an internist are apparently much less likely to be prescribed this important medication than those seen by a rheumatologist.

According to a Canadian study that followed nearly 30,000 RA patients over a five-year period, 80 percent of those seen by a rheumatologist had used a DMARD, compared to only 53 percent of those seen by an internist and 14 percent of those seen by a family practitioner. So seeing a rheumatologist may mean better treatment for many arthritis sufferers, particularly those with RA.

For referrals to rheumatologists in your area, contact your health insurance company or the American Board of Medical Specialties, which is on the Web at www.abms.org.

Primary Care Physician

Even though you may be seeing a rheumatologist, you still need to maintain a relationship with your primary care physician, who is most likely the first health care professional you see when troubled by joint pain. Your primary care doctor (a family practitioner, internist, or geriatric specialist) continues to be responsible for your overall health and well-being, even though he may refer you to a rheumatologist or other specialists.

The primary care physician's role is crucial. Many rheumatologists and other specialists don't provide regular health maintenance, which is essential for arthritis patients. Important examples include cancer screenings like pap smears, breast exams, and mammograms, which are especially important because many of the drugs used to treat arthritis and related conditions increase the risk of cancer. Paying attention to the prevention and treatment of heart disease is also vital, as more and more research suggests that patients with inflammatory arthritis of any kind are at increased risk of heart problems. Your primary care physician can also treat any coexisting diseases (keeping tight control of blood pressure in a lupus patient with kidney disease helps the person's kidneys survive longer), and primary care physicians also can provide vaccines. (Most patients who are taking immunosuppressants should get a yearly flu shot.) Patients receiving the best care often have close communication between their rheumatologist and their primary care physician.

For referrals to primary care physicians in your area, contact your health insurance company or the American Medical Association, which is on the Web at www.ama-assn.org. In the upper-left corner, find the word Patient and click **Go**. Then click on **Doctor Finder**, and then **Search for a Physician**.

Pharmacist

Your pharmacist can do a lot more than just fill your prescriptions. These highly educated professionals are walking encyclopedias when it comes to information on interactions between drugs, drugs and foods, or drugs and herbs or supplements. They can give suggestions for maximizing drug effectiveness and minimizing or avoiding side effects. They automatically keep track of all medications you're taking (assuming you get all of your medications from the same pharmacy), and they can look for potential problems or overdoses. Some pharmacists can even check your blood pressure, screen you for osteoporosis or high cholesterol, or administer flu shots. Bring your medication-related questions to your pharmacist, who is a goldmine of free, accurate, and trustworthy information.

Physical Therapist or Exercise Physiologist

A physical therapist or exercise physiologist can help you put together a program of exercises to strengthen the muscles supporting your painful joints. They show you how to do the exercises correctly, without inflicting more joint damage. Either one can also help you increase joint and muscle flexibility, restore range of motion, and pump up your endurance without putting undue strain on your joints. One difference between the two is that the services of the physical therapist may be covered by your insurance.

Although you won't need the services of either of these professionals forever, it does take several weeks to get you on track with a good exercise program and to supervise your exercising and stretching to make sure that you're not doing more harm than good to your body. You may also find techniques using heat, cold, or water therapy that can help you manage pain and improve your mobility. For referrals to physical therapists in your area, contact your health insurance company or the American Physical Therapy Association, which is on the Web at www.apta.org. To find an exercise physiologist, see www.exercisejobs.com. Enter **Exercise Physiologist** under Job Category and type in your state.

Occupational Therapist

An occupational therapist (OT) can show you how to overcome arthritis-related movement limitations through the use of special techniques or assistive devices that can ease the performance of daily activities. The OT will interview you and watch you in action, and then come up with recommendations that can make it easier for you to get dressed, groom yourself, get around, shop, do housework, drive, or work. He may also design special splints or supports for you and show you techniques to reduce joint stress and help prevent further joint damage.

For referrals to occupational therapists in your area, contact your health insurance company or the American Occupational Therapy Association, which is on the Web at www.aota.org.

Registered Dietitian

If you have osteoarthritis and are overweight, nutrition therapy can be an important component in your recovery. OA of the knee is often a direct result of carrying too much weight, and losing as little as 5 pounds can do much to prevent arthritis of the weight-bearing joints or, at least, dramatically reduce the symptoms. But losing weight, as we all know, is a lot easier said than done, and getting the help of a professional may be well worth the cost. A good dietitian can help you figure out how to eat regular, well-balanced meals consisting of standard size portions; distinguish between eating/food-related behaviors and feelings/psychological problems; and help you gradually lose weight and keep it off.

For referrals to dietitians in your area, contact your health insurance company or the American Dietetic Association, which is located on the Web at www.eatright.org and click on **Find a Nutrition Professional**.

Social Worker

A social worker can help you solve personal and family problems, locate community resources, recommend support groups or other special services, and help you deal with serious illness or disability. He can also help you apply for public assistance, find a home health care worker, access after-hospital services such as meals-on-wheels or hospital equipment, and locate valuable community resources.

Several different kinds of social workers are available, but the ones who may be of most use to you are those specializing in clinical, health care, or gerontology social work. Clinical social workers offer psychotherapy and counseling. Healthcare social workers can help you and your family cope with chronic illness and work through the paperwork and red tape involved in applying for health care benefits. Gerontology social workers can advise those who are over 65 about senior citizen housing, transportation, and long-term care options.

For referrals to social workers in your area, contact your health insurance company or the National Association of Social Workers, which is located on the Web at www.naswdc.org and click on **Find a Social Worker**.

Chiropractor

A chiropractor manipulates the spine to relieve nerve pressure that can be caused by poor posture, stress injury, disease, or lack of exercise. By applying controlled and directed forces to your spine using massage, acupressure, trigger point therapy, and myofascial release, or by applying a precise, measurable force to specific points on your body with a tool called an activator, the chiropractor can help relieve pain, release stress, improve joint alignment, and increase joint function. A chiropractor may also be able to increase your range of motion by manipulating your joints.

For referrals to chiropractors in your area, contact your health insurance company or the American Chiropractic Association, which is located on the Web at www.amerchiro.org.

Mental Health Professional

A mental health professional can help you cope with the depression, anger, anxiety, relationship problems, or other emotional fallout that you may experience due to chronic illness. She can help you understand the origins of your emotional troubles, find new ways of handling these problems, and address coexisting conditions, such as alcoholism, drug abuse, or prescription drug dependence.

Although anyone can call herself a "therapist" and set up a practice, a licensed mental health professional (psychologist, social worker, or psychiatrist) is your best bet. Social workers have a master's or doctoral degree in social work, and psychologists hold a master's degree or a doctoral degree in psychology. Both must perform thousands of hours of supervised counseling before they can be licensed. Psychiatrists are physicians and are therefore the only mental health professionals who can prescribe medication. But most mental health professionals can refer you to a psychiatrist if medication is needed.

For referrals to mental health professionals in your area, contact your health insurance company or the National Register of Health Service Providers in Psychology, which is on the Web at www.nationalregister.com, or the National Association of Social Workers on the Web at www.naswdc.org.

Massage Therapist

If you have arthritis, your other muscles may be working overtime to favor the joints that hurt. A good massage therapist can help ease the pain that can settle in the muscles doing double duty. Massage may also relieve some of your arthritis pain by easing tension in the muscles surrounding your painful joints and improving joint range of motion. In general, by increasing circulation, helping your body release the metabolic byproducts that can irritate nerve endings, pumping up endorphin levels, and relieving tension, massage can be an effective way of helping you let go of pain, stress, and the extra tension in locked-up muscles.

But don't turn your body over to just anybody. Find a massage therapist who's skilled in treating arthritis patients. Some kinds of massage may be too rough or painful for certain kinds of arthritis, so consult your doctor first. And if you're having an arthritis flare, you've got an infection or a fever, or you're coming down with an illness, avoid a massage because it will increase circulation and can therefore increase inflammation.

To find referrals for a massage therapist in your area, contact the American Massage Therapy Association on the Web at www.amtamassage.org.

Chapter 23

Ten Crackerjack New Treatments

In This Chapter

▶ Unveiling breakthrough treatments

▶ Undergoing advanced surgery for carpal tunnel syndrome

▶ Injecting cartilage cells from goats to grow new cartilage in damaged joints

▶ Shoring up diseased bones with crushed glass particles

*1*n the not-too-distant future, physicians may be able to diagnose arthritis by looking at a map of the patient's genes and treating the ailment through subtle genetic manipulation. In fact, doctors may be able to prevent arthritis by studying an infant's genetic code and tweaking it to ensure that the young one's joints never begin the process of deterioration.

We're certainly not there yet, but medical researchers have developed a host of new treatments. Some are modern twists on older therapies; others are entirely new ideas.

Anti-TNF Drugs for Rheumatoid Arthritis

If you have rheumatoid arthritis (RA), your immune system turns on your body, which is one reason that doctors use drugs that suppress the immune system (disease modifying antirheumatic drugs, or DMARDs) to control this disease. But this approach is a rather broad one, interfering with the immune system's helpful actions, as well as its harmful ones. So a new family of drugs, called *biologic response modifiers* or BRMs, has been devised to address this problem by focusing on very specific parts of the immune system, trying to spare the "good" parts of the immune response while stifling the "bad" ones.

When overproduced, one of the "bad" parts of the immune system, called *tumor necrosis factor* (TNF), can cause severe inflammation and tissue damage. Large amounts of TNF often go hand-in-hand with autoimmune diseases like RA, and a special subgroup of the BRMs called the "anti-TNF" drugs can help calm inflammation and ward off tissue damage.

Three of these anti-TNF drugs — etanercept, infliximab, and adalimumab — have made new strides in relieving RA symptoms and controlling the disease. Designed for those with moderate to severe RA who haven't been helped by the standard disease-modifying medicines, these drugs calm down the body's immune system and decrease the effects of TNF, which helps slow the progression of RA. Here's an overview of each:

✔ **Etanercept** is injected just beneath the skin twice weekly to help the body regulate TNF and slow disease progression. In studies of etanercept, a little more than 60 percent of patients enjoyed a 20 percent or greater improvement in joint pain, joint swelling, and other symptoms. The medicine works fairly quickly, so many patients are able to handle daily chores with greater ease within two weeks. Etanercept is currently approved as a treatment for RA, JRA, ankylosing spondylitis, and psoriatic arthritis.

✔ **Infliximab,** when combined with a standard medication for RA, methotrexate, showed dramatic improvement in RA symptoms compared with methotrexate used alone. Fifty-two percent of those getting the combination of drugs enjoyed significant reduction in swollen and tender joints, compared to 17 percent on methotrexate alone. The improvement in symptoms occurred within two to six weeks (as opposed to months with methotrexate) and remained after one year. Infliximab has also been found to significantly reduce long-term damage. It's given intravenously once every eight weeks, although the dose is occasionally increased to once every four to six weeks. Infliximab is currently approved as a treatment for RA and Crohn's disease.

✔ **Adalimumab,** like infliximab, rapidly reduces the pain, tenderness, and swelling of joints seen in RA, and sustains those results over the long-term. It also helps to slow or prevent the progressive destruction of the joints. Clinical trials involving more than 2,400 patients have shown that treatment with adalimumab significantly improves physical function and the health-related quality of life, and surveys of nearly 2,500 patients have also shown that the drug is generally safe and well-tolerated. Adalimumab is currently approved as a treatment for RA.

The anti-TNF medications can bring about dramatic results, but they are also costly and can produce some serious side effects. A very small percentage of patients who were apparently prone to infections developed deadly diseases, such as tuberculosis, while taking these medications. Because of the possibility of developing tuberculosis, every single patient must have a TB skin test (called PPD), and in some cases, a chest X-ray before beginning treatment with anti-TNFs. Other side effects caused by these drugs include reactions at the injection site and headaches.

Rituximab for Rheumatoid Arthritis

Rituximab (brand name Rituxan), is an anti-cancer drug administered by infusion that is approved by the FDA for the treatment of non-Hodgkin's lymphoma. Recently, it was also shown to have excellent potential as a treatment for RA. Rituximab belongs to a class of drugs called the *monoclonal antibodies*, which act like little "smart bombs." They zero in on a targeted protein on the surface of certain cells and then attack and kill that cell, while sparing the healthy cells that surround it. Rituximab goes after immune cells called B-cells, which may be the driving force behind the autoimmune reaction that causes RA. Treatment with rituximab kills about 90 percent of these errant B cells and preserves the stem cells that "give birth" to new, healthy B cells.

A study of 161 RA patients, published in the *New England Journal of Medicine* in 2004, shows rituximab's exciting potential as a treatment for this disease. Just two infusions of rituximab, either taken alone or combined with a standard RA drug, relieved RA symptoms for as long as six months in up to 40 percent of the patients. Only 13 percent of those taking methotrexate (the most widely used RA drug) enjoyed similar results.

Rituximab is not yet approved for use as an RA treatment, and much more study is needed. But it may be the forerunner of a new wave of focused treatments that zero in on the causes of arthritis and other joint diseases.

The "Mini-Open" Surgical Technique for Carpal Tunnel Syndrome

A new ten-minute surgical procedure, done on an outpatient basis, may provide excellent relief from the pain of advanced carpal tunnel syndrome (compression of the nerve and tendons that pass through the carpal tunnel, a corridor between the ligaments and bones in the wrist). Carpal tunnel syndrome causes pain, numbness, and tingling in the thumb, index, and middle fingers that can move all the way up to the arm and shoulder.

Splints, medications to reduce pain and inflammation, and steroid injections into the afflicted nerve are standard treatments. But those who don't respond to these treatments may opt for surgery. In the past, a longer, more complex surgery was used, but today a new surgery called the *mini-open technique* is becoming more popular. This technique allows better access to important structures in the wrist and sidesteps the pain and complications that come from making incisions in the more painful area of the palm of the hand. A tiny 2-centimeter incision is made in the palm, through which specially designed surgical instruments are inserted, allowing the surgeon to "open up" the carpal tunnel and relieve nerve compression. Most patients can use the affected hand the same day for regular activities like brushing teeth, and physical therapy is almost never needed. In most cases, the mini-open surgery cures the problem permanently.

Etoricoxib for RA, OA, and Gout

In December 2003, a new medication called etoricoxib was submitted for FDA approval as a treatment for osteoarthritis, rheumatoid arthritis, and acute gouty arthritis. Widely available in Europe and Mexico, etoricoxib is a COX-2 inhibitor. As described in Chapter 8, NSAIDs relieve inflammation by interfering with an enzyme called COX (cyclooxygenase). But it turns out that there are *two* of these COX enzymes: COX-1 helps keep your stomach healthy (among many other things), and COX-2 plays a role in the inflammation process. The standard NSAIDs inhibit both COX enzymes, the "good" and the "bad." As a result, your joints may feel better, but your stomach feels worse.

The new COX-2 inhibitors (including etoricoxib, rofecoxib, celecoxib, and valdecoxib) are designed to spare the COX-1 "healthy stomach" enzymes while going after the "inflammatory" COX-2 enzymes. So, like the NSAIDs, they relieve pain and inflammation, but they're less likely to leave you with a raw, burning stomach or stomach ulcers (although some people do develop gastrointestinal bleeding and ulcerations while taking COX-2 inhibitors). Etoricoxib, which is a more selective COX-2 inhibitor, goes even further than the other "coxibs," targeting the COX-2 enzymes 100 times more often than the COX-1 enzymes. Although yet to be proven, the theory is that this should make etoricoxib even easier on your stomach.

Studies of RA patients show that etoricoxib reduces joint tenderness, swelling, and RA disease activity, working just as well as or better than a standard RA treatment: the NSAID naproxen. Not only that, in a quality-of-life study, etoricoxib significantly improved pain relief, physical functioning, social functioning, and the patients' general perception of health when compared to patients who were using naproxen. Yet the risk of developing kidney complications (a possibility with certain OA and RA drugs) was low. It also causes significantly less gastrointestinal blood loss than ibuprofen does.

When etoricoxib was compared to the commonly used OA medication diclofenac, it provided an equal amount of pain relief but worked faster, providing much greater relief within the first four hours. As an added bonus, etoricoxib is taken only once a day, compared with diclofenac's three times a day.

In patients with acute gouty arthritis, etoricoxib relieved joint pain, inflammation, and tenderness as quickly and effectively as the standard gout medication, indomethacin, but with fewer side effects.

Although the COX-2 inhibitors may be a great idea for patients who have a history of stomach ulcers or suffer from gastrointestinal side effects when taking traditional NSAIDs, it's important to remember that many people do well with traditional NSAIDS, which are quite a bit cheaper. And some people taking etoricoxib experience dizziness and headaches. Those who are pregnant or have liver disease, gastrointestinal bleeding or ulcers, asthma, inflammatory bowel disease, or congestive heart failure should not take this drug.

Bosentan for Scleroderma

Scleroderma, a disease that causes the body to produce too much collagen and store it in body tissues in harmful ways, has no cure. Thick, hardened, and rough skin with lumpy calcium deposits, joint swelling and locking, problems swallowing, and organ impairment are just a few of the devastating effects of this disease. One serious complication of scleroderma is a lung disorder called pulmonary arterial hypertension (PAH), which is characterized by abnormally high blood pressure in the arteries between the heart and the lungs. PAH causes shortness of breath and significantly reduces your ability to exercise or exert yourself. PAH is caused by changes in the lining of the blood vessels that service the lungs that make it harder to deliver nutrients and take away wastes from these vital organs. It's a rare disease, but it's also fatal.

In the past, scientists thought that these unhealthy changes in the blood vessels were permanent. But in July 2003, a report of the long-term results of a medication called bosentan showed that these blood vessel changes could actually be reversed. Bosentan, the first FDA-approved oral treatment for PAH, works by blocking a hormone that constricts the blood vessels. It was shown to improve blood vessel health, allowing many (but not all) patients to walk farther and function better overall. This improvement in walking distance continued for as long as seven months after treatment was stopped. Bosentan also prevented the painful, debilitating hand ulcers often seen in those with scleroderma and significantly improved their hand function.

Another reason that bosentan is considered a breakthrough in the treatment of PAH is that it's taken orally. In the past, most PAH patients had to use a medication that was continuously infused through a central venous line, so they were forced to carry around an infusion pump. Bosentan does have two significant risks: It can cause birth defects and liver toxicity. Anyone who is pregnant, may become pregnant, or who has liver disease should not take this medication.

MMF for Lupus-Related Kidney Problems

Mycophenolate mofetil (MMF) is an immunosuppressive drug that has been used for several years to help prevent the rejection of organ transplants. But several recent studies have shown that MMF is also a promising treatment for the kidney inflammation seen in lupus patients. In the past, these patients were generally treated with a very toxic chemotherapy drug, cyclophosphamide, subjecting them to serious side effects, including irreversible sterility, bone marrow suppression, and an increased risk of cancer. But MMF, which has far fewer side effects (there is often some bone marrow suppression), appears to reduce kidney inflammation and send it into remission in some patients. MMF is also effective as a maintenance therapy for patients who were treated with cyclophosphamide and are already in remission. This is great news for lupus patients with kidney disease. At last, a treatment that is generally well-tolerated and safe!

MMF has also been used successfully to treat lupus-related skin lesions, psoriatic arthritis, inflammatory arthritis, rheumatoid arthritis, and scleroderma, although it's not yet been approved for such purposes. Remember that MMF *does* weaken your immune system, although it seems to be safer than the other immunosuppressive drugs. MMF is usually taken twice a day in capsule or liquid form, and common side effects include nausea, vomiting, loss of appetite, abdominal pain, diarrhea, anemia, and low white blood cell count.

Cartilage Self-Transplants and Tissue Engineering

It would be nice if we could simply pop in a new "slab" of cartilage every time a joint went bad. Of course we can't, but doctors have figured out a way to use cartilage from a healthy joint to buff up a joint with cartilage that has seen better days.

The concept is simple: Use an arthroscope to take a small sample of cartilage from a healthy joint, "wash" this cartilage clean, and then let it grow and multiply in the laboratory. At the appropriate time, open up the damaged joint with an arthroscope and "plant" the cultured cartilage into the bad joint. If all goes well, the new, healthy cartilage will grow and multiply in the new location, replacing the diseased cartilage and restoring the damaged joint to health. And you don't have to worry about tissue rejection, because it's your very own tissue.

Cartilage self-transplantation is primarily performed on the knee. So far, the results are promising, with up to 80 percent of patients reporting improved joint function several months or years later.

Researchers from Johns Hopkins University are currently working on a new approach to the problem of old or worn-out cartilage. It involves harvesting cartilage stem cells (cells that have the ability to multiply) from adult goats, adding them to a nutrient-rich fluid, and injecting the fluid under the skin. When an ultraviolet light or a visible laser is shined through the skin, the liquid hardens into a solid material called a *hydrogel*. In theory, this gel can then be injected into the joint, where the stem cells regenerate and eventually replace the damaged cartilage. Bone stem cells could work the same way to replace damaged bone tissue.

Although studies involving humans are years away, researchers hope that replacing joint parts with living tissue instead of metal or plastic parts will provide better, more long-lasting results.

Glass Therapy to Repair Bone and Treat RA

Although still in developmental stages, crushed glass particles and tiny glass spheres form the basis of two new treatments for diseased bones and joints. By crushing particles of glass and mixing them with a polymer, researchers at the University of Missouri-Rolla are attempting to create a solution that can be injected into broken or diseased bones to fill up the spaces or cracks. Just as caulk fills cracks in your windowsill, this solution is designed to shore up broken or diseased bones, making them stronger and better able to function.

Another development in the pipeline is tiny biodegradable glass beads made of radioactive material, which can be injected into a joint to irradiate diseased tissue, such as that seen in RA. By delivering the radiation only to the diseased tissue, healthy tissues remain unaffected. The glass beads (which have a diameter ⅕ to ⅒ the size of a human hair) will eventually dissolve. This procedure has been used in many studies to perform a nonsurgical *synovectomy* (removal of a diseased joint lining). However, now that we have better medications for prevention and treatment of joint lining disease, (specifically the disease modifying antirheumatic drugs — see Chapter 8), the need for synovectomies may be less and less. The niche for glass therapy may be as a way to handle stubborn cases of RA, rather than as a first line of treatment.

Therapeutic Tape for Osteoarthritis Pain

Researchers in Australia recently found that using special therapeutic taping techniques on knees affected by OA significantly reduced knee pain and disability, and the benefits lasted as long as three weeks after removal of the tape! The study included 87 patients with OA of the knee who were randomly assigned to one of three groups. The therapeutic tape group had their knees taped in a special way with hypoallergenic tape topped with rigid strapping tape. The control group had their knees taped in the same fashion, using hypoallergenic tape only, and those in the third group didn't have their knees taped.

After three weeks, 73 percent of those in the therapeutic tape group had reduced knee pain, compared with 49 percent of those in the control group and only 10 percent of those who had no taping. The therapeutic tape group had significant improvements in pain, disability, and quality of life compared with the no-tape group.

Although no one is quite sure why therapeutic taping works, researchers think it may be because it helps improve joint alignment and helps "take a load off" inflamed tissues.

The therapeutic taping technique is easy to learn, inexpensive, and may be an effective way of self-managing OA of the knee. If you're interested in finding out more about therapeutic tape, contact a physical therapist. (See Appendix B.)

Improvements in Hip Replacement Materials and Techniques

Every year, approximately 435,000 Americans have joint replacement surgery to give a new lease on life to a joint damaged by severe arthritis. But even though this surgery can improve joint function, increase range of motion, and reduce pain dramatically, many people put it off for years or even decades. That's because the joint replacements themselves tend to wear out or come loose over time. Until recently, hip replacement implants were made of metal and plastic, and the plastic wore down over time, sometimes even causing joint infection. Revision surgeries to install a new replacement were often required after as little as ten years. So in order to reduce the number of surgeries they'd need over a lifetime, young people or those who were particularly active were usually warned to wait as long as possible before going under the knife. Yet delaying joint replacement surgery can be a bad idea. Studies have shown that those who delay their joint replacement surgery until the decline in joint function is severe have the worst surgical outcomes.

Luckily, there may no longer be a need to delay, thanks to recent improvements in the quality and durability of the materials used in hip replacements. New implants made completely of metal can increase the life of joint replacements substantially and reduce the risk of joint infection. That means that scores of young people, baby boomers, and active adults who would have been considered unsuitable for joint replacement surgery in the past can now enjoy the benefits of an artificial hip much sooner.

And we have even more good news: Hip surgery itself has become less damaging to the surrounding tissues and requires less time for recovery, thanks to a new, minimally invasive form of hip surgery that was pioneered in 2001. The incision is only 4 to 6 inches long (a far cry from the standard 10 to 12 inches!), which means that fewer muscles and other body tissues must be cut. That's because the ball-and-stem portion of the artificial joint can be folded before insertion, making it able to fit into a much smaller opening. The stem is also shorter and narrower than the older varieties, so less drilling is required to make the shaft in the bone. This translates to less bone and tissue damage and a much faster recovery time.

Although the shaft portion has gotten smaller, in some new implants, the hip-ball portion has gotten larger. Although a traditional hip replacement has a hip-ball that is about the diameter of a nickel (26 to 28 millimeters), in two new prostheses (the Conserve® Total Femoral Head and the Conserve® Plus) the hip-ball is about twice that size (up to 54 millimeters). These larger hip-balls more closely match the size of a natural femoral ball, allowing greater range of motion and reducing the risk of dislocation.

Part VI
Appendixes

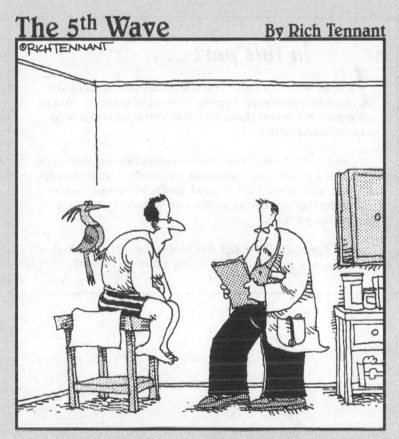

"Bursitis? Well, maybe. But, like that pain in your shoulder, it could be a lot of things."

In this part . . .

In Appendix A, we give you a glossary that defines the most frequently used terms relating to arthritis. You'll probably encounter these terms as you read and talk to others about arthritis.

Appendix B is a list of resources — associations where you can find a practitioner, get more information, find support groups, and more. A lot of good, free information can be found on the Internet as well, so we've listed Web sites whenever possible.

And in Appendix C, we tell you how to take stress off your joints by reaching and maintaining a healthy weight.

Appendix A

Glossary

• •

Acupressure (Shiatsu): A Japanese form of massage that aims to restore health by normalizing the flow of energy and blood in the body.

Acupuncture: A part of traditional Chinese medicine that uses the insertion of very fine needles to help balance the flow of energy in the body.

Acute pain: Pain that typically strikes severely and suddenly, builds, and then fades away. It occurs in response to injury, inflammation, surgery, and so on, and usually doesn't last long.

Alternative medicine: Healing techniques that fall outside of the realm of conventional, Western medicine.

Ankylosing spondylitis: A disease that causes inflammation and stiffness of the spine and its joints and that can result in the fusing or "locking" of those joints.

Antioxidants: Substances manufactured by the body and found in foods and supplements that help control the oxidation and free radical activity that can damage body tissue and cause or worsen certain disease states.

Aromatherapy: An alternative healing system based on the belief that inhaling certain aromas or scents can help the body heal itself.

Arthritis: A group of diseases (formerly called rheumatism) that strikes the joints and/or nearby tissues. The word arthritis means *joint inflammation,* although not all forms of arthritis cause inflammation.

Arthrodesis: Surgically immobilizing a joint so that the bones grow together and "lock" into position. This procedure is sometimes performed in cases of rheumatoid arthritis.

Arthroplasty: Surgical reconstruction of a joint using a combination of natural tissues and artificial parts; most commonly performed on the hip and knee.

Arthroscopy: Visual examination of the inside of a joint performed by using a special "scope" that is passed through a small incision. Arthroscopy can be used to diagnose certain types of joint disease and in some cases, make repairs surgically.

Autologous chondrocyte implantation: The transplantation of healthy cartilage cells from a normal joint to a damaged one, so that they can grow and supplement or replace ailing cartilage.

Ayurvedic healing: An ancient Indian healing art that uses diet, exercise, internal cleansing, herbs, massage, crystals, aromatherapy, color therapy, gems, and other modalities to eliminate illness and restore balance to the body.

Bee venom therapy: The use of bee venom to relieve pain and inflammation. The venom may be delivered via the sting of a live bee or through an injection.

Biofeedback: A method for helping one learn to exert some control over certain physiological functions, such as muscle tension or blood pressure. During a biofeedback session, you're hooked up to a machine that provides audio and visual feedback, as for example, muscle tension increases or decreases. Feedback from the machines shows you how certain body functions change as you relax.

Biomechanics: In a non-technical sense, it is the study of the way the body deals with its own weight — for example, the impact of walking or running on the weight-bearing joints. Using proper biomechanical techniques, one can greatly minimize the stress placed on the joints while moving, lifting, or even sitting.

Borrelia burgdorferi: The bacteria that causes Lyme disease, transmitted to humans by infected ticks.

Bursitis: A painful condition resulting from inflammation of the bursae, the fluid-filled pouches that keep certain joints moving smoothly. Shoulder joints are likely targets of bursitis.

Calcium pyrophosphate dihydrate crystals: Crystals that can accumulate in a joint and cause the symptoms of pseudogout.

Capsaicin: The hot part of chili peppers. Capsaicin fights pain by stimulating nerve cells to release large amounts of substance P, which sensitizes the receptors that originate the pain signals. When the cells run out of substance P, pain signals subside.

Carpal tunnel syndrome: A condition caused by pressure on the median nerve as it runs through the *carpal tunnel,* a narrow opening between the ligaments and bones in the wrist. Symptoms include pain, weakness, tingling, burning, and muscle atrophy.

Cartilage: Connective tissue found in the joints and elsewhere in the body. Joint cartilage helps protect bone ends that would otherwise rub against each other and produce pain and other problems.

Chiropractic: A healing system based on the belief that disease arises when spinal vertebrae are out of alignment and press on nerves. Chiropractic healing techniques include spinal manipulation and possibly exercise, nutrition, massage, and other modalities.

Chondroitin sulfate: A supplement that, studies suggest, can relieve symptoms of osteoarthritis. Often used in conjunction with glucosamine, chondroitin sulfate helps pull water into the cartilage and fight cartilage-eating enzymes that can damage this precious tissue.

Chronic pain: Pain that lasts weeks or months, that accompanies long-term disease, or that keeps recurring. It may continue long after the apparent cause has disappeared and can significantly reduce the quality of life.

Complementary medicine: Nonstandard healing approaches designed to work with conventional Western medicine.

Corticosteroids: A group of hormones naturally produced by the body that have wide ranging effects on metabolism, water balance, and organ function. The man-made versions have powerful anti-inflammatory properties but also have some serious side effects.

COX-2 Inhibitors: A relatively new form of NSAID with the same pain-relieving and anti-inflammatory benefits as other NSAIDs, but with fewer side effects.

Deep tissue massage: The application of strong pressure to the muscles using fingers, hands, or elbows to relieve chronic tension in the muscles.

Dermatomyositis: A disease that produces muscle pain plus skin rashes and other problems.

DHEA (dehydroepiandrosterone): A hormone that the body uses to make testosterone, estrogen, and other hormones, DHEA is sometimes used by alternative healers to treat lupus and other ailments. Sometimes called the mother of all hormones, it is produced primarily in the adrenal glands.

Discoid lupus erythematosus: A "limited" form of lupus that may produce a rash and other skin problems, weakening of the immune system, and other symptoms, but isn't as severe as systemic lupus erythematosus.

DMARDs: Disease-modifying, antirheumatic drugs used for rheumatoid arthritis, psoriatic arthritis, and other forms of the disease. DMARDs appear to work by altering the behavior of the immune system.

DMSO (dimethyl sulfoxide): A form of alternative therapy, DMSO is a clear liquid that may be applied to the skin, injected, or swallowed in hopes of reducing arthritis pain and inflammation.

Fibromyalgia: A disease characterized by inflammation of the connective tissue, including the ligaments, tendons, and muscles. Symptoms include chronic achy pain, stiffness, disturbed sleep, depression, and fatigue.

Glucosamine: A supplement that studies suggest can relieve symptoms of osteoarthritis. Often used in conjunction with chondroitin sulfate, glucosamine is used by the body to manufacture proteoglycans, which draw water into the cartilage and keep it moist.

Gonococcal arthritis: The most common form of infectious arthritis, caused by the *gonococci* bacterium.

Gout: A type of arthritis caused by an accumulation of uric acid crystals in the joint, often the bunion joint of the large toe. Symptoms of gout include terrible pain, joint stiffness and swelling, and possibly fever, chills, and an elevated heart rate.

Herbalism (phytotherapy): The use of the roots, bark, stems, flowers, or other parts of selected plants to relieve the symptoms of illness and/or strengthen the body.

Holistic medicine: An approach to healing and health based on treating a patient's mind, body and spirit, rather than simply trying to counteract the disease or relieve symptoms.

Homeopathy: An alternative healing system developed in the eighteenth century, based on the belief that "like cures like." Thus, for example, patients suffering from nausea would be treated with very small doses of a substance that can cause nausea when given in large amounts to healthy people.

Hydrotherapy: The use of water, both hot and cold or in the form of steam, ice, compresses, and so on to relieve symptoms and help the body heal itself.

Immunosuppressants: Drugs that dampen the immune system. These may be used to treat rheumatoid arthritis, lupus, and other diseases in which the immune system is malfunctioning.

Infectious arthritis: Arthritis that is caused by the invasion of bacteria, viruses, or fungi.

Joint: The place where two bones meet. Joints can be moveable or fixed. There are gliding joints such as the spinal vertebrae, hinge joints such as the elbows, saddle joints such as the wrist, and ball-and-socket joints such as the hip.

Juvenile rheumatoid arthritis (JRA): The most common form of arthritis to strike children, producing pain or swelling in the joints, fever, anemia, and other symptoms.

Lyme disease: A disease caused by the *borrelia burgdorferi* bacteria, which is transmitted to humans through the bite of an infected tick. Lyme disease can produce a large bull's-eye shaped rash at the bite site, swelling and pain in the joints, fever, fatigue, muscle aches, nausea, swollen lymph nodes, and other symptoms.

Mediterranean diet: The standard diet consumed by people living in the Mediterranean areas of Greece, Italy, southern France, and parts of Spain, made up of plenty of fresh vegetables, fruits, whole-grain breads, pasta and cereal, nuts and legumes, plus good amounts of olive oil. This diet may help ease RA-related pain and swelling.

MSM (methylsulfonylmethane): A breakdown product of DMSO, MSM is an anti-inflammatory used by some alternative practitioners to treat arthritis.

Naturopathy: A healing art based on the belief that all diseases have natural causes and that the body has very strong, natural healing powers. Naturopathic physicians use diet, herbs, exercise, stress reduction, acupressure, and other modalities to help increase the body's healing prowess.

NSAIDs: Nonsteroidal anti-inflammatory medications designed to reduce pain and inflammation, often prescribed for various forms of arthritis.

Occupational therapist: A licensed professional who can help you cope with the day-to-day problems of living with arthritis (and other ailments) by finding easier ways for you to accomplish tasks, designing splints, recommending assistive devices, teaching you ways to protect your joints, and so on.

Omega-3 fatty acids: Sometimes called fish oil because their major source is certain types of fish, these substances can help reduce inflammation and other symptoms of rheumatoid arthritis, and possibly other forms of arthritis.

Omega-6 fatty acids: Found primarily in salad or cooking oils, these fatty acids can increase the inflammatory response. The exception is an omega-6 called gamma-linolenic acid (GLA), which helps calm inflammation. GLA is found in evening primrose oil, as well as black currant seed oil and borage seed oil.

Orthopedist: A medical doctor specializing in diagnosing and treating problems of the bones, joints, muscles, and related tissues.

Osteoarthritis: A type of arthritis caused by the breakdown of cartilage, most often in the hips, knees, and other weight-bearing joints. Osteoarthritis may be due to injury, obesity, metabolic errors, heredity, or other factors.

Osteotomy: A surgical procedure during which a piece of bone is removed to improve joint alignment. It is sometimes used to treat osteoarthritis or ankylosing spondylitis.

Paget's disease: A disease in which the body inappropriately breaks down and rebuilds bone, resulting in weaker bones, bone deformity, and other problems. Many patients with Paget's disease are middle aged or older.

Physical therapy: The use of massage, exercise, hydrotherapy, electrical stimulation, and other modalities to help relieve pain, increase range of motion, strengthen muscles, and stimulate healing.

Polarity therapy: An alternative healing art based on the idea that the body contains energy systems that must be kept in balance. Polarity therapists attempt to find and release energy blockages by touching specific points on the body, and sometimes use gentle massage.

Polymyalgia rheumatica: A rheumatic condition characterized by severe, sudden stiffness in major joints, plus headaches, difficulty swallowing, coughing, and other symptoms.

Polymyositis: A disease that produces inflammation of the muscles and loss of strength. There may also be joint pain, weight loss, Raynaud's phenomenon, and other symptoms. Polymyositis is like dermatomyositis, without the skin problems.

Pseudogout: A from of arthritis similar to gout, but caused by the accumulation of calcium pyrophosphate dihydrate crystals (rather than uric acid crystals) in the affected joint.

Psoriatic arthritis: Striking about 5 percent of those who have the skin condition known as psoriasis, psoriatic arthritis can cause inflammation, swelling, and sometimes joint deformity.

Raynaud's phenomenon: A disease in which arterial spasms cause pain, burning, tingling, numbness, and/or discoloration, primarily in the fingers and toes. Raynaud's disease is the more common and often milder form; Raynaud's phenomenon is triggered by another ailment, such as lupus or scleroderma.

Reactive arthritis: A disease that may develop after an infection, reactive arthritis can produce mild to severe pain in the joints, inflammation of the eyelid, eyeball, and urethra, and other problems.

Reflexology: An alternative healing system based on the idea that specific areas of the feet are linked to parts of the body. Manipulating the point on the foot corresponding to the lungs, for example, is believed to help relieve some of the symptoms of asthma.

Reiki: A Japanese healing art in which the practitioner channels energy into the patient by laying his hands lightly on or directly above the patient's body to help restore the body's flow and balance of energy.

Rheumatoid arthritis: The second most common form of arthritis, rheumatoid arthritis is brought about when the immune system attacks the body. The result can be joint pain and inflammation, generalized soreness and stiffness, fever, difficulty sleeping, and joint deterioration. The disease can also attack the lungs, blood vessels, and other parts of the body.

Rheumatoid factor (RF): An antibody found in some 80 percent of those with rheumatoid arthritis. Its presence strongly suggests that one has rheumatoid arthritis, although it's possible to have RF and not develop the disease.

SAMe (S-adenosyl-L-methione): A product of body metabolism, SAMe (pronounced *sammy*) is sometimes used in supplement form to combat depression and the symptoms of osteoarthritis.

Scleroderma: An autoimmune disease in which the body produces and stores excess collagen, resulting in damage to the skin, joint pain and swelling, difficulty swallowing, digestive difficulties, injury to the blood vessels, and damaged organs.

Sjögren's syndrome: A disease that produces dryness of the eyes and mouth and certain other parts of the body. Depending on the extent of the dryness and which parts of the body are affected, problems can range from the manageable to the very serious. A fair number of those with Sjögren's syndrome also develop arthritis, but this arthritis is most often a separate entity.

Soft tissue rheumatism: An old term indicating inflammation or pain in the bursae, tendons, ligaments, and other tissues surrounding and/or supporting the joints. Carpal tunnel syndrome is an example of soft tissue rheumatism.

Swedish massage: The gentle kneading and stroking of muscles, connective tissue, and skin to relieve stress and soothe pained muscles.

Synovectomy: A surgery in which an overgrown, inflamed joint lining is removed; it may be performed for rheumatoid arthritis.

Synovial membrane: Part of the capsule surrounding certain joints, this membrane releases a lubricating fluid into the joint.

Systemic lupus erythematosus: An autoimmune disease that tends to attack women of childbearing age. Systemic lupus erythematosus can cause a variety of symptoms, including joint pain and inflammation, fever, rash, hair loss, anemia, weakness of the immune system, depression, and nervous system disorders. It can be fatal.

Tendonitis: Inflammation of a tendon, characterized by pain to the touch or upon movement. The upper arms, hands, fingers, and backs of the ankles are common targets of tendonitis.

TENS: Transcutaneous electrical nerve stimulation — the use of mild electrical currents to deliver small jolts to painful areas of the body. The electricity overrides pain signals.

Trigger finger: The locking of a finger in a bent position caused by swelling and inflammation of a tendon.

Trigger point therapy: Prolonged, deep tissue pressure applied to specific, tender, and hard points on muscles to relieve tension and pain. The therapy may include injections of local anesthetic into trigger points.

Urethritis: An inflammation of the *urethra,* the tube urine passes through to get from the bladder to the outside of the body.

Uric acid crystals: The offending agents in gout that accumulate in the joint, causing pain and other symptoms.

Vasodilators: Medications that relax blood vessels and help blood flow more freely.

Appendix B
Resources

• •

Organizations

Acupuncture/Acupressure

American Academy of Medical Acupuncture, 4929 Wilshire Blvd., Suite 428, Los Angeles, CA 90010; phone 323-937-5514; Web site www.medical acupuncture.org/index.html

National Certification Commission for Acupuncture and Oriental Medicine (NCCAOM), 11 Canal Center Plaza, Suite 330, Alexandria, VA 22314; phone 703-548-9004; Web site www.nccaom.org

Alexander Technique

Alexander Technique International, 1692 Massachusetts Ave., Third Floor Cambridge, MA 01238; phone 888-668-8996; Web site www.ati-net.com

American Society for the Alexander Technique, P.O. Box 60008, Florence, MA 01062; phone 800-473-0620; Web site www.alexandertech.org

Alternative Medicine

National Center for Complementary & Alternative Medicine (NCCAM) Clearinghouse, P.O. Box 7923, Gaithersburg, MD 90898; phone 888-644-6226; Web site nccam.nih.gov/health

Aromatherapy

National Association for Holistic Aromatherapy (NAHA), 4509 Interlake Ave. N., #233, Seattle, WA 98103-6773; phone (888) ASK-NAHA or 206-547-2680; Web site www.naha.org

Arthritis Information and Management

American College of Rheumatology, 1800 Century Place, Suite 250, Atlanta, GA 30345-4300; phone 404-633-3777; Web site www.rheumatology.org

American Juvenile Arthritis Organization, 1330 West Peachtree St., Atlanta, GA 30309; phone 800-283-7800 or 404-872-7100; Web site www.arthritis. org/communities/juvenile_arthritis/about_ajao.asp

Arthritis Foundation, P.O. Box 7669, Atlanta, GA 30357-0669; phone 800-283-7800 or 404-872-7100 or call your local chapter; Web site www.arthritis.org

Fibromyalgia Network, P.O. Box 31750, Tucson, AZ 85751-1750; phone 800-853-2929; Web site www.fmnetnews.com

Lupus Foundation of America, Inc., 2000 L St., N.W., Suite 710, Washington, DC 20036; phone 202-349-1155; Web site www.lupus.org

The Myositis Association, 1233 29th St. NW, Suite 402, Washington, DC 20036; phone 202-887-0082; Web site www.myositis.org

National Institute of Arthritis and Musculoskeletal and Skin Diseases (NIAMS) Information Clearinghouse, National Institutes of Health, 1 AMS Circle, Bethesda, MD 20892-3675; phone 877-226-4267 (toll free) or 301-495-4484; Web site www.nih.gov/niams

The National Psoriasis Foundation, 6600 SW 92nd Ave., Suite 300, Portland, OR 97223-7195; phone 800-723-9166 (toll free) or 503-244-7404; Web site www.psoriasis.org

The Paget Foundation, 120 Wall St., Suite 1602, New York, NY 10005-4001; phone 800-237-2438 (toll free) or 212-509-5335; Web site www.paget.org

Scleroderma Foundation, 12 Kent Way, Suite 101, Byfield, MA 01922; phone 800-722-4673 or 978-463-5843; Web site www.scleroderma.org

Sjögren's Syndrome Foundation, Inc., 8120 Woodmont Ave., Bethesda, MD 20814; phone 800-475-6473 (toll free; voice mail only); Web site www.sjogrens.org

Spondylitis Association of America (SAA), P.O. Box 5872, Sherman Oaks, CA 91413; phone 800-777-8189 or 818-981-1616; Web site www.spondylitis.org

Bee Venom Therapy

American Apitherapy Society, 5390 Grande Road, Hillsboro, OH 45133; phone (937)364-1108; e-mail aasoffice@in-touch.net, Web site www.apitherapy.org

Biofeedback

The Association for Applied Psychophysiology and Biofeedback, 10200 W. 44th Ave., Suite 304, Wheat Ridge, CO 80033-2840; phone 303-422-8436; Web site www.aapb.org

Biomechanics Experts

American Academy of Osteopathy, 3500 DePauw Blvd., #1080, Indianapolis, IN 46268; phone 317-879-1881; Web site www.academyofosteopathy.org

Chiropractors

American Chiropractic Association (ACA), 1701 Clarendon Blvd., Arlington, VA 22209; phone 800-986-4636; Web site www.amerchiro.org

ChiroWeb – Everything Chiropractic for Chiropractors, Students, Patients and Health Care Consumers, Dynamic Chiropractic, P.O. Box 4109, Huntington Beach, CA 92605-4109; phone 714-230-3150; Web site www.chiroweb.com

DMSO/MSM

Dr. Stanley Jacob, DMSO Research Institute, L225, 3181 S.W. Sam Jackson Park Rd., Portland, OR 97201-3098; Dr. Jacob can be contacted by e-mail at Jacobs@ohsu.edu; for information about treatment, contact Dr. Jeffrey Tyler at 503-255-4256; Web site www.dmso.org

Feldenkrais Method

The Feldenkrais Guild of North America (FGNA), 3611 SW Hood Ave., Suite 100, Portland, OR 97239; phone 800-775-2118 or 503-221-6612; Web site www.feldenkrais.com

Help for Caregivers

Family Caregiver Alliance, 690 Market St., Suite 600, San Francisco, CA 94104; phone 800-445-8106 (toll free) or 415-434-3388; Web site www.caregiver.org

National Family Caregivers Association, 10400 Connecticut Ave., #500, Kensington, MD 20895-3944; phone 800-896-3650; Web site www.nfcacares.org

Homeopathic Medicine

Homeopathic Educational Services, 2124B Kittredge St., Berkeley, CA 94704; phone 510-649-0294; Web site www.homeopathic.com

National Center for Homeopathy, 801 N. Fairfax St., Suite 306, Alexandria, VA 22314; phone 703-548-7790; Web site www.homeopathic.org

Hypnotherapists

American Council of Hypnotist Examiners (ACHE), 700 So. Central Ave., Glendale, CA 91204-2011; phone 818-242-1159; Web site www.sonic.net/hypno/ache.html

National Guild of Hypnotists, Inc. P.O. Box 308, Merrimack, NH 03054-0308; phone 603-429-9438; Web site www.ngh.net

Massage Therapists

The American Massage Therapy Association, 820 Davis St., Suite 100, Evanston, IL 60201-4444; phone 847-864-0123; Web site www.amtamassage.org

Associated Bodywork & Massage Professionals, 1271 Sugarbush Dr., Evergreen, CO 80439-9766; phone 800-458-2267 or 303-674-8478; e-mail expectmore@abmp, Web site www.abmp.com

National Certification Board for Therapeutic Massage & Bodywork, 8201 Greensboro Dr., Suite 300, McLean, VA 22102; phone 800-296-0664 or 703-610-9015; Web site www.ncbtmb.com

Medical Societies

American Academy of Orthopaedic Surgeons, 6300 North River Rd., Suite 200, Rosemont, IL 60018–4262; phone 800-346-2267 or 847-823-7186; Web site www.aaos.org

American Academy of Physical Medicine and Rehabilitation, One IBM Plaza, Suite 2500, Chicago, IL 60611-3604; phone 312-464-9700; Web site www.aapmr.org

American Board of Medical Specialties, 1007 Church St., Suite 404, Evanston, IL 60210-5913; phone 847-491-9091; Web site www.abms.org can provide you with referrals to physicians who are board-certified in orthopedic surgery, pain management, rheumatology, surgery, and other specialties

American Board of Surgery, 1617 John F. Kennedy Blvd., Suite 860, Philadelphia, PA 19103-1847; phone 215-568-4000; Web site www.absurgery.org

American Medical Association, 515 N. State St., Chicago, IL 60610-4320; phone 800-621-8335 or 312-464-5000; Web site www.ama-assn.org

American Occupational Therapy Association, 4720 Montgomery Ln., P.O. Box 31220, Bethesda, MD 20824-1220; phone 800-377-8555 or 301-652-2682; Web site www.aota.org

American Physical Therapy Association, 1111 N. Fairfax St., Alexandria, VA 22314-1488; phone 703-684-2782; Web site www.apta.org

The Mind/Body Connection

Academy for Guided Imagery, 30765 Pacific Coast Hwy., #369, Malibu, CA 90265; phone 800-726-2070; Web site www.academyforguidedimagery.com

The Mind/Body Medical Institute, 824 Boylston St., Chestnut Hills, MA 02467; phone 617-991-0102; Web site www.mbmi.org

Naturopathic Medicine

The American Association of Naturopathic Physicians, 3201 New Mexico Ave. NW, Suite 350, Washington, DC 20016; phone 866-538-2267 (toll free) or 202-895-1392; Web site www.naturopathic.org

Bastyr University, 14500 Juanita Dr. NE, Kenmore, WA 98028-4966; phone 425-823-1300; Web site www.bastyr.edu

The Homeopathic Academy of Naturopathic Physicians, 1412 W. Washington St., Boise, ID 83702; phone 208-336-3390; Web site www.hanp.net

Nutritional Counseling

The American Dietetic Association, 120 South Riverside Plaza, Suite 2000, Chicago, IL, 60606-6995; phone 800-877-1600; Web site www.eatright.org

Pain Management

American Academy of Pain Management, 13947 Mono Way, #A, Sonora, CA 95370; phone 209-533-9744; Web site www.aapainmanage.org

American Chronic Pain Association, P.O. Box 850, Rocklin, CA 95677; phone 800-533-3231; Web site www.theacpa.org

American Pain Society, 4700 West Lake Ave., Glenview, IL 60025; phone 847-375-4715; Web site www.ampainsoc.org

Polarity Therapy

American Polarity Therapy Association, P.O. Box 19858, Boulder, CO 80308; phone 303-545-2080; Web site www.polaritytherapy.org

Psychotherapy

American Psychological Association, 750 First St., NE, Washington, DC 20002-4242; phone 800-374-2721 (toll free) or 202-336-5700; Web site www.apa.org

Association for Applied and Therapeutic Humor, 1951 W. Camelback Rd., Suite 445, Phoenix, AZ 85015; phone 602-995-1449; Web site http://aath.org

National Register of Health Service Providers in Psychology, 1120 G St., NW, #330, Washington, DC 20005; phone 202-783-7663; Web site www.nationalregister.com

Reiki

The International Association of Reiki Professionals, P.O. Box 104, Harrisville, NH 03450; phone 603-881-8838; Web site www.iarp.org

Reflexology

Reflexology Association of America, 4012 Rainbow Blvd., Suite K-PMB# 585, Las Vegas, NV 89103-2059; phone 978-779-7955; Web site www.reflexology-usa.org

Social Workers

National Association of Social Workers, 750 First St., NE, Suite 700, Washington DC 20002; phone 202-336-8200; Web site www.naswdc.org

Support Groups Online

National Mental Health Consumer Self-Help Clearinghouse, 1211 Chestnut St., #1207, Philadelphia, PA 19107; phone 800-553-4539 or 215-751-1810; Web site www.mhselfhelp.org; for information about how to start your own self-help group

SupportPath.Com, www.SupportPath.com; source for arthritis-related message boards and online chat

Therapeutic Touch

Nurse Healers — Professional Associates International (The Official Organization of Therapeutic Touch), 3760 South Highland Dr., Suite 429, Salt Lake City, UT 84106; phone 801-273-3399; Web site www.therapeutic-touch.org

The Trager Approach

Trager International, 24800 Chagrin Blvd., Suite 205, Beachwood, OH 44122; phone 216-896-9383; Web site www.trager.com

Assistive Devices — Mail-Order Catalogs

Access With Ease, 1755 Johnson, P.O. Box 1150, Chino Valley, AZ 86323; phone for information 928-636-9469, to order 800-531-9479; e-mail kmjc@northlink.com, Web site http://stores.yahoo.com (under Search type in **Access With Ease**); products to help prevent falls and eliminate bending, kneeling, and stooping

AliMed, 297 High St., Dedham, MA 02026; phone 781-329-2900 or 800-225-2610; e-mail for information info@alimed.com, to order cust_serv@alimed.com, Web site www.alimed.com; medical and ergonomic products

Dr. Leonard's Healthcare Products, 100 Nixon Ln., P.O. Box 7821, Edison, NJ 08818-7821; phone 800-785-0880; Web site www.drleonards.com; daily living aids

Don Kreb's Access to Recreation, 8 Sandra Ct., Newbury Park, CA 91320; phone 800-634-4351; e-mail dkrebs@accesstr.com, Web site www.accesstr.com; daily living aids, all-terrain wheelchairs, wheelchair ramps, shower lifts, and many other items

IMAK Products Corporation, 2515 Camino del Rio South, #240, San Diego, CA 92108; for information, phone 619-291-9990, to order 800-231-8226; e-mail customercare@imakproducts.com, Web site www.imakproducts.com; gloves, splints, cushions, and ergonomic products

Life With Ease, P.O. Box 302, 1329 Route 103, Newbury, NH 03255; 800-966-5119; e-mail for information questions@lifewithease.com, to order order@lifewithease.com, Web site www.lifewithease.com; ergonomic products, supports, daily living aids

Maxi-Aids and Appliances for Independent Living, 42 Executive Blvd., Farmingdale, NY 11735; for information, phone 631-752-0521, to order 800-522-6294; e-mail sales@maxiaids.com, Web site www.maxiaids.com

PHS West, Inc., 11283 River Rd. NE, Hanover, MN 55341; phone 888-639-5438; e-mail info@phswest.com, Web site www.phswest.com; motorized carts

Sammons Preston Rolyan, U.S.A., 4 Sammons Ct., Bolingbrook, IL 60440-5071; phone 630-226-1300; e-mail spr@ablityone.com, Web site www.sammonsprestonrolyan.com; daily living aids, wheelchairs, exercise equipment, splints

SoftFLEX Computer Gloves, Four Points Products, Inc., 4230 Winding Willow Dr., Tampa, FL 33618; phone 800-216-8415; e-mail info@softflex.com, Web site www.softflex.com

Books

The Arthritis Cure. Theodosakis, J., Adderly, B., Fox, B. New York, NY: St. Martin's Press, 1997. Discusses the use of glucosamine and chondroitin sulfate to ease OA pain and help repair cartilage

Eighty-Eight Easy-To-Make Aids for Older People and for Special Needs. Caston, D., Point Roberts, WA: Hartley and Marks, Inc., 1988. Although this book is out of print, new and used copies are available at www.amazon.com

Books from the Arthritis Foundation

To find the following titles, see your local Arthritis Foundation chapter or go to its Web site at www.arthritis.org, click on **Store** and then **Books**.

250 Tips for Making Life With Arthritis Easier

All You Need to Know About Back Pain

All You Need to Know About Joint Surgery

Good Living With Fibromyalgia Workbook

Guide to Alternative Therapies

Guide to Good Living With Fibromyalgia

Guide to Good Living With Osteoarthritis

Guide to Good Living With Rheumatoid Arthritis

Guide to Managing Your Arthritis

Guide to Pain Management

Raising a Child With Arthritis: A Parent's Guide

Tips for Good Living With Arthritis

Audio Tapes

Walk With Ease. Provides motivation to get you started on a walking program and keep you going. See your local Arthritis Foundation chapter or go to its Web site at www.arthritis.org, click on **Store** and then **Audio/Video.**

Videos

To find the following videos, see your local Arthritis Foundation chapter or go to its Web site at www.arthritis.org, click on **Store** and then **Audio/Video.**

Fibromyalgia Interval Training (FIT). These warm-water exercises, which are performed in both shallow and deep water, are designed to help those with fibromyalgia ease their pain, stiffness, and fatigue.

People with Arthritis Can Exercise (PACE) I. Basic strengthening, stretching, and cardio-fitness exercises to help you tone up and regain your range of movement. Led by Jan Stephenson, champion golfer.

People with Arthritis Can Exercise (PACE) II. A more advanced version of PACE I, led by Jan Stephenson, with the same goals in mind.

Pool Exercise Program (PEP). By exercising in water (no deeper than chest level), you can get a great workout while putting little or no strain on your joints.

Appendix C
Weight Loss and Management Guide

*E*ven if you're eating a balanced diet, getting plenty of omega-3s, and avoiding danger foods, you need to take one more step — the one that puts you up on a scale. And if what you see when you look at the dial doesn't look good, you need to lose weight.

If you're overweight or obese, one of the best things you can do for your aching joints is to lose weight. Cutting away the extra pounds takes a tremendous burden off those joints that have to bear your weight, such as your hip and knee joints. Not only does it take the pressure off, but strong evidence suggests that dropping down to your ideal weight can stave off the appearance of at least one form of arthritis.

The Framingham Study used X-rays to track the development of arthritis in women. The researchers found that in overweight women of normal height, every 11 pounds of weight loss reduced the risk of knee OA by 50 percent. And a study sponsored by the Arthritis Foundation found that older and overweight women could lower their risk of developing osteoarthritis of the knee — significantly — by reducing their weight.

Figuring Out Whether You're Too Heavy

On average, adult Americans have packed on an additional 8 pounds in the past decade, and we're continuing to grow. Medical experts agree that being slim is better, especially where arthritis is concerned. But what's slim? Unfortunately, we're not very good at knowing when enough is enough. In general, women tend to think they're too heavy, and men usually assume they're doing okay.

For years, people have looked at height-weight charts to see if they should drop a few pounds, but these charts were only rough guidelines. In 1998, a division of the National Institutes of Health issued a new set of guidelines based on the body mass index (BMI), a comparison of height and weight. Now you just look for one number, your BMI, to see whether you need to lose weight. Here are the standards:

✔ If your BMI is 24 or less, you're fine.

✔ If it's between 24 and 29, you're overweight. Those extra pounds are beginning to challenge your health and put extra pressure on your joints.

✔ If it's over 30 you're obese. Your weight is or likely will cause health problems.

So you want your BMI to be no more than 24, and certainly less than 29. The formula for determining BMI is simple: Multiply your weight in pounds by 703 and divide the answer by your height in inches squared. Well, maybe it's not so simple. Table C-1 will help you skip the figuring and get a fairly good idea of where you stand.

Table C-1		Body Mass Index Chart	
Height	Weight That Gives a Healthy BMI of 24	Weight That Puts You in the Overweight BMI Range	Weight That Gives an Obese BMI of 30
5'0"	123	124-153	154
5'1"	127	128-158	159
5'2"	131	132-163	164
5'3"	135	136-168	169
5'4"	140	141-174	175
5'5"	144	145-179	180
5'6"	149	150-185	186
5'7"	153	154-191	192
5'8"	158	159-196	197
5'9"	162	163-202	203
5'10"	167	167-208	209
5'11"	172	173-214	215

Height	Weight That Gives a Healthy BMI of 24	Weight That Puts You in the Overweight BMI Range	Weight That Gives an Obese BMI of 30
6'0"	177	178-220	221
6'1"	182	283-226	227
6'2"	187	187-233	234

The BMI isn't an absolutely perfect guide to weight. It only compares height to weight; it doesn't take into account that fact that some people appear "fatter" and get higher BMIs because they have lots of muscles. For others, the reverse can be true because they don't have much muscle. Still, BMI is a good starting point.

Losing Weight the Safe and Healthy Way

The bad news is that we can't provide you with a quick, simple, guaranteed way to lose weight. The gimmicks don't work, and the fad diets don't live up to their promises. Oh yes, you'll lose weight on most any fad diet, primarily because they all get you to restrict your intake one way or another. And many of them cause you to quickly lose lots of water weight. But most people quickly gain back all the water weight — and all the other weight as well. The overwhelming majority of people who drop pounds on fad diets gain them back — plus a few more. And to make matters worse, a fair number of fad diets are nutritionally unbalanced: Eating what these diets recommend for long periods of time can lead to trouble.

The good news is that you *can* lose weight without sacrificing nutrition or health. We can't go into great detail on losing weight, because this isn't a diet book. Fortunately, many books present safe, sensible, and effective diets, including *Dieting For Dummies* by the American Dietetic Association and Jane Kirby (Wiley).

Most people already know how to lose weight. Notwithstanding the hype in the fad diet books, the basic principles for healthy people are simple: Eat a well-rounded diet emphasizing fresh vegetables, whole grains, and fruits; keep your fat content down to reasonable levels; enjoy sweets as occasional treats; and burn lots of calories through physical activity and exercise. In short, burn more calories than you take in.

Aiming for long-term benefits

Don't diet. "Dieting" is a bad word, because it means giving up favorite foods and eating a lot of stuff you don't like, or starving yourself. It's a short-term fix to be discarded as soon as possible.

Instead, eat for lifelong good health. Focus on the slow, steady, and permanent weight loss that comes when your diet and activity/exercise habits are in alignment.

Eating fruits and vegetables

Eat a variety of vegetables, fruits, and whole grains to ensure that you get all the numerous nutrients in foods. No single food or food group gives you all you need, for there's no such thing as a magic food. Eat fewer meat, poultry, and dairy products, but when you do, eat many different kinds.

Limiting your intake of certain foods

Take it easy on cholesterol, saturated fat, sugar, and salt.

Eat sweets sparingly. Many people have found that the more they cut back, the less they crave these foods. Don't look upon it as depriving yourself: Just cut back a little bit at a time. You may be surprised to find that your desire falls off with your consumption.

Read the labels on your food cans and packages carefully. You may be surprised at how many calories food makers squeeze into some foods you thought were fairly "lite."

Using psychological strategies to get through

Put smaller portions on your plate. That way, you can clean your plate without stuffing yourself.

Avoid places and settings that normally cue to you overeat. For example, if you always gobble down plates and plates of fried chips and gooey, fatty cheese dip when you meet your friends at the Mexican restaurant for an after-work drink, try going somewhere else.

Don't shop when you're hungry, because the growl in your stomach will tempt you to buy sweets and fattening foods.

Set a reasonable goal. Don't try to lose 30 pounds a month or squeeze into that teensy bathing suit by next week. People who lose weight that fast usually put it back on almost as rapidly. If you stick to a good eating and exercise plan and only lose a quarter or a half pound a week, you're doing well.

Don't be too hard on yourself if you don't meet all your goals exactly on schedule. You're only human; you're allowed some leeway. And besides, you're eating for life; you're in it for the long haul. You don't have to sprint, but just stay on the right track.

When you do something great, reward yourself with something other than food.

Understanding that it's not just what you eat . . .

Remember that what you do or do not eat is only half the equation. You must also burn up calories with physical activity and exercise.

Eat slowly. It takes a while for your brain to catch up with what you're eating, so it's possible to eat more than you want or need to when you shovel it in. Take your time, and let your brain register the fact that you've eaten. You'll eat less that way.

"Pre-eat" a little bit before going to parties, movies, and other places where you can't get healthful food. If you eat a small portion of health-enhancing food before you go out, you won't be tempted to overdo the popcorn and chocolate after you're there. Instead, you can enjoy a little taste, as a special treat.

Eyeballing those portions

Many diets suggest specific portion sizes, such as 3 ounces of fish or ½ cup of vegetables or 8 ounces of milk. But because few of us carry little food scales or measuring cups, we're often forced to estimate. Eyeball estimations can be difficult, because most people tend to underestimate the portion size of foods they enjoy eating and overestimate those they don't like. (Ever notice how ½ cup of ice cream looks like nothing, but ½ cup of beets looks like way too much?)

Table C-2 offers some tips developed by Sheldon Margen and Dale Ogar for eyeballing food portion sizes. The tips are easy to remember, or if you like, you can cut the table out and carry it in your wallet or pocketbook.

Table C-2	Visual Food Portion Guidelines
Quantity	*Visual Aid*
How big is a 3-ounce serving?	About the size of a deck of cards.
What's one serving of pancake or waffle?	A pancake or waffle the size of a 4-inch CD.
How much is 1 teaspoonful?	About the size of the tip of your thumb.
What's ½ cup serving of veggies, rice, pasta, or cereal?	Cooked, a mound about the same size as a small fist (or baseball).
How big is a small baked potato?	Roughly the size of a computer mouse.
What's a medium apple or orange?	One about the size of a baseball.
What's an ounce of cheese?	About the size of four dice.

Index

• C •

caffeine, 228
Calcarea carbonica-ostrearum (homeopathic remedy), 261
Calcimar (medication), 122
calcitonin-salmon, 122
calcium, 16, 57, 320
CAM. *See* complementary alternative treatment
can opener, 230
cantaloupe, 156
capsaicin
    definition, 149, 320
    overview, 171–172, 255
car rental, 293
cardiovascular exercise. *See* endurance exercise
caretaker, 224
carpal tunnel syndrome. *See also* repetitive motion injury
    definition, 321
    overview, 19, 81
    symptoms, 81
    treatment, 81, 309–310
carrier oil, 278
cartilage
    autologous chondrocyte implantation, 138
    cause of breakdown, 30–32
    components, 28
    definition, 321
    illustration of damage, 28, 29
    overview, 11–12, 27–28
    primary versus secondary osteoarthritis, 30–31
    repair process, 32
    rheumatoid arthritis process, 40–41
    transplant, 312–313
    water content, 12
case-history game, 244
cat posture, 190
Cataflam (medication), 127
catechin, 162
cat's claw, 252
Causticum (homeopathic remedy), 261
CBC (Complete Blood Count), 103
CBT (cognitive behavioral therapy), 222
Cefazolin (medication), 120–121

Celebrex (medication), 115
celebrity sufferers, 25
celecoxib, 115
celery seed, 253
cement, 135
centaury, 252
cephalexin hydrochloride, 120–121
certification
    CAM practitioner, 242, 243
    doctor, 88–89, 90
chair exercise, 193–196
Chamomilla (homeopathic remedy), 261
chicken, 168
children, 21, 84
child's pose, 192–193
Chinese medicine, 263–266
Chinese Thunder God Vine (herbal medicine), 253
chiropractic medicine
    benefits, 269
    definition, 241, 321
    doctor selection, 269–270, 305
    overview, 268–269
    resources, 329
ChiroWeb (professional organization), 329
Chlamydia trachomatis bacteria, 71
choline magnesium trisalicylate, 126–127
chondrocytes, 28, 31
chondroitin sulfate, 173–175, 321
chopsticks, 33
chronic pain, 142–144, 321
Cimicifuga racemosa (homeopathic remedy), 261
circulation, 147
citrus fruit, 157
classical homeopathy, 258–259
Clinoril (medication), 116
clothing, 73, 77, 232
cognitive behavioral therapy (CBT), 222
ColBenemid (medication), 116
colchicine, 56
colchicum, 98
cold pack, 36, 48, 147
collagen
    hydrolysate, 168
    overview, 28
    primary osteoarthritis, 31
    scleroderma process, 68–69
color, finger, 76

sex, 228–229
typical arthritis symptoms, 19–20
pain management
chronic pain, 143–145
clinic, 144
food, 156–163
medication, 152
noninvasive therapies, 145–152, 314
positive thinking, 219–223
resources, 332
supplements, 164–169
surgery, 152
pantothenic acid, 175
papaya, 157
paraffin wax treatment, 147
passive movement, 149
pauciarticular JRA, 58
The PDR Pocket Guide to Prescription Drugs, 93
Pediapred (medication), 123
pellagra, 169
pelvis
exercise, 184–185, 187–188
posture, 207
Pen Vee (medication), 123
Penicillamine, 123
penicillin, 123
Pentids (medication), 123
People with Arthritis Can Exercise (PACE) video, 200, 336
pericarditis, 43
personality, doctor, 91
pet, 73
pharmacist, 144, 303
pharmacy, 298–299
phone, 230
PHS West, Inc. (assistive device supplier), 334
physical exam, 99–100
physical therapist
chronic pain management, 144
exercise goals, 178
exercise program design, 197
job description, 151
overview, 303
physical therapy
ankylosing spondylitis treatment, 63
definition, 324
recovery plan, 140

rheumatoid arthritis treatment, 47
scleroderma treatment, 70
physician. *See* doctor
pillow, 227
Pipracil (medication), 123
piroxicam, 118
Plaquenil (medication), 123–124
pleurisy, 43
polarity therapy, 273–274, 324, 332
polka, 195
polyarticular JRA, 58
polymyalgia rheumatica, 18, 78–80, 324
polymyositis, 19, 83–84, 324
pool exercise, 148, 180, 336
positive thinking, 219–223
postoperative care, 139
posture
biomechanics, 202–203
body components, 204–208
correct stride, 209–210
ergonomics, 203–204
lifting technique, 211–212
sleeping, 211
potassium ion, 145
prayer, 223–224
prednisolone sodium phosphate, 123
prednisone, 83–84, 117
pregnant women, 51, 226
pretzel posture, 191
primary care physician, 302–303
primary osteoarthritis, 30–31
probenecid-colchicine, 116
processed meat, 163
programmed relaxation, 220–221
prolotherapy, 285–286
pronation, 205
Prosorba therapy, 124
prostaglandin, 160
protein, 105
proteoglycans, 28, 31
pseudogout, 16, 57, 324
psoriatic arthritis
definition, 324
overview, 16, 61
symptoms, 61
treatment, 61
zinc, 169
psychologist, 144, 305–306, 332

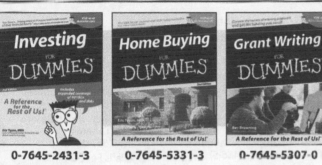
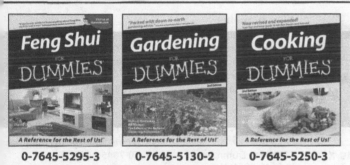
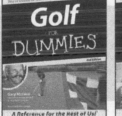
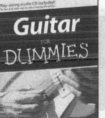
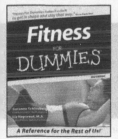
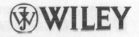

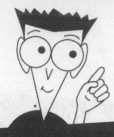

FOR DUMMIES®

A world of resources to help you grow

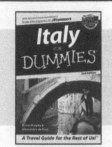
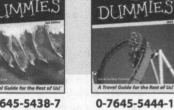
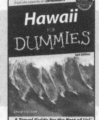
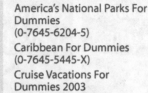
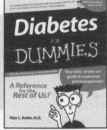
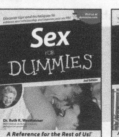
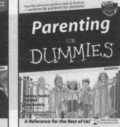

FOR DUMMIES®

Plain-English solutions for everyday challenges

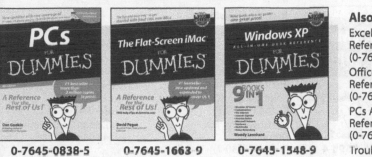
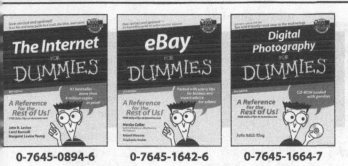
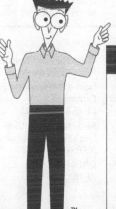

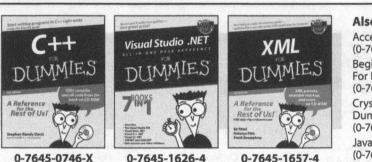
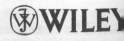